AF597692

Robotic Surgery of the Head and Neck

Gregory A. Grillone • Scharukh Jalisi
Editors

Robotic Surgery of the Head and Neck

A Comprehensive Guide

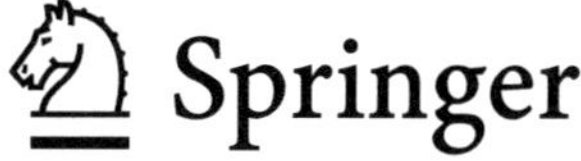

Editors
Gregory A. Grillone, MD
Professor and Vice Chairman
Department of Otolaryngology—Head and Neck Surgery
Boston Medical Center
Boston University School of Medicine
Boston, MA, USA

Scharukh Jalisi, MD
Department of Otolaryngology—Head and Neck Surgery
Division of Head and Neck Surgical Oncology and Skullbase Surgery
Boston Medical Center
Boston University School of Medicine
Boston, MA, USA

ISBN 978-1-4939-1546-0 ISBN 978-1-4939-1547-7 (eBook)
DOI 10.1007/978-1-4939-1547-7
Springer New York Heidelberg Dordrecht London

Library of Congress Control Number: 2014953588

Printed on acid-free paper

Springer is part of Springer Science+Business Media (www.springer.com)

To my patients, students, residents, and mentors, who have all taught me so much
To my wife, Diane, and my children, Gregory James and Deanna Rose, for their constant support, love, and patience
To my parents and sister, who taught me that anything is possible with hard work and dedication
To Charles W. Vaughan, who always taught me to think "outside the box"

Gregory A. Grillone

To my parents for their diligence in raising me and making me human,
To my teachers for their selflessness in educating me,
To my children, Omar and Zahan, for enriching our lives, and
To my wife, Moushmi, for her unwavering support, patience, and love.

Scharukh Jalisi

Foreword

I recall when I was a surgical intern, one of my senior residents said to me something like this: "Well, you know that surgery exists only to the extent that there are limitations in what medical science can do to provide cures for patients." That seemed to me to be a rather negative comment, hard to grasp, and a bit of a downer for me to hear as I was about to begin the lengthy training that would prepare me to become an otolaryngologist. But, after thinking a bit more about the comment, I realized that there was truth in the concept that surgical removal or repair of parts of the human body meant that the disease or dysfunction affecting those parts of the body had not been eradicated or rectified with medical therapy or by other means such as radiation therapy. Hence, to restore patients to health, a surgeon physically removes the diseased parts of the body or reconstructs the malfunctioning parts of the body, aiming, to the extent possible, to preserve portions of the body that surround the disease but are unaffected by the disease. In the past two decades, surgical techniques have evolved toward minimally invasive approaches. Robotic surgery is the latest technologic advancement that expands the capabilities of surgeons. The robot enables a surgeon to have a magnified close-up view of the operative site and to do things that cannot be done without the advantage of the mechanical aspects of the robotic device. Robotic surgery is not only minimally invasive, but it can be maximally effective because the robot arms and pincer graspers can get to locations within the head and neck that are difficult to visualize and virtually inaccessible to the hands of the surgeon. Accordingly, what is most notable about this book is that the methods described herein have the potential to make surgery of the head and neck more elegant and effective than it has ever been. The authors of all of the chapters have provided concise and easily readable instructions on how to perform all types of robotic surgery in the head and neck. There is a reason that I am particularly gratified that this book has been edited by two otolaryngologists who were residents in the Boston University Otolaryngology Residency Program and who are now on the faculty of the Boston University School of Medicine. Fifty years ago, lasers had not yet been used for surgery. Here at the Boston University School of Medicine, three pioneering young otolaryngologists, M. Stuart Strong, Charles W. Vaughan, and Geza Jako, worked with a physicist, Thomas Polanyi, to construct the first carbon dioxide laser that could be used for laryngeal surgery. That was a revolutionary innovation that offered otolaryngologists, for the first time, the ability to view the larynx through a microscope and ablate with a laser and with pinpoint accuracy lesions within the larynx. This book on robotic surgery of the head and neck, in some ways, shows that surgical innovation continues among faculty members where such innovation got a jump start when the carbon dioxide laser was harnessed here for use in head and neck surgery nearly 50 years ago.

Boston, MA, USA Kenneth M. Grundfast

Preface

> "The world as we have created it is a process of our thinking. It cannot be changed without changing our thinking."
>
> —Albert Einstein

The concept of minimally invasive surgery has been of interest to physicians since the time of Hippocrates, but it was not until the twentieth century that technological advancements, such as the operating microscope, fiberoptics, rigid endoscopes, and lasers, allowed surgeons to begin performing operations through natural body orifices or through small incisions in the skin. In the field of modern Otolaryngology a major paradigm shift occurred in the early 1970s when Drs. Stuart Strong, Geza Jako, Charles Vaughan, and Thomas Polanyi combined the operating microscope, carbon dioxide laser, specially designed laryngoscopes, and microlaryngeal instruments to perform transoral surgery for benign diseases of the larynx and pharynx. Over the next several decades this approach was expanded to include malignant disease of these anatomic areas as well. Another paradigm shift in our field occurred with the introduction of functional endoscopic sinus surgery, developed by Drs. Messerklinger and Stamberger in Europe and popularized in the United States by Dr. David Kennedy in the 1980s. These advancements did require sacrificing certain advantages long held sacred by surgeons. In the case of transoral laser procedures surgeons had to give up the ability to see around corners and to utilize wrist action, required for important functions like sewing. In the case of functional endoscopic sinus procedures, surgeons were forced to give up two-handed surgery and stereoscopic vision. Despite these limitations, these pioneering advancements have changed forever the fundamental way we approach surgical diseases in these anatomic areas and have resulted in reduced morbidity for our patients compared to treating these same diseases with more conventional "open" techniques.

We believe that current and future advances in robotic technology will likely lead to the next major paradigm shift in minimally invasive surgery of the head and neck. Robotic technology allows two-handed, wristed manipulation of surgical instruments while preserving binocular vision and the ability to see around corners. While currently available systems lack haptic feedback and are too large to be used in smaller anatomic areas of the head and neck, we believe these limitations will eventually be overcome as robotic technology advances.

In the 5 years since the DaVinci Robotic Surgical System (Intuitive Surgical, Inc.) was approved by the FDA for use in the head and neck, it has been applied to a variety of anatomic areas and disease processes in the head and neck. The intent of this text is to provide a comprehensive overview of robotic surgery for the practicing otolaryngologist-head and neck surgeon including anatomic considerations, operating room setup, and indications and technique for both transoral and transcutaneous robotic procedures currently performed in the head and neck.

Boston, MA, USA

Gregory A. Grillone
Scharukh Jalisi

Acknowledgments

I would like to thank Maria Smilios, Developmental Editor, and Rebekah Amos, Editor for Clinical Medicine, at Springer Science+Business Media, LLC for their unwavering support and assistance in the preparation of this text. As with any project, this was a team effort and so I would like to thank my coeditor, Dr. Scharukh Jalisi, and all of the authors for contributing their time and knowledge to the development of this book.

I would like to thank Gregory Weinstein in the Department of Otolaryngology—Head and Neck Surgery at the University of Pennsylvania for giving me the opportunity to learn the intricacies of transoral robotic surgery.

I would also like to acknowledge my colleagues Kenneth Grundfast and Steven Zeitels and my early mentors M. Stuart Strong, Stanley Shapshay, the late Werner Chasin, and Charles Vaughan, who sadly passed away this past year. They have all had an indelible impact on my development as an otolaryngolgist and for that I am extremely grateful.

Gregory A. Grillone, MD

I would like to thank Maria Smilios, Developmental Editor, and Rebekah Amos, Editor for Clinical Medicine, at Springer Science+Business Media, LLC for their support and assistance in the preparation of this text. I would like to thank all others involved in the preparation of this book and especially my coeditor, Dr. Gregory Grillone, and all of the authors for contributing their time and knowledge to the success of this book.

I would like to thank Dr. Gregory Grillone in the Department of Otolaryngology—Head and Neck Surgery at the Boston University for sowing the “seed” for transoral robotic surgery in me.

I would also like to acknowledge my mentors Kenneth Grundfast, James Netterville, Brian Burkey, Stanley Shapshay, Robert Dolan, John Gooey, and Charles Vaughan who made me a thoughtful surgeon.

Scharukh Jalisi, MD, MA, FACS

Contents

Contributors

Eelam Adil, MD, MBA Department of Otology and Laryngology, Harvard Medical School, Boston, MA, USA

Department of Otolaryngology and Communication Enhancement Boston Children's Hospital, Boston, MA, USA

Donald J. Annino Jr., MD, DMD Brigham and Women's Hospital, Division of Otolaryngology, Boston, MA, USA

Asit Arora, MBBS, MRCS, DOHNS Department of Surgery and Cancer, Imperial College London, St. Mary's Hospital Campus, London, UK

Christopher Brook, MD Department of Otolaryngology—Head and Neck Surgery, Boston University Medical Center, Boston, MA, USA

Iacopo Dallan, MD Ear Nose and Throat Unit, Azienda Ospedaliero-Universitaria Pisana, Pisa, Italy

William S. Duke, MD Department of Otolaryngology, Georgia Regents University, Augusta, GA, USA

Mohamed Eesa, MD Department of Otolaryngology—Head and Neck Surgery, University of Zagazig, Ash Sharqiyah, Egypt

George Garas, BSc, MBBS, MRCS, DOHNS Department of Surgery and Cancer, Imperial College London, St. Mary's Hospital Campus, London, UK

Eric M. Genden, MD Otolaryngology—Head and Neck Surgery, The Icahn School of Medicine at Mount Sinai, New York, NY, USA

The Head Neck, and Thyroid Center, The Mount Sinai Medical Center, New York, NY, USA

Laureano A. Giraldez-Rodriguez, MD Department of Otolaryngology—Head and Neck Surgery, Icahn School of Medicine at Mount Sinai, New York, NY, USA

Gregory A. Grillone, MD Department of Otolaryngology—Head and Neck Surgery, Boston University School of Medicine, Boston Medical Center, Boston, MA, USA

Scharukh Jalisi, MD, MA, FRCS Department of Otolaryngology—Head and Neck Surgery, Division of Head and Neck Surgical Oncology and Skullbase Surgery, Boston University Medical Campus, Boston, MA, USA

Jeffrey S. Jumaily, MD Department of Otolaryngology—Head and Neck Surgery, Boston University School of Medicine, Boston Medical Center, Boston, MA, USA

Georges Lawson, MD Department of Otolaryngology—Head and Neck Surgery, Louvain University Hospital of Mont-Godinne, Yvoir, Belgium

Bao Anh Le, BS Tufts University Dental School of Medicine, Boston, MA, USA

Lance Maggiacomo, RN, BSN Department of Surgery, Boston Medical Center, Boston, MA, USA

Abie Mendelsohn, MD Department of Head & Neck Surgery, David Geffen School of Medicine at UCLA, Los Angeles, CA, USA

Brett Miles, DDS, MD Department Otolaryngology Head and Neck Surgery, Department Oral and Maxillofacial Surgery, Icahn School of Medicine at Mount Sinai, New York, NY, USA

Filippo Montevecchi, MD Department of Special Surgery, Otolaryngology—Head and Neck Surgery Division, Oral Surgery Unit, University of Pavia in Forlì, G.B. Morgagni L. Pierantoni Hospital, Forlì, Italy

Eric J. Moore, MD Professor-Otolaryngology/Head and Neck Surgery, Mayo Clinic, Rocherster, NY, USA

Prachi Nene, BA Division of Head and Neck Surgical Oncology and Skullbase Surgery, Department of Otolaryngology—Head and Neck Surgery, Boston University Medical Campus, Boston, MA, USA

Hiep T. Nguyen, MD Department of Urology, Boston Children's Hospital, Boston, MA, USA

Shaheer Piracha, MD Department of Otolaryngology, Boston University, Boston, MA, USA

Reza Rahbar, DMD, MD Department of Otology and Laryngology, Harvard Medical School, Boston, MA, USA

Department of Otolaryngology and Communication Enhancement Boston Children's Hospital, Boston, MA, USA

Marc Remacle, MD, PhD Department of Otolaryngology—Head and Neck Surgery, Louvain University Hospital of Mont-Godinne, Yvoir, Belgium

Matthew S. Russell, MD, FACS Department of Otolaryngology—Head and Neck Surgery, University of California, San Francisco, CA, USA

David J. Terris, MD, FACS Department of Otolaryngology, Georgia Regents University, Augusta, GA, USA

Tom Thomas, MD, MPH Center for Head and Neck Oncology, Dana Farber Cancer Institute, Boston, MA, USA

Neil Tolley, MD, FRCS (Eng & Ed), DLO Department of Surgery and Cancer, Imperial College London, St. Mary's Hospital Campus, London, UK

Claudio Vicini, MD Department of Special Surgery, Otolaryngology—Head & Neck Surgery Division, Oral Surgery Unit, University of Pavia in Forlì, G.B. Morgagni L. Pierantoni Hospital, Forlì, Italy

Bharat B. Yarlagadda, MD Department of Otolaryngology—Head and Neck Surgery, Boston University School of Medicine, Boston, MA, USA

History and Overview of Robotic Surgery in Otolaryngology—Head and Neck Surgery

Bharat B. Yarlagadda, Matthew S. Russell, and Gregory A. Grillone

Introduction

Surgical robots are commonly utilized in multiple surgical specialties but have only relatively recently been used routinely in Otolaryngology—Head and Neck Surgery. The high levels of instrument maneuverability, magnification, and excellent visualization make modern surgical robots ideal for certain confined spaces of the head and neck including the oropharynx, hypopharynx, and larynx. This chapter outlines the basic principles of robotic surgery and technology and provides a brief history of the technological developments that led to the robotic devices currently in use. In addition, the use of robotics in specific head and neck subsites is reviewed including the oropharynx, larynx, thyroid, and skull base.

B.B. Yarlagadda, M.D.
Department of Otolaryngology—Head and Neck Surgery, Boston University School of Medicine, Boston, MA, USA

M.S. Russell, M.D., F.A.C.S
Department of Otolaryngology—Head and Neck Surgery, University of California, San Francisco, CA, USA
e-mail: mrussell@ohns.ucsf.edu

G.A. Grillone, M.D. (✉)
Department of Otolaryngology—Head and Neck Surgery, Boston University School of Medicine, Boston Medical Center, Boston, MA, USA
e-mail: Gregory.Grillone@bmc.org

Robotic and robotic-assisted surgery has existed in various forms for the past 20 years, but these systems have gained favor over recent years in multiple surgical specialties [1–3]. This was spurred by advantages over open, endoscopic, and microscopic techniques including increased range of motion (six degrees of freedom) of the surgical instruments, binocular endoscopic vision, tremor control, motion scaling, and force feedback [4]. Neurosurgery and orthopedic surgery were early adopters of robotic technology, which allowed for very precise preplanned surgical manipulation for applications such as drilling and electrode placement as well as bone milling for joint replacement surgery [5, 6]. Popularity of robotic systems has, of course, increased with uses in urologic and cardiothoracic procedures as well [1–3]. Since approval by the United States Food and Drug Administration (FDA) in 2009, the use of robotics in otolaryngology has seen major advancements. This chapter explores the current and future applications of these surgical robotic systems in the field of Otolaryngology—Head and Neck surgery.

Capabilities of Surgical Robotic Systems

As the roles and complexity of surgical robotic systems advance, it will be useful for surgeons to have a basic understanding of the general principles of robotics. Camarillo et al. have described a role-based classification of robotic systems

G.A. Grillone and S. Jalisi (eds.), *Robotic Surgery of the Head and Neck: A Comprehensive Guide*, DOI 10.1007/978-1-4939-1547-7_1, © Springer Science+Business Media New York 2015

Table 1 Role-based classification for robotic systems. Adapted from Camarillo et al. [7]

Passive role	Robotic assistance is limited in scope, and generally aims to assist the surgeon with a specific noninvasive task. Inherently, these systems are low risk
Restricted (semi-active)	The robotic system is more integrated into the surgical procedure, and is involved in more invasive tasks such as stereotactic localization or hand stabilization. These systems receive direct input from the surgeon and tend to limit action. Inherent risk is moderate
Active role	The robot is intimately involved in the surgical procedure. There is a greater freedom of function and movement, and the robot is generally in direct contact with the patient while the surgeon operates the machine remotely

(Table 1) that will facilitate the interdisciplinary discourse between engineers and medical professionals [7]. Current technology and techniques allow employment of robotics in the "Active Role." Below is a brief discussion of relevant engineering terminology.

Degrees of Freedom Maneuverability of surgical instruments becomes increasingly difficult in more confined spaces and with nonlinear trajectories (not in the surgeon's line of sight). Each degree of freedom allows movement in an additional dimension. One degree of freedom allows for unidirectional motion, for instance, along a linear trajectory. Conventional endoscopic and microscopic procedures in otolaryngology and other surgical fields generally provide four degrees of freedom. Surgical robotic systems such as the da Vinci system (Intuitive Surgical, Mountain View, USA) provide six degrees of freedom. The effect is that of a "wristed" distal end of the surgical instrument that moves much like the human wrist, allowing the head of the instrument to "turn corners" and operate beyond the traditional line-of-site limitation. This effect has potential benefits in small, narrow, anatomic regions commonly encountered in otolaryngology.

Workspace and Resolution Workspace refers to the area that a robot can physically access. This is limited by the length and maneuverability of the surgical arms. Also, configurations of the surgical arms are limited by interference between the arms outside of the surgical field. Resolution deals with the magnitude of robotic arm movement. Smaller surgical fields will require more precise movement, and will therefore require finer resolution of robotic movement.

Inertia and Stiffness Inertia and stiffness are greater concerns in the engineering world than in the surgical world, and are important when calculating the forces needed to accelerate or decelerate the robotic arms. Robotic arms that need to move quickly will either need to be lighter or have a larger motor to generate greater force.

Speed and Force Much like the transmission of an automobile, robots have a transmission that alters the gear ratio between the motor and the surgical arm. This allows forces to be scaled up or down, changing the resolution of the robotic arm movement. Like in an automobile, there is a trade-off between speed and force. In lower gears, there is an emphasis on force, whereas in the higher gears the purpose is speed. Speed and force are not mutually exclusive, but can be limited by expense.

Dynamic Range The ratio of the highest and lowest force produced by a robot is known as the force dynamic range. The human hand has a high dynamic range, which can be difficult to replicate mechanically.

Advantages and Disadvantages of Robotic Systems

Advantages

Image Guidance and Stereotactic Orientation of the Surgical Instrument Stereotactic image guidance systems are widely used in clinical practice today. In the broadest sense, image guidance can be considered "robotic," though the combination of robotic systems discussed here with image guidance is an even more powerful tool than either independently. Planning complex surgical trajectories preoperatively using imaging data can be coupled with robotic systems that carry out the surgical maneuvers in an active-role system.

Instrument Stabilization and Tremor Control Studies monitoring the precision of the human hand demonstrate decreased reliability within 100 µm of a target for senior surgeons [7]. Accuracy further deteriorates due to the natural development of intention tremor with fatigue. Instrument stabilization can increase precision to 10 µm, which can be maintained over time with a computer-assisted robot to subtract intention tremor from the surgeon's movements independent of fatigue. In addition, robotic systems can filter the natural 200 Hz eye motion to stabilize the visual field [8].

Binocular Endoscopic Vision While open and microscopic procedures do allow binocular vision, endoscopic and laparoscopic technology typically suffers from loss of three-dimensional vision and depth perception. The da Vinci system employs stereoscopic video telescopes [8, 9]. Two 5 mm cameras sit within a 12 mm laparoscopic arm. Zero degree and 30° stereoscopic video telescopes are available providing a magnified 60° field of view, or a narrower field of view with higher magnification, depending on the nature of the operative field.

Motion Scaling Engineers and surgeons interested in microscopic robotic surgery have hypothesized that scaling the surgeon's hand movements would improve technical abilities and outcomes by converting gross hand movements into fine surgical motion. The da Vinci system can be used in a 1:1 or 4:1 mode although little is known about how beneficial motion scaling is in improving accuracy.

Telepresence and Telementoring Telepresence refers to the ability of the surgeon to operate at a site that is remote from the patient. Early in the development of surgical robotic, the United States Department of Defense and the National Aeronautics and Space Administration, NASA, became interested in exploring this technology to decrease wartime morbidity and mortality by allowing the surgeon at a base hospital to operate on wounded soldiers in the field and astronauts in orbit, respectively. Telementoring is a logical extension of telepresence and refers to the ability to disseminate new surgical techniques to surgeons anywhere in the world.

Disadvantages

Expense The cost-effectiveness of robotic surgery has often been questioned. Expenses must consider both upfront and maintenance costs. Despite increasing utilization in the head and neck, a dedicated otolaryngologic device is usually economically unfeasible for most centers. Collaboration between surgical departments as well as research grants can help defray some of the cost burden of individual specialties while disbursing economic risk.

Size Studies by Hockstein et al. demonstrated the feasibility of laryngologic surgery using 5 mm diameter instruments [10]. According to their preliminary work this is the maximum diameter capable of operating in the extreme confines of otolaryngologic surgery. Five millimeter robotic instrumentation has only recently become available, spurring the use of this technology in otolaryngologic applications. Future development of even smaller instruments may have additional benefits for accessibility and maneuverability.

Loss of Force Feedback/Haptics One drawback of currently available robotic technology is loss of tactile perception of the tissue being manipulated. Experienced robotic surgeons often feel that this is largely compensated for by the improved visual information provided by the stereoscopic camera. Although sensory substitution methods, such as a visual color scale on the monitor, provide some improvements, there remains a need to develop true haptic feedback between operator and machine.

Specific Surgical Robotic Systems

Specific systems range from highly specialized, task-limited instruments to larger telerobotic surgical systems capable of multitasking application. It is important, therefore, to introduce a few of the individual systems that are in use today, with specific emphasis on ones with applications in otolaryngology. The systems are discussed in order of increasing robot responsibility as described above by the role-based classification. The first systems were basic, single function devices. After FDA approval in 2009 for use in the head and neck, active telerobotic systems have come to dominate the field in various otolaryngologic applications.

One of the first commercially available applications of surgical robotics was AESOP, Automated Endoscopic System for Optimal Positioning (Computer Motion, Santa Barbara, USA). AESOP offers a steady platform for a laparoscope that could be controlled by a surgeon via foot pedal and later voice activation, eliminating the need for an assistant to maintain a steady image with proper orientation. The AESOP system later became integrated into the Zeus surgical robotic system.

Robotic drilling and milling platforms are available for certain surgical applications. ROBODOC (Curexo Technology, Fremont, CA), used in orthopedic surgery, was the first such device approved by the FDA [4]. Its function is to mill femur shafts during total hip arthroplasty to improve accuracy and reliability over hand reaming. Neuromate (Integrated Surgical Systems, Sacremento, CA) is the modern derivative of neurosurgical robots used to place probes, electrodes, and drills under stereotactic guidance into the brain. The newest version of Neuromate uses ultrasonic stereotactic registration obviating the need for painful head frames.

Telerobotic systems have drastically changed the size and complexity of surgical robotics. These systems provide a complete interface between the surgeon and the patient and have changed the nature of robotics from adjunctive to inherent in the surgical process. This "master–slave" configuration converts the surgeons hand movements at the "master" console into a digital signal that is sent to the "slave" robotic arms and converted to movement of the surgical instruments. The digital signals are processed and relayed through a computer system [8, 9]. Previously, the two major competing systems in telerobotic and telepresence surgery were the da Vinci surgical system and the Zeus system (Computer Motion Inc, Santa Barbara, USA). In 2003, a corporate merger between Intuitive Surgical and Computer Motion eventually led to phasing out of the Zeus platform in favor of the da Vinci system.

The da Vinci console is designed to completely engross the surgeon in the surgical field. The console hood acts as "blinders" so the surgeon is unable to see the remainder of the operating theater. The advantage is, in theory, to make the surgical movements more intuitive with fewer distractions. The 3D endoscopic technology incorporates two small cameras in a single endoscope. The da Vinci system isolates the images from each camera which are then independently fed to left and right visual fields in the surgical console.

The da Vinci system allows for the use of up to four arms, one which holds the endoscope, two that hold the left- and right-hand instruments, and a fourth arm which can be used to hold a retractor. Given the confines of head and neck operative fields, in most cases only two arms are used in addition to the endoscopic camera. The surgeon has control of the instrument arms and the endoscopic camera and can toggle between these with the use of foot pedals. Additional instrumentation such as a suction and forceps are provided by the surgical assistant who stands at the head of the bed.

One barrier that robotic technology was able to overcome is the fulcrum effect with laparoscopic instruments. As the length of surgical instruments increased to accommodate minimally invasive surgery the body wall trocar system created a fulcrum point that affected the movement of surgical instruments so that the surgeon's hand motion was the reverse of the motion at the distal end of the laparoscopic instrument. Because the hand movements in a telerobotic system are not directly connected to the instruments the controllers can be designed to "grasp" the surgical instruments at any point along the robotic arm. The da Vinci system overcomes the nonintuitive fulcrum effect by virtually "holding" the instruments at their distal end. In addition, the ends of the robotic arms are "wristed" allowing human wrist-like movement within the surgical field. The real effect is a serially oriented six degrees of freedom robotic arm that allows pitch, yaw, roll, and in-out movement of the robotic arm at the instrument tip. In addition, instruments with grasping or cutting abilities add a seventh degree of freedom [8]. The Zeus system on the other hand was designed to virtually hold the instruments much like a surgeon would in laparoscopic surgery. This resulted in maintenance of the fulcrum effect with only four degrees of freedom in the surgical arms without the articulating instrument tips.

Applications of Surgical Robotics

History and General Principles

Studies by Hockstein et al. described the feasibility of using the da Vinci robot to access and manipulate the structures of the oropharynx, hypopharynx, and larynx [10, 11]. Their first study evaluated the technical aspects of operating within the confines of the oral cavity and upper airway using presently available da Vinci surgical equipment [10]. The four variables in this study included: (1) Retractor: Lindholm laryngoscope versus McIvor mouthgag. (2) Endoscope: 0° 2D scope versus 30° 3D scope. (3) Surgical instrument diameter: 8 mm versus 5 mm. (4) Positioning of the robotic arms in relation to the "patient."

Using an airway management mannequin, they demonstrated that the combination of these variables that allowed for the greatest visualization and surgical access was a McIvor mouthgag with tongue blade, 30° 3D endoscope, and two 5 mm instruments, with the operating table rotated 30–45° relative to the robotic arms. This allowed for visualization of the hypopharynx, supraglottis, glottis, and anterior commissure. Other studies validated use of different mouth gags, such as the Crowe-Davis or the Feyh–Kastenbauer, rather than a traditional tubed laryngoscope. Furthermore, by minimizing the size of the surgical arms they were able to manipulate the laryngeal structures, and suture between the vocal fold without difficulty.

Subsequently, Hockstein et al. performed proof-of-principle dissections on a human cadaver using the previously noted surgical setup [11]. Six procedures were performed and timed: (1) Bilateral true vocal cord stripping, (2) Rotation of a mucosal flap from the epiglottis to the anterior commissure, (3) Partial vocal cordectomy, (4) Arytenoidectomy, (5) Partial epiglottectomy and thyrohyoid dissection, and (6) Partial resection of the base of tongue with primary closure. Though they did not compare these procedures with conventional open or laser surgeries, they reported greater ease of operation with the wristed instruments, tremor stabilization, and binocular vision compared to the author's prior experience. Also, they noted the length of operation was comparable to conventional techniques with a similar safety profile in terms of hemostasis and risk of patient injury [12].

From these initial experiments, the practice of transoral robotic surgery (TORS) was popularized. The results of institutional patient trials at the University of Pennsylvania were presented to the Food and Drug Administration, leading to the 2009 approval of the da Vinci system for treatment of head and neck benign disease and select T1 and T2 malignancies. Since that time, there has been a flurry of publications from multiple institutions detailing the use of surgical robotics in otolaryngologic applications. A review of the literature shows not only technical descriptions of robotic use, but also recent manuscripts regarding the clinical outcomes, comparisons to traditional approaches, as well as discussion of the logistical roadblocks to implementing robotic techniques into existing surgical programs.

There are several general principles of robotic head and neck surgery performed with the da Vinci system regardless of the involved anatomic subsite, as outlined by Newman et al. [13].

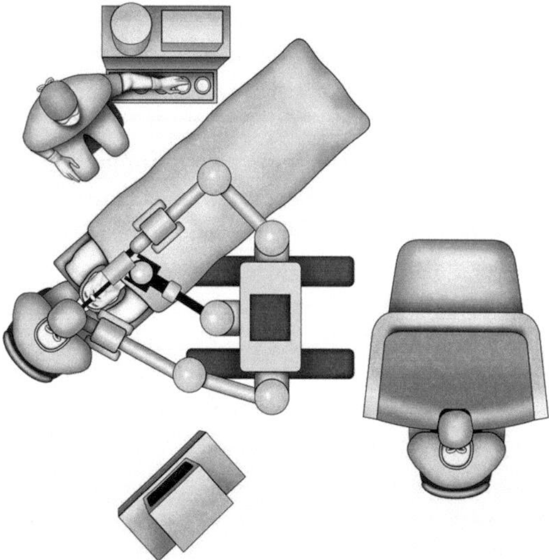

Fig. 1 Diagram of the operating room setup of the da Vinci system with primary surgeon at the console and assistant at the head of the patient. Reprinted from Hockstein NG and BW O'Malley, Transoral robotic surgery, Operative Techniques in Otolaryngology—Head and Neck Surgery, 2008, with permission from Elsevier [13]

These include issues of airway management, intra-operative patient safety measures, and room setup (Fig. 1).

Laryngology

Laryngology has benefited tremendously from the introduction of the microscope, microscopic instrumentation, and the CO_2 laser into clinical practice. By coupling the operating microscope to the laser, Strong, Jako, and Vaughan showed that a variety of lesions could be excised or ablated from laryngeal cancers to vocal cord papillomas [14]. One major disadvantage of microinstruments and also the CO_2 laser is that they cannot turn corners and are restricted to line-of-sight working corridors. Overcoming this obstacle is seen as the primary advantage of using surgical robots in the upper airway.

Transoral laryngeal surgery significantly predates the use of robotics in otolaryngology. Partially in response to a trend toward functional organ preservation in the treatment of laryngeal malignancy, transoral endoscopic partial laryngectomy techniques were developed to spare patients from both total laryngectomy and the morbidity of open partial laryngeal surgery such as the need for tracheostomy and feeding tubes. These techniques were pioneered by the work of Drs. Stuart Strong and Charles Vaughn as well as Wolfgang Steiner among others [15, 16]. Indications for partial laryngectomy are contingent on loco-regional staging and are out of the scope of this chapter. However, it is important to note that the use of robotics in laryngeal surgery, as well as other head and neck subsites, simply represents an alternate technical method, with unique advantages and drawbacks, for achieving the outcomes previously described by the proponents of transoral partial laryngectomy techniques.

Laryngeal TORS has been described for benign disease such as respiratory papillomatosis and laryngeal schwannoma, but the vast majority of the literature concerns the treatment of supraglottic squamous cell carcinoma. Weinstein et al. reported three cases of TORS resection of T2 and T3 supraglottic tumors with successful surgical exposure and access as well as achievement of negative margins [17]. TORS total laryngectomy has also been described, but experience with this technique is limited [18].

Several series reporting experience with TORS supraglottic laryngectomy (TORS-SL) are now available. Exposure is facilitated by the routine use of transnasal intubation to keep the endotracheal tube posterior in the field and the use of the Feyh–Kastenbauer retractor. Clinical outcomes are encouraging. Mendelsohn and colleagues report a series of 18 patients who underwent TORS-SL for T1 and T2 supraglottic tumors [19]. Negative margins were obtained in all patients and no local recurrences on 2-year follow-up. Ozer and colleagues report largely similar results in a series of 13 patients [20]. All achieved negative margins but one patient required conversion to an open approach due to extensive pre-epiglottic space invasion (Fig. 2).

TORS laryngeal procedures will benefit from continued advances in robotic technology such as smaller instrumentation with improved articulation. Current drawbacks of the da Vinci setup include limited maneuverability due to a narrow working corridor and inherent line-of-site restrictions

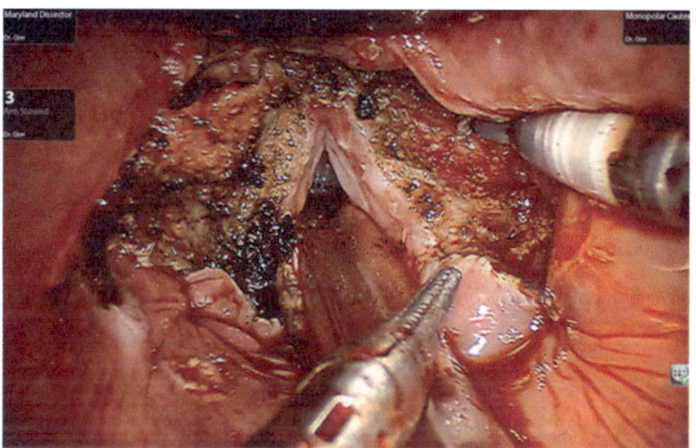

Fig. 2 View of the operative field during TORS supraglottic partial laryngectomy with a 30° telescope. The endotracheal tube is visible in the glottis at the bottom of the figure. Reprinted from Ozer E, et al, Clinical outcomes of transoral robotic supraglottic laryngectomy. Head and Neck, 2012, with permission from John Wiley and Sons [20]

of rigid instrumentation. A highly flexible robotic system, initially developed at Carnegie Mellon University and now at Medrobotics Corporation (Raynham, MA), attempts to overcome these shortcomings. It features a single arm with 50 cylindrical links that advance in a follow-the-leader mechanism. There are approximately 10° of rotation between each link allowing the arm to conform to complex three-dimensional spaces with no extrinsic support mechanism. Two working channels allow for the use of flexible instrumentation. Proof-of-concept experiments have been performed in cardiac surgery and laryngoscopic applications [21].

Head and Neck Surgery

The surgical management of oropharyngeal malignancy has traditionally involved significant morbidity to the patient. Operative approaches often necessitated mandibulotomy, lip splitting, tracheostomy, and reconstruction with tissue transfer techniques. Patients who elect to undergo upfront chemoradiation often contend with toxicities such as severe xerostomia, mucositis, and dysphagia. Minimally invasive techniques have developed in parallel with the transoral approaches to the larynx described elsewhere in this chapter. The advent of TORS provides another tool for use in the transoral approach.

The first report of the oropharyngeal application of TORS involved the robotic resection of a vallecular cyst [22]. After FDA approval of the use of the Da Vinci system for oropharyngeal malignancy in 2009, several case series have studied the use and outcome of the application to the tonsil and tongue base. Successful use of TORS is contingent on adequate visualization and the ability to place appropriate retractors, which may be difficult in the presence of trismus, obesity, or a large tongue. Weinstein and colleagues have described several contraindications for oropharyngeal TORS: unresectable nodal disease, mandibular invasion, necessity to resect greater than 50 % of the tongue base, necessity to resect greater than 50 % of the posterior pharyngeal wall, carotid artery involvement, and fixation of the tumor to the prevertebral fascia [23].

A majority of TORS defects are allowed to close successfully via secondary intention. However, certain defects may require reconstructive measures in order to achieve, for example, maintenance of velopharyngeal competence, coverage of the great vessels, separation from the cervical deep spaces, and maintenance of mucosal sensation. De Almeida and colleagues have reported on a variety of methods for reconstruction using the robotic system such as the posterior pharyngeal wall musculomucosal flap or the pyriform sinus mucosal flap [24]. In the post-radiation setting or when tissue bulk is required, free tissue transfer may be necessary. Mukhija and colleagues report an early experience with robotic inset of radial forearm free flaps while Selber et al. demonstrate the use of the robot to perform the arterial anastomosis as well [25, 26]. Selecting a reconstructive method depends on the involved subsites and goal of the reconstruction.

Weinstein and colleagues have reported a multi-institutional series of 177 patients undergoing TORS with a focus on safety and margin status [27]. The majority of tumors were located in the oropharynx (78.5 %) with the remainder located in the larynx or hypopharynx. An elective perioperative tracheostomy rate of 12.4 % was encountered while only a total of four patients (2.3 %) remained with a tracheostomy at 12 months follow up. For patients undergoing primary TORS treatment, a gastrostomy dependency of 5 % was encountered. Positive surgical margins were noted in 3.8 % of patients with oropharyngeal tumors, a rate that the authors feel compares favorably with other transoral or open techniques.

Perioperative complications are relatively uncommon. In the Weinstein study of 177 TORS cases, there was no postoperative fatality, catastrophic hemorrhage, or emergent airway compromise [27]. Other perioperative events such as pneumonia, myocardial infarction, or acute respiratory distress syndrome did occur, but according to an independent analyst, no event was judged to be related to the robot itself. The management of the perioperative airway is certainly a concern, and a certain rate of elective tracheostomy may be observed. Bourdeaux et al. reported two patients requiring postoperative re-intubation due to airway edema [28]. This experience resulted in the practice of elective intubation up to 48 h postoperatively to allow for adequate resolution of the edema prior to extubation.

Thus far, the use of robotics has been described as an additional tool with which to implement existing treatments and surgical procedures. However, there is growing evidence that the use of robotics, particularly in oropharyngeal cancer, is actually changing treatment paradigms. The TORS approach offers the ability to achieve local tumor control with negative margins and minimal morbidity, allowing the surgeon to offer ipsilateral staging neck dissection. The pathologic information from the neck dissection, as Weinstein and colleagues have noted, may allow de-intensification, or altogether avoidance, of adjuvant chemotherapy and radiation [29]. Although the data are relatively preliminary, the locoregional control and rate of cure of surgical therapy for early stage disease aims to rival that of upfront chemo-radiation, without the inherent morbidities of the nonsurgical modalities.

In addition to the treatment of aerodigestive malignancy, there are multiple other applications for surgical robotics in head and neck surgery. Oropharyngeal surgery for the treatment of obstructive sleep apnea has been described, with an emphasis on addressing lingual tonsillar hypertrophy allowing the surgeon to address an area that is difficult to access by traditional means [30]. In addition, the TORS approach has been used to access extraoral sites. For instance, transpalatal TORS approaches to the parapharynx and infratemporal fossa for resection of neoplasia have been published [31]. Further, cervical incisions have been designed for robotic arm entry and access to perform procedures such as neck dissection, thyroidectomy (as described below), and infratemporal fossa dissection [32, 33]. Additional novel approaches and applications continue to populate the literature.

Thyroidectomy

As the incidence of thyroid cancer increases, in part due to earlier detection and more sensitive diagnostic modalities, the number of thyroid lobectomies and total thyroidectomies will increase as well. Multiple techniques have been developed over the years with the goal of minimizing or eliminating the neck incision classically associated with thyroid surgery. This has included the use of smaller incisions with placement of endoscopes through the cervical incision to improve visualization. Multiple endoscopic remote access techniques have been developed to remove the incision from the midline of the neck including lateral neck ports, transaxillary ports, inframammary and areolar access, as well as various combinations of these. In South Korea, a cultural emphasis on cervical cosmesis has resulted in some centers gaining considerable experience with the remote access approaches, particularly the endoscopic transaxillary approach [34]. Specialized retractors can eliminate the need for gas insufflation and allow working room for the placement of robotic arms. In 2009, a group from the Yonsei University in Seoul reported the first large series of patients undergoing robotic transaxillary approach to thyroidectomy [35]. The technique has gained popularity given the obvious benefit of a lack of a cervical incision.

In brief, the transaxillary approach involved creation of a working space starting at the axilla and coursing over the pectoralis muscle [36]. The space is extended superiorly over the clavicle to encounter the strap muscles, which are lifted off of the gland. An additional port is created via a paramedian chest wall incision into which a grasping device is inserted. The use of this approach requires awareness of potential harm to anatomic structures usually not at great risk during conventional thyroid surgery including the carotid artery, jugular vein, esophagus, and brachial plexus.

Several limitations exist to proliferation of the robotic thyroidectomy technique in the United States. Most importantly, the steep learning curve can be prohibitive and few centers in the country offer the procedure. The successful TORS thyroid surgeon must have training and experience with both conventional and endoscopic thyroid procedures. A training paradigm has been proposed which includes live and video case observations, cadaver dissection, and proctored surgical experiences [36]. Further challenges include the fact that the body habitus of the average American patient is different from that in Korea and can create difficulties in exposure of the surgical field [37]. Finally, the equipment cost must be considered, which would include the fixed cost of specialized retractors in addition to the robot itself.

Rhinology

The telescopes, cameras, and instrumentation used in endoscopic sinus surgery have advanced to the point that there are very few applications in which the addition of robotic technology would be of significant benefit. However, researchers are demonstrating benefits of robotics in the region of the skull base. Several groups have already developed advanced transnasal endoscopic approaches to the anterior and middle skull base in order to address areas previously accessible only through craniotomy and craniofacial resection. This includes treatment of benign and malignant pathologies such as meningioma, esthesioneuroblastoma, and sellar tumors. These advances have been spurred by development of reconstructive techniques such as the vascularized nasoseptal flap. A group from the MD Anderson Cancer Center performed cadaveric studies with robotic access obtained through a Caldwell Luc approach with wide middle meatus antrostomies [38]. The da Vinci system was then used to perform sinus surgery as well as resection of the cribriform plate with sharp dissection of the skull base. In addition, the group at the University of Pennsylvania has noted that the da Vinci system may be used to provide access to the middle and lower clivus and provides potential for resection of intradural tumors of this region [39]. This study showed that performance of tremor-free dural closure was possible with the use of the robotic arms' multiple degrees of motion. Further development of specialized instruments, especially for bony work, is required to optimize the use of the da Vinci robot at the skull base, but the current work appears promising. Force feedback and torque sensor technology can also have important roles in skull base work, especially at the bone dural interface [40].

Otology

The precise and delicate nature of surgery of the middle ear is, in theory, the ideal type of surgery to apply the advantages of robotic systems such as tremor control, force feedback, and image-guided localization. Prior studies have shown high levels of precision and accuracy with robotic milling of cadaveric temporal bones embedded in methylmethacrylate blocks [41]. The main drawback of robotic temporal drilling was found to be the use of a cylindrical drilling pattern. Three-dimensional paths could theoretically be constructed, analogous to techniques used in intensity-modulated radiation therapy for cancer treatment. Other applications include the incorporation of haptic feedback mechanism, especially to assist with surgery at the skull base [42]. Recently, a group from Vanderbilt University has applied these principles to perform an entire mastoidectomy using the Mitsubishi RV-3S (Mitsubishi Electric & Electronics USA, Inc., Cyprus, CA) robot programmed to a pre-drilling CT scan [43]. The authors noted that mastoidectomy could be performed rapidly on cadaveric specimens, in under 20 min, with high reproducibility and accuracy.

The main benefit of the rapidity of performing ablative bony work would be to allow the surgeon to concentrate on finer portions of the procedure without the fatigue and tremor associated with milling during the early stages of a complex surgical procedure.

Robotic technology has also been used in the percutaneous placement of cochlear implants. A group at Vanderbilt University has developed a proprietary technology in which a microstereotactic frame is anchored to a cadaveric temporal bone and acts as a fiducial marker for image guidance [44]. This frame is calibrated to CT scan images and an optimally safe trajectory to the cochlea is calculated. A microsurgical drill and implant insertion tool are deployed in order to insert the cochlear electrode without the need for mastoidectomy or facial recess drilling. The procedure was found to be accurate and reproducible, but subject to registration errors that currently limit clinical applicability. The authors note that there are potential future endeavors including applying the technology to other procedures such as petrous apex drainage and deep brain stimulation.

Summary

Surgical robotic technology has been in use for over two decades and ranges from single-armed stereotactic drills to complex telerobotic systems with the potential for performing complete operations with the surgeon at great distance from the patient. This technology holds great promise for overcoming natural human limitations such a hand tremor and fatigue as well as allowing the surgeon to perform minimally invasive procedures in an intuitive, three-dimensional field.

The application of robotic technology in otolaryngology is still in its infancy, but a number of research groups have proven that robotic surgery is feasible in the head and neck. With miniaturization of instrumentation and further research into novel applications of this technology in otolaryngology, robotic systems may allow surgeons of the future to better perform procedures currently practiced and invent new techniques not feasible due to human limitations. Beyond feasibility, much work still needs to be done to evaluate whether robotic surgery is beneficial over traditional open, endoscopic, and microscopic techniques.

Development of surgical robotic technology for clinical use will require close collaboration between engineers and clinical and research otolaryngologists who each bring their unique expertise to the field of robotic surgery.

References

1. Falk V, Diegeler A, Walther T, et al. Total endoscopic computer enhanced coronary artery bypass grafting. Eur J Cardiothorac Surg. 2000;17:38–45.
2. Nifong LW, Chu VF, Bailey BM, et al. Robotic mitral valve repair: experience with the da Vinci system. Ann Thorac Surg. 2003;75:438–42.
3. Tewari A, Kaul S, Menon M. Robotic radical prostatectomy: a minimally invasive therapy for prostate cancer. Curr Urol Rep. 2005;6:45–8.
4. Lanfranco AR, Castellanos AE, Desai JP, Meyers WC. Robotic surgery: a current perspective. Ann Surg. 2004;239:14–21.
5. Kwoh YS, Hou J, Jonckheere EA, Hayati S. A robot with improved absolute positioning accuracy for CT guided stereotactic brain surgery. IEEE Trans Biomed Eng. 1988;35:153–60.
6. Davies B. A review of robotics in surgery. Proc Inst Mech Eng H. 2000;214:129–40.
7. Camarillo DB, Krummel TM, Salisbury Jr JK. Robotic technology in surgery: past, present, and future. Am J Surg. 2004;188:2S–15.
8. Ballantyne GH, Moll F. The da Vinci telerobotic surgical system: the virtual operative field and telepresence surgery. Surg Clin North Am. 2003;83:1293–304.
9. Marescaux J, Rubino F. The ZEUS robotic system: experimental and clinical applications. Surg Clin North Am. 2003;83:1305–15.
10. Hockstein NG, Nolan JP, O'malley Jr BW, Woo YJ. Robotic microlaryngeal surgery: a technical feasibility study using the daVinci surgical robot and an airway mannequin. Laryngoscope. 2005;115:780–5.
11. Hockstein NG, Nolan JP, O'malley Jr BW, Woo YJ. Robot-assisted pharyngeal and laryngeal microsurgery: results of robotic cadaver dissections. Laryngoscope. 2005;115:1003–8.
12. Hockstein NG, Weinstein GS, O'malley Jr BW. Maintenance of hemostasis in transoral robotic surgery. ORL J Otorhinolaryngol Relat Spec. 2005;67:220–4.
13. Newman JG, Kuppersmith RB, O'malley Jr BW. Robotics and telesurgery in otolaryngology. Otolaryngol Clin North Am. 2011;44:1317–31. viii.

14. Vaughan CW, Strong MS, Jako GJ. Laryngeal carcinoma: transoral treatment utilizing the CO_2 laser. Am J Surg. 1978;136:490–3.
15. Ambrosch P, Kron M, Steiner W. Carbon dioxide laser microsurgery for early supraglottic carcinoma. Ann Otol Rhinol Laryngol. 1998;107:680–8.
16. Strong MS. Laser excision of carcinoma of the larynx. Laryngoscope. 1975;85:1286–9.
17. Weinstein GS, O'malley Jr BW, Snyder W, Hockstein NG. Transoral robotic surgery: supraglottic partial laryngectomy. Ann Otol Rhinol Laryngol. 2007; 116:19–23.
18. Lawson G, Mendelsohn AH, Van DV, Bachy V, Remacle M. Transoral robotic surgery total laryngectomy. Laryngoscope. 2013;123:193–6.
19. Mendelsohn AH, Remacle M, Van DV, Bachy V, Lawson G. Outcomes following transoral robotic surgery: supraglottic laryngectomy. Laryngoscope. 2013; 123:208–14.
20. Ozer E, Alvarez B, Kakarala K, Durmus K, Teknos TN, Carrau RL. Clinical outcomes of transoral robotic supraglottic laryngectomy. Head Neck. 2012;35: 1158–61.
21. Rivera-Serrano CM, Johnson P, Zubiate B, et al. A transoral highly flexible robot: novel technology and application. Laryngoscope. 2012;122:1067–71.
22. McLeod IK, Melder PC. Da Vinci robot-assisted excision of a vallecular cyst: a case report. Ear Nose Throat J. 2005;84:170–2.
23. Weinstein GS, O'malley Jr BW, Snyder W, Sherman E, Quon H. Transoral robotic surgery: radical tonsillectomy. Arch Otolaryngol Head Neck Surg. 2007;133:1220–6.
24. de Almeida JR, Park RC, Genden EM. Reconstruction of transoral robotic surgery defects: principles and techniques. J Reconstr Microsurg. 2012;28:465–72.
25. Mukhija VK, Sung CK, Desai SC, Wanna G, Genden EM. Transoral robotic assisted free flap reconstruction. Otolaryngol Head Neck Surg. 2009;140:124–5.
26. Selber JC. Transoral robotic reconstruction of oropharyngeal defects: a case series. Plast Reconstr Surg. 2010;126:1978–87.
27. Weinstein GS, O'malley Jr BW, Magnuson JS, et al. Transoral robotic surgery: a multicenter study to assess feasibility, safety, and surgical margins. Laryngoscope. 2012;122:1701–7.
28. Boudreaux BA, Rosenthal EL, Magnuson JS, et al. Robot-assisted surgery for upper aerodigestive tract neoplasms. Arch Otolaryngol Head Neck Surg. 2009;135:397–401.
29. Weinstein GS, Quon H, O'malley Jr BW, Kim GG, Cohen MA. Selective neck dissection and deintensified postoperative radiation and chemotherapy for oropharyngeal cancer: a subset analysis of the University of Pennsylvania transoral robotic surgery trial. Laryngoscope. 2010;120:1749–55.
30. Lee JM, Weinstein GS, O'malley Jr BW, Thaler ER. Transoral robot-assisted lingual tonsillectomy and uvulopalatopharyngoplasty for obstructive sleep apnea. Ann Otol Rhinol Laryngol. 2012;121:635–9.
31. Kim GG, Zanation AM. Transoral robotic surgery to resect skull base tumors via transpalatal and lateral pharyngeal approaches. Laryngoscope. 2012;122: 1575–8.
32. Byeon HK, Ban MJ, Lee JM, et al. Robot-assisted Sistrunk's operation, total thyroidectomy, and neck dissection via a transaxillary and retroauricular (TARA) approach in papillary carcinoma arising in thyroglossal duct cyst and thyroid gland. Ann Surg Oncol. 2012;19:4259–61.
33. McCool RR, Warren FM, Wiggins III RH, Hunt JP. Robotic surgery of the infratemporal fossa utilizing novel suprahyoid port. Laryngoscope. 2010;120: 1738–43.
34. Kang SW, Jeong JJ, Yun JS, et al. Gasless endoscopic thyroidectomy using trans-axillary approach; surgical outcome of 581 patients. Endocr J. 2009;56:361–9.
35. Kang SW, Jeong JJ, Yun JS, et al. Robot-assisted endoscopic surgery for thyroid cancer: experience with the first 100 patients. Surg Endosc. 2009;23: 2399–406.
36. Holsinger FC, Terris DJ, Kuppersmith RB. Robotic thyroidectomy: operative technique using a transaxillary endoscopic approach without CO_2 insufflation. Otolaryngol Clin North Am. 2010;43:381–8.
37. Lin HS, Folbe AJ, Carron MA, et al. Single-incision transaxillary robotic thyroidectomy: challenges and limitations in a North American population. Otolaryngol Head Neck Surg. 2012;147:1041–6.
38. Hanna EY, Holsinger C, DeMonte F, Kupferman M. Robotic endoscopic surgery of the skull base: a novel surgical approach. Arch Otolaryngol Head Neck Surg. 2007;133:1209–14.
39. Lee JY, O'malley Jr BW, Newman JG, et al. Transoral robotic surgery of the skull base: a cadaver and feasibility study. ORL J Otorhinolaryngol Relat Spec. 2010;72:181–7.
40. Steinhart H, Bumm K, Wurm J, Vogele M, Iro H. Surgical application of a new robotic system for paranasal sinus surgery. Ann Otol Rhinol Laryngol. 2004;113:303–9.
41. Kavanagh KT. Applications of image-directed robotics in otolaryngologic surgery. Laryngoscope. 1994;104:283–93.
42. Federspil PA, Geisthoff UW, Henrich D, Plinkert PK. Development of the first force-controlled robot for otoneurosurgery. Laryngoscope. 2003;113: 465–71.
43. Danilchenko A, Balachandran R, Toennies JL, et al. Robotic mastoidectomy. Otol Neurotol. 2011;32: 11–6.
44. Kratchman LB, Blachon GS, Withrow TJ, Balachandran R, Labadie RF, Webster III RJ. Design of a bone-attached parallel robot for percutaneous cochlear implantation. IEEE Trans Biomed Eng. 2011;58:2904–10.

Anatomic Considerations in Transoral Robotic Surgery

Bharat B. Yarlagadda and Gregory A. Grillone

Introduction

Classic approaches to the head and neck are well described in the surgical literature. These "external" or "open" approaches correspond to traditional anatomic dissections and are thus very familiar to head and neck surgeons. In contrast, the anatomy of the larynx and pharynx from a transoral robotic (TORS) standpoint must be approached from an "inside-out" perspective. Thorough knowledge of this anatomic perspective is necessary for achieving appropriate oncologic resection as well as avoiding potentially catastrophic complications.

The transoral approach to the pharynx and larynx has been described in the past, especially in the setting of transoral laser microsurgery (TLM). Wolfgang Steiner and colleagues have described several such approaches and procedures [1]. Although laryngoscopic exposure is considerably different than that achieved with the TORS approach, many of the anatomic details and considerations overlap.

Anatomic considerations of the TORS approach can be viewed from a perspective of (1) myofascial layers of the surgical field and (2) neurovascular structures that traverse the field. Given the confined space of dissection, three-dimensional understanding is critical. In addition, familiarity with this anatomic region of the head and neck from a trans-cervical standpoint is important for understanding the TORS perspective.

Tonsil and Lateral Pharyngeal Wall

The oropharynx is that portion of the pharynx extending from the level of the soft palate to the level of the epiglottis. Subsites of the oropharynx include the soft palate, base of tongue, posterior pharyngeal wall, and the lateral pharyngeal wall including the palatine tonsils. Stratified squamous epithelium comprises the surface of this portion of the pharynx, including the lining of the crypts within the lymphoid tissue of the base of tongue and palatine tonsils. This architecture is postulated to allow access to human papillomavirus, which is known to mediate the development of squamous cell carcinoma [2]. Given the interest and ability to treat such neoplasm with surgery, this anatomic area is of particular interest to the TORS surgeon.

The anatomy of the tonsil is well known to head and neck surgeons (Fig. 1). The squamous

B.B. Yarlagadda
Department of Otolaryngology—Head and Neck Surgery, Boston University School of Medicine, Boston, MA, USA
e-mail: yarlagb@gmail.com

G.A. Grillone (✉)
Department of Otolaryngology—Head and Neck Surgery, Boston University School of Medicine, Boston Medical Center, 820, Harrison Ave, FGH Building, 4th Floor, Boston, MA 02118, USA
e-mail: Gregory.Grillone@bmc.org

G.A. Grillone and S. Jalisi (eds.), *Robotic Surgery of the Head and Neck: A Comprehensive Guide*,
DOI 10.1007/978-1-4939-1547-7_2, © Springer Science+Business Media New York 2015

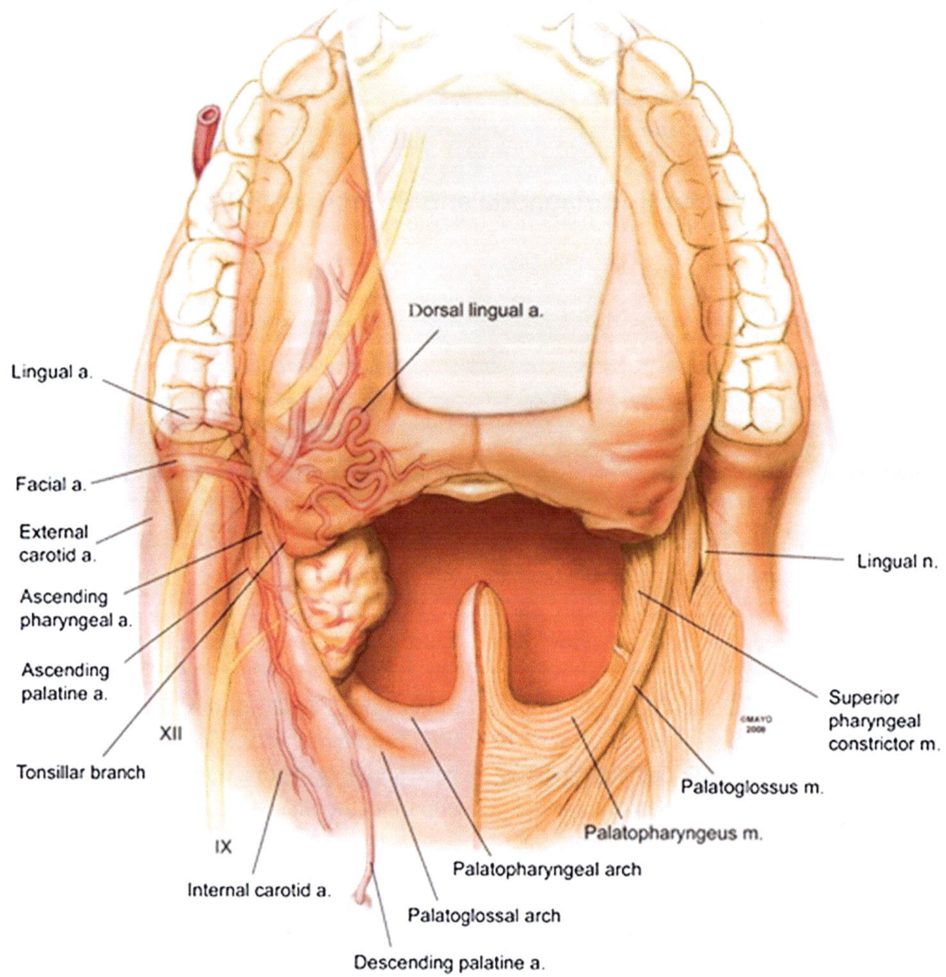

Fig. 1 A transoral view of the oropharynx demonstrating the arrangement of the superficial muscles of the lateral oropharyngeal wall and tonsillar fossa as it would appear with a surgical retractor in place. The vascular and neural supply to this region is outlined. From Moore, EJ, et al. Transoral robotic surgery of the oropharynx: Clinical and anatomic considerations. Clinical Anatomy, 2012. Reprinted with permission [11]

epithelium lined lymphoid tissue sits in the tonsil fossa, which is bordered anteriorly by the palatoglossus and posteriorly by the palatopharyngeus. The lateral border of the tonsil is bounded by fascial layers comprising the tonsillar capsule and the medial border of the peri-tonsillar space. Just deep to this lies the pharyngobasilar fascia. This layer of fascia, attached superiorly to the occipital and temporal bones, which is thickened at the level of the tonsil fossa, thins and disappears as it traverses inferiorly and is attached anteriorly to the pterygomandibular raphe [3]. Lateral to this is the superior pharyngeal constrictor muscle, which, along with the overlying pharyngobasilar fascia, forms the bed of the tonsillar fossa. Inferiorly, the muscular bed may be formed by the middle constrictor muscle overlapping the superior constrictor. In instances where a large gap exists between these constrictors, portions of the stylopharyngeus will then form the bed [4]. These muscles, as will be discussed, are critical landmarks for TORS pharyngeal surgery. On the deep, or lateral, surface of the superior constrictor muscle is the buccopharyngeal fascia.

Finally, access to the parapharyngeal space is achieved through dissection lateral to the bucco-pharyngeal fascia.

The parapharyngeal space is a well-known potential space in the shape of an inverted pyramid extending from the skull base to the greater cornu of the hyoid bone [3, 5]. This space is bounded anteriorly by the pterygomandibular raphe on the lingual surface of the mandibular ramus; laterally by the deep lobe of the parotid, pterygoid muscles, and stylomandibular ligament; medially by the buccopharyngeal fascia; and posteriorly by the retropharyngeal space. The pre- and post-styloid compartments are divided by fascial condensations arising from the stylohyoid ligament, although this boundary varies by author. Pre-styloid contents include the deep lobe of the parotid and fat tissue whereas the post-styloid contents consist of neurovascular structures including the carotid sheath and sympathetic chain. Performance of TORS tonsillectomy does not routinely involve deep dissection of the parapharyngeal space. However, intimate knowledge of this space is a requisite for safe and effective TORS surgery as the internal carotid artery (ICA) and external carotid artery (ECA) branches are encountered, and in addition, displacement or effacement of the parapharyngeal fat is indicative of the extent and resectability of tonsillar tumors.

The stepwise surgical procedure of TORS radical tonsillectomy and the nuances thereof are have been previously described and are discussed elsewhere [6, 7]. However, further consideration of muscular and vascular anatomy can be appreciated in the context of the operation itself. Radical TORS tonsillectomy begins with a vertical incision through the pterygomandibular raphe. Dissection proceeds along the fascia of the medial pterygoid muscle and the surgeon enters the plane between the superior constrictor muscle and the buccopharyngeal fascia. The styloglossus and stylopharyngeus muscles are encountered and represent important anatomic landmarks in the procedure.

The styloglossus muscle arises from the inferior aspect of the styloid process and broadens as it descends, running deep to the medial pterygoid muscle before blending with the fibers of the intrinsic tongue muscles [3]. This muscle is located anterior and lateral to the stylopharyngeus and is encountered first. The stylopharyngeus originates from the medial aspect of the styloid process and courses medial and posterior to the styloglossus [3]. After running between the external and internal carotid arteries, the stylopharyngeus fans out and inserts into the pharynx between the superior and middle pharyngeal constrictors, spreading out between the middle constrictor and the pharyngobasilar fascia (Fig. 2). As noted previously, in instances where there is an anatomic dehiscence between the superior and middle pharyngeal constrictors, the stylopharyngeus will fill the space and form that portion of the tonsil bed. The styloglossus and stylopharyngeus muscles provide a key landmark as a sheath that separates the neurovascular structures of the parapharynx from the surgical bed and lumen of the oropharynx (Fig. 3). The neurovascular structures are lateral and inferior to the plane of the styloglossus, and thus the styloglossus often represents the deep boundary of dissection. Although they are carefully transected during performance of radical tonsillectomy, and in some cases are resected for

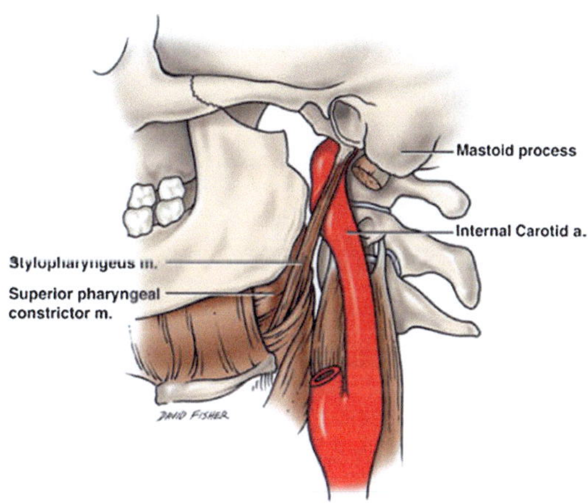

Fig. 2 External view of the musculature of the lateral oropharyngeal area and styloid apparatus. Note the course of the stylopharyngeus muscles as it starts lateral to the internal carotid artery at the level of the styloid, but at its insertion at the level of the oropharynx, lies medial to both the internal and external carotid arteries. From Tubbs RS, et al. Compression of the cervical internal carotid artery by the stylopharyngeus mucle. J Neurosurg. 2010. Reprinted with permission [8]

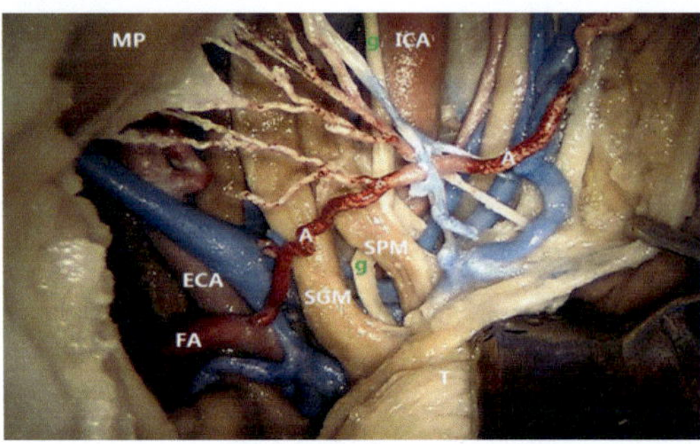

Fig. 3 Transoral view of the parapharyngeal space contents after removal of the superior constrictor muscle in a cadaveric dissection. Note the styloglossus and stylopharyngeus slings protecting the lateral contents including the major cervical vessels. In this anatomic variant, the ascending pharyngeal is seen arising from the facial artery rather than directly from the external carotid artery. *A* ascending pharyngeal artery, *MP* medial pterygoid muscle, *ICA* internal carotid artery, *ECA* external carotid artery, *FA* facial artery, *SGM* styloglossus muscle, *SPM* stylopharyngeus muscle, *g* glossopharyngeal nerve, *T* tongue. From Wang, C, et al. A description of arterial variants in the transoral approach to the parapharyngeal space. Clinical Anatomy. 2014. Reprinted with permission [9]

oncologic purposes, structures medial to these muscles must be respected.

The lingual nerve may be encountered if dissection is continued inferiorly and anteriorly at this location (Fig. 4). This main branch of V3 is joined by the chorda tympani at the level of the posterior border of the medial pterygoid muscle and provides general sensation and taste to the anterior two-thirds of the tongue as well as parasympathetic innervation to the submandibular and sublingual salivary glands. The nerve courses anteriorly and inferiorly between the lingual surface of the mandible and the lateral surface of the medial pterygoid. At the anterior aspect of the medial pterygoid, the lingual nerve runs lateral to the superior constrictor muscle and thus may be near the field of dissection. Dissection of the nerve itself is usually not necessary in routine radical tonsillectomy, buts its location in this region should be noted to avoid injury.

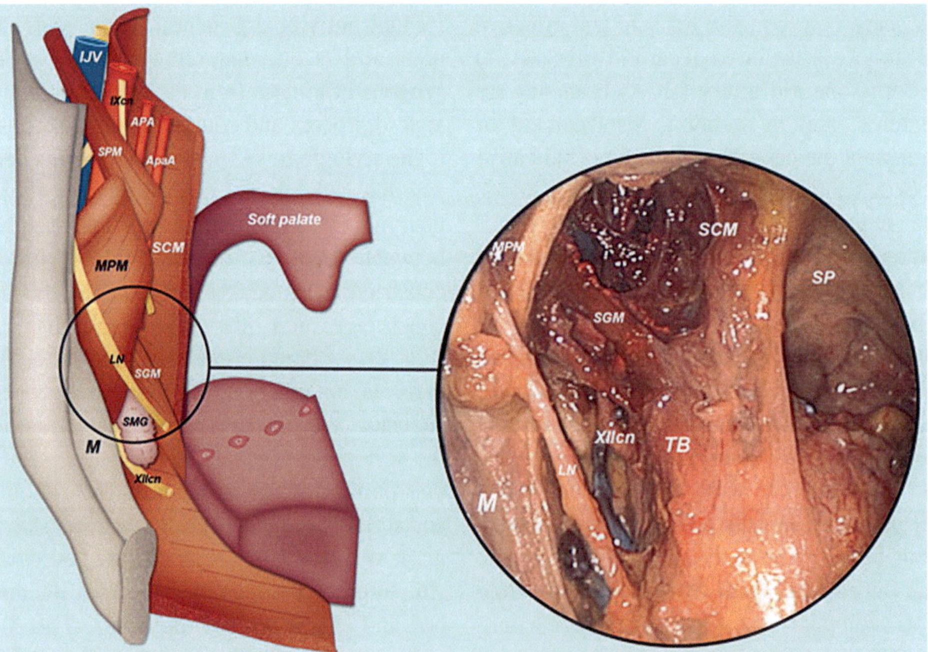

Fig. 4 A schematic drawing and correlating cadaver dissection depicting an anterior–posterior view of the dissected lateral pharyngeal wall. *APA* ascending pharyngeal artery, *ApaA* ascending palatine artery, *IJV* internal jugular vein, *LN* lingual nerve, *M* mandible, *MPM* medial pterygoid muscle, *SCM* superior constrictor muscle, *SGM* styloglossus muscle, *SMG* submandibular gland, *SP* soft palate, *SPM* stylopharyngeus muscle, *TB* tongue base, *IXcn* glossopharyngeus nerve, *XIIcn* hypoglossal nerve. From Dallan, I, et al. Transoral endoscopic anatomy of the parapharyngeal space: A step-by-step logical approach with surgical considerations. Head and Neck. 2010. Reprinted with permission [5]

The second important nervous structure to consider in TORS tonsillectomy is the glossopharyngeal nerve (CN IX). This nerve is responsible for providing sensation in the oropharynx, motor innervation to the stylopharyngeus, and autonomic innervation to the parotid gland and carotid body. After exiting the skull base via the jugular foramen, CN IX runs inferiorly, coursing medial to the styloid process between the stylopharyngeus and styloglossus muscles, laying on the lateral aspect of the stylopharyngues. As it courses toward the middle constrictor muscle, it sends terminal branches to the tonsil and posterior one-third of the tongue. The main trunk of the nerve may be very close to the tonsil fossa especially if there is dehiscence between the middle and superior pharyngeal constrictors. Transection of the lingual and tonsillar branches of CN IX occurs during the course of a TORS extirpation. This, as well as potential damage to the main nerve itself, is likely responsible for postoperative dysgeusia noted in patients undergoing routine tonsillectomy as well as TORS operations [10].

As dissection continues medial to the parapharyngeal fat, the surgeon will encounter and must control the arterial supply to the surgical field. Vascular supply to the tonsil and lateral pharyngeal wall is based on the branches of the ECA [11]. The blood supply to the tonsil includes the ascending palatine and tonsillar branches of the facial artery, the ascending pharyngeal artery, and branches from the lingual artery, ascending palatine artery, and internal maxillary artery. During routine tonsillectomy, these branches are easily controlled with cautery. However, dissection deep to the superior constrictor muscles during radical tonsillectomy encounters blood vessels of a higher caliber that may require ligation with surgical clips to avoid hemorrhage. In addition, several variations and aberrant courses of these vessels will be discussed.

The dominant arterial supply to the tonsil is the tonsillar branch of the facial artery. The facial artery, along with the lingual and ascending pharyngeal arteries, lies approximately 5- to 8-mm deep to the styloglossus muscle [12]. The tonsillar branch has a variable course and can run between, anterior, or posterior to the styloglossus and stylopharyngeus muscles. Application of surgical clips facilitates control of this dominant branch. Another consideration related to the facial artery relates to the main trunk of the vessel. After originating from the ECA in the neck, the artery courses superiorly before turning anteriorly to supply the submandibular gland and face. Tumors with anterior and inferior extension can approximate the artery at either the horizontal portion or the anterior turn, and troublesome bleeding may be encountered [13].

The pharyngeal venous plexus is encountered inferomedially when dissecting lateral to the superior constrictor muscle. These venous branches are encountered medial to the branches of the external carotid artery (ECA) within the space between the stylopharyngeus and the superior constrictor muscle [5, 12]. Terminal drainage of this plexus is to the internal jugular vein. The vessels of this plexus are highly variable in their course and redundancy and can often be controlled readily with monopolar or bipolar electrocautery.

Thus, hemostasis is readily achieved in TORS radical tonsillectomy with knowledge and anticipation and control of the known arterial supply. Further, several maneuvers have been described in order to protect the patient from vascular injury and hemorrhage encountered during TORS radical tonsillectomy. This includes, for example, ligation of the lingual artery or placement of cotton patties medial to the carotid sheath to protect the sheath contents via a cervical approach, prior to the TORS procedure [7, 11]. Whether or not such methods are used, intimate knowledge of the vasculature and anatomic variations is needed to avoid complications. In addition, advanced TORS approaches are currently under investigation including dissection of the parapharyngeal space and infratemporal fossa which require knowledge of vascular aberrations.

The ascending palatine artery contributes to the blood supply of the tonsil and lateral pharyngeal wall. This artery branches from the facial artery and crosses the styloglossus muscle prior to entering the prestyloid parapharyngeal space. In one described variant, the ascending palatine

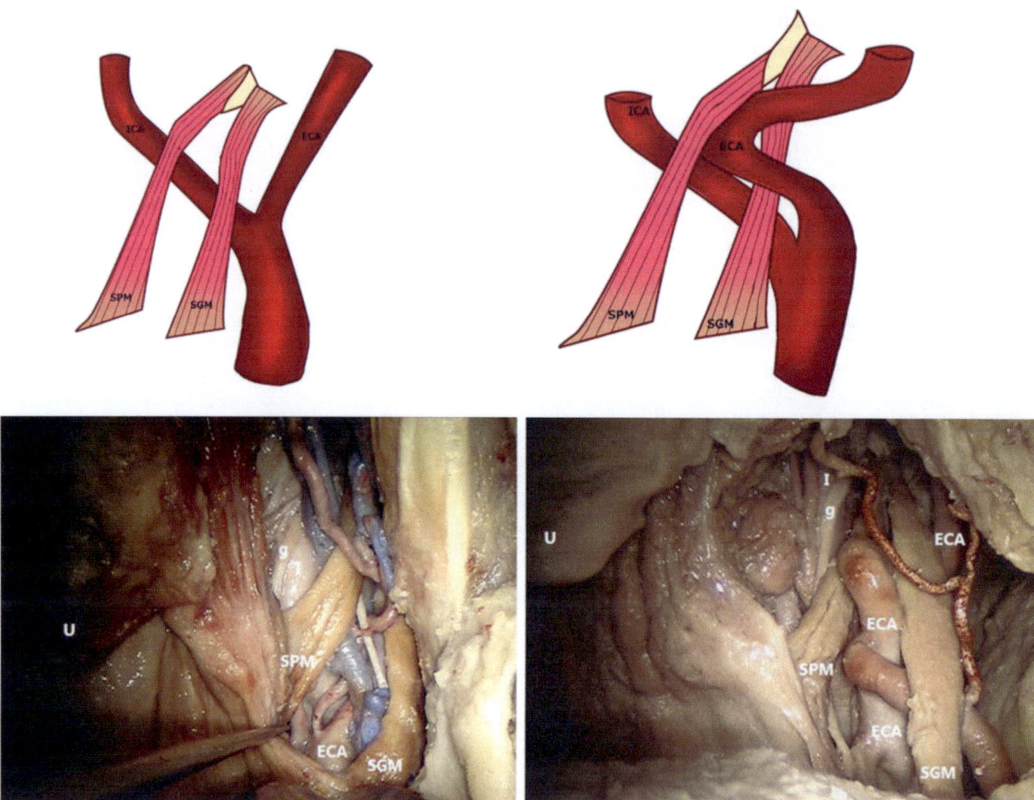

Fig. 5 Depicted in the left column is the normal arrangement of the external carotid artery in relation to the stylopharyngeus and styloglossus muscles. In the right column, the external carotid is coursing medially through a dehiscence between the two muscle bellies. *S* styloid process, *g* glossopharyngeal nerve, *I* internal carotid artery, *ECA* external carotid artery, *SGM* styloglossus muscle, *SPM* stylopharyngeus muscle, *P* medial pterygoid muscle, *U* uvula, *IJV* internal jugular vein, *D* digastric muscle. From Wang, C, et al. A description of arterial variants in the transoral approach to the parapharyngeal space. Clinical Anatomy. 2014. Reprinted with permission [9]

courses between the styloglossus and stylopharyngeus [9]. If encountered, this artery can be controlled with clips or cautery. The ascending pharyngeal artery is a more robust artery providing blood supply to the same region. This originates from the medial surface of the ECA near the carotid bifurcation, but has been known to originate from the ICA or the occipital artery [9]. The artery ascends vertically lateral to the pharyngeal wall towards the skull base. A mean distance of between 5- and 8-mm was noted between the ascending pharyngeal artery, as well as other ECA branches, and the styloglossus muscle [12]. Control of this artery with appropriate clipping from a transoral approach or ligation from a cervical approach is critical.

The ECA has a fairly consistent relationship with the lateral pharyngeal wall. When measured at the C2–C3 vertebral interspace, the ECA lies approximately 1.8 cm lateral to the lateral pharyngeal wall [12]. This distance may of course be altered by the mass effect of tumor and should be noted preoperatively. In cadaveric studies, Wang and colleagues noted the presence of an aberrant ECA in a minority of specimens [9]. In 92 % of cases, the ECA ran deep to and was protected by the styloglossus muscle. Thus, the main trunk of ECA was exposed to injury when dissection proceeded deep to the styloglossus and stylopharyngeus muscle slings. However, in the remaining 8 %, the ECA perforates a dehiscence in the fascial plane between the styloglossus and stylopharyngeus, and thus lies in close relationship to the constrictor musculature (Fig. 5). This creates a situation of potential injury during TORS radical tonsillectomy as well as parapharyngeal space dissection (Fig. 5). In addition, as seen in cadaveric dissection, completion of TORS radical tonsillectomy in a patient with this variation may leave the ECA exposed through the pharyngeal defect and require reconstruction for coverage.

A potentially catastrophic complication of TORS radical tonsillectomy may be ICA injury and this should be avoided at all costs. The cervical ICA normally runs vertically through the neck to the skull base without branching. As one reaches adulthood, the distance between the ICA and the tonsillar fossa approaches 25 mm [14]. Thus, dissection lateral to the constrictor muscle, especially in a blunt manner, can be performed safely under normal circumstances. The styloglossus and styloparyngeus muscles serve as landmarks for the location and therefore protection of the ICA. Although the styloglossus originates lateral to the ICA, it courses medially and, along with the stylopharyngeus, is medial to the ICA at the level of the oropharynx. Thus, transection of these muscles can be performed, if needed, in the presence of a known parapharyngeal fat pad that can be bluntly dissected away to protect the ICA.

However, between 10 and 40 % of the general population may have some aberration of the cervical ICA that alters this course and relation to the oropharynx [15]. Tortuosity, kinking, or coiling of the ICA must be assessed with preoperative imaging. These variants are associated with decreased distance between the ICA and tonsil fossa as well as loss of integrity in the tunica media and adventitia [16]. In addition, the presence of a submucosal or retropharyngeal carotid artery must be ruled out. This is a contraindication to TORS radical tonsillectomy due to a high risk of catastrophic vascular injury.

The remaining steps of TORS radical tonsil resection include a soft palate incision, and floor of mouth and base of tongue resection depending on the extent of the tumor, as well as an incision through the superior constrictor muscle and overlying mucosa posteriorly. At the completion of the procedure, the wound bed is comprised of the buccopharyngeal fascia and the styloglossus and stylopharyngeus muscles. Thus, care is taken to preserve the buccopharyngeal fascia if possible while the lateral surface of the constrictor muscle is dissected away during the surgery. The presence of these structures prevents communication into the neck via the parapharyngeal space and protects the carotid vasculature from exposure into the neck. If this barrier is excised for oncologic purposes, reconstruction can be performed for protection of the parapharyngeal contents, such as suturing of the fascial edges or use of a mucosal advancement flap for coverage of the defect [7].

Lymphatic drainage of the tonsillar region involves levels IIa, IIb, III, and IV of the neck as well as the retropharyngeal nodes. Classically defined by Rouviere and described in modern literature, the retropharyngeal nodes are divided into the poorly defined medial nodes that are often absent in adults, and the lateral nodes which are more pertinent to tumors of the oropharynx [13, 17]. Although there is generally one lateral retropharyngeal node on each side, up to three may be present. The location of the lateral nodes is fairly consistent and is anterior to the prevertebral fascia at the level of C1 and medial to the ICA and cervical sympathetic chain. The surgical resection of the lateral retropharyngeal nodes via the TORS approach has been described, and is performed after completion of robotic oropharyngectomy [18].

Although the data continue to evolve, it does not appear that lateral retropharyngeal nodal resection is universally required in tonsillar squamous cell carcinoma. Data have shown that when patients with early stage disease (T1 or T2 and N0-N2a) and no retropharyngeal involvement on preoperative imaging undergo routine retropharyngeal dissection, the rates of histologically confirmed metastasis are zero [17]. High quality multi-modality imaging is required for this purpose: either fine-cut computed tomography or magnetic resonance imaging combined with positron emission tomography. Thus surgery of the pharynx and tonsil alone may be sufficient in the appropriate patient.

Base of Tongue

The tongue is divided by the circumvallate papilla into two major units, the base of tongue and the oral tongue. The dorsal and posterior aspect of

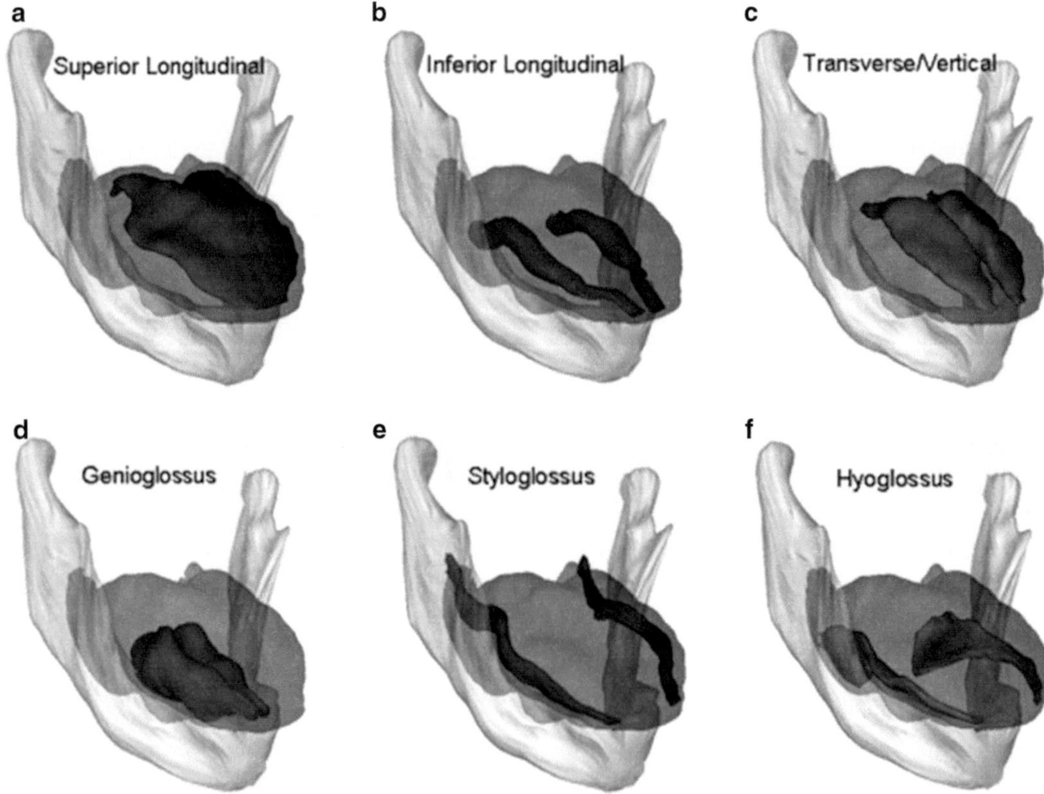

Fig. 6 Depiction of the intrinsic (**a**, **b**, **c**) and extrinsic (**d**, **e**, **f**) muscles of the tongue. Although depicted separately, these muscles have extensive overlap and interdigitation. From Sanders I, et al. A three-dimensional atlas of human tongue muscles. Anat Rec. 2013. Reprinted with permission. [20]

the tongue base comprises the anterior wall of the oropharynx. Like the lateral oropharyngeal wall, transoral robotic surgery greatly facilitates surgical access to the tongue base. Successful robotic surgery of the tongue base, as with other regions, is contingent on knowledge of the neurovascular anatomy. Preservation of at least one tongue base neurovascular bundle is necessary for survival and function of the remaining tongue.

Posterior to the tongue base lies the epiglottis. A median and two lateral glossoepiglottic folds connect these two structures. The valleculae represent the depression between the median and lateral folds. Even further laterally are the glossotonsillar folds, created by the palatoglossus muscle, which are continuous with the palatoglossal arch that runs anterior to the palatine tonsils.

The tongue and tongue base are comprised of intrinsic and named extrinsic muscles. The intrinsic muscles are bundles of interlacing fibers separated by connective tissue septa, which is particularly well formed at the midline. The superior fibers lie submucosally and run along the entire dorsum of the tongue, splaying laterally. The inferior longitudinal fibers course between the genioglossus and hyoglossus muscles. Transverse and vertical fibers contribute to the remainder of tongue bulk and run, respectively, from the septum to the lateral surface and from the dorsal to lateral surface of the tongue [19].

The extrinsic muscles of the tongue include the genioglossus, the hyoglossus, and the styloglossus muscles (Fig. 6). Some consider the palatoglossus to be included in this group but other authors exclude this muscle due to its innervation by the pharyngeal plexus rather than the hypoglossal nerve [19]. The genioglossus arises from the upper part of the mental spine on the lingual surface of the mandibular symphysis. It extends in a fan-like manner to insert onto the tongue along its length towards the hyoid. The styloglossus muscle has been previously described. The hyoglossus muscle originates from the lateral body and greater cornua of the hyoid bone. The fibers extend superiorly and anteriorly to interdigitate with the syloglossus and instrinsic tongue muscles. The importance of the hyoglossus muscle is due to its relationship with the neurovasculature of the region. The hypoglossal nerve and lingual vein run along the lateral aspect of this muscle as they enter the tongue. Also lateral to the hyoglossus muscle is the lingual nerve and submandibular duct. The lingual artery runs on the deep surface of the hyoglossus muscle, sandwiched between this and the genioglossus muscle. It is in this location that the TORS surgeon will encounter the lingual artery and must obtain control to prevent troublesome hemorrhage.

The lingual nerve provides general sensation and taste to the anterior two-thirds of the tongue. Fibers of general sensation include those transmitting touch, pain, and temperature. These fibers derive from the trigeminal ganglion and are a component of the V3 distribution. Taste fibers are derived from the geniculate ganglion of the facial nerve and travel with the lingual nerve by way of chorda tympani. The chorda tympani nerve joins the lingual nerve at the level of the posterior border of the medial pterygoid muscle. The lingual nerve then runs anteriorly between the mandible and the lateral surface of the medial pterygoid muscle continuing forward, lateral to the styloglossus and then the hyoglossus muscles. It courses around the submandibular duct and runs upward into the tongue between the sublingual gland and genioglossus muscle. It is at the anterior border of the medial pterygoid that the nerve is exposed to risk during TORS tongue base procedures, as described previously.

Motor innervation is provided by the hypoglossal nerve. After exiting the skull base, the hypoglossal nerve descends between the ICA and internal jugular vein. It courses forward and crosses over superficial to both carotid vessels. It is tethered at the forward turn by branches of the occipital artery which feed the sternocleidomastoid muscle. The nerve then passes lateral to the hyoglossus muscle and over the greater cornu of the hyoid bone. It continues deep to the mylohyoid muscle and divides into terminal branches which course upwards on the lateral surface of the genioglossus to enter the tongue musculature. It is in this area, as the nerve runs lateral to the hyoglossus and above the hyoid bone, that it is at greatest risk of injury during TORS tongue base resection. Resections of the tongue base extending deep towards the greater cornu of the hyoid, as well as resection of the hyoglossus, expose the nerve to direct or thermal injury during resection and cautery.

The lingual artery is the second branch arising anteriorly from the ECA. Within the curvature early after its origin from the ECA, the tonsillar branch is given off, and the artery runs anteriorly, above the hyoid and medial to the hypoglossal nerve (Fig. 7). It courses deep to the superior border of the digastric tendon and then medial to the hyoglossus muscle. There are variable collateral patterns between the lingual and facial artery after the takeoff of lingual artery from the ECA. Thus, ligation above the level of the hyoid is suggested if interruption of the vessel is desired [19]. For this purpose, the artery can be found just deep to the plane of Lesser's Triangle—the space bounded by the hypoglossal nerve and the two bellies of the digastric muscle and tendon. At the posterior border of the hyoglossus, the lingual artery gives off the dorsal lingual branches. At the anterior border of the muscle, the lingual artery divides into its terminal branches, the deep lingual and sublingual arteries. These arteries have more robust anastomoses distally towards the tongue tip as compared to more posterior areas. Thus, from the perspective of TORS, the hyoglossus muscle and hyoid bone provide useful landmarks for the location of the lingual artery. Resection deep to the superior constrictor muscle at the level of the greater cornu of the hyoid bone will expose lingual artery as it sits medial to the hyoglossus muscle (Fig. 8).

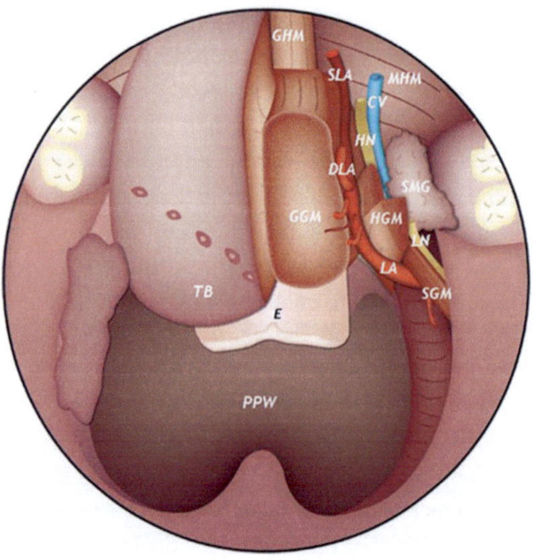

Fig. 7 A schematic reconstruction demonstrating the anatomy of the tongue base and surrounding structure from the perspective of a TORS approach. The lingual artery courses between the hyoglossus and genioglossus muscles. *TB* tongue base, *GGM* genioglossus muscle, *HGM* hyoglossus muscle, *MHM* mylohyoid muscle, *GHM* geniohyoid muscle, *SGM* styloglossus muscle, *SMG* submandibular gland, *LN* lingual nerve, *IXcn* glossopharyngeal nerve, *HN* hypoglossal nerve, *CV* comitant vein, *LA* lingual artery, *DLA* dorsal lingual artery, *SLA* sublingual artery, *E* epiglottis, *PPW* posterior pharyngeal wall. From Dallan, I, et al. Anatomical landmarks for transoral robotic tongue base surgery: comparison between endoscopic, external, and radiological perspectives. Surgical and Radiologic Anatomy. 2013. Reprinted with permission [21]

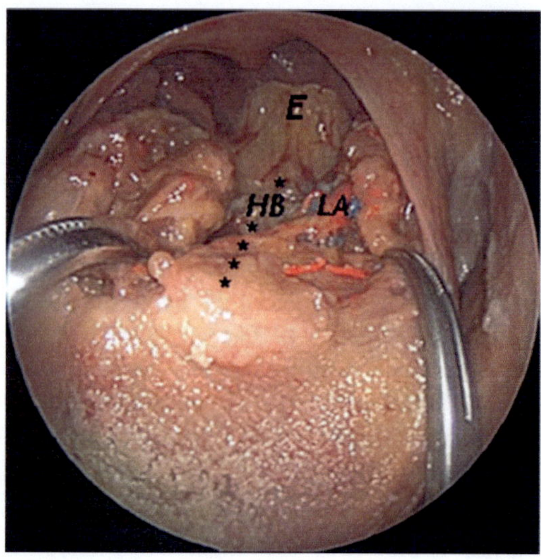

Fig. 8 An endoscopic transoral tongue base dissection demonstrates the exposure of the lingual artery at the level of the hyoid bone. *E* epiglottis, *HB* hyoid bone, *LA* lingual artery, *Black asterisks*—midline. From Dallan, I, et al. Anatomical landmarks for transoral robotic tongue base surgery: comparison between endoscopic, external, and radiological perspectives. Surgical and Radiologic Anatomy. 2013. Reprinted with permission [21]

Analysis of the relevant anatomy from a cervical perspective appears to indicate that TORS tongue base resection is safely and readily performed towards the midline, but one will encounter critical structures as one approaches the lateral aspect of the dissection towards the glossotonsillar folds. This, of course, is true from a transoral perspective as well. The submucosal vessels of the dorsal lingual anastomoses are first encountered with the anterior and horizontal tumor cuts. As the surgeon dissects through the intrinsic muscles and the genioglossus, the dorsal lingual artery itself is visualized laterally, especially as one approaches the hyoid bone at the level of the glossoepiglottic space [21]. This can be traced laterally to identify the main lingual artery trunk running medial to the hyoglossus. Standard cervical landmarks used to identify this "lateral" neurovascular bundle do not apply to the TORS approach. Variations in the volume of lingual lymphoid tissue and the bulk of the tongue itself confound the distance to the arteries and nerves of interest. Lauretano and colleagues noted that on average in cadavers, the neurovascular bundle lie 2.7 cm inferior and 1.6 cm lateral to the foramen cecum [22]. Kokot and colleagues noted the bundle to be on average 2.2 cm inferior and 1.3 cm lateral to the foramen cecum [13]. The hypoglossal nerve was approximately 1.6 cm lateral to the foramen cecum, and its distance from the lingual artery was variable. However, these measurements may not apply in the live patient, especially in light of distortion due to retraction and tumor effect. Regardless, the surgeon should be aware and obtain control of the lingual artery at the lateral aspect of the dissection as the vessel enters the tongue musculature.

Supraglottic Larynx

The transoral view of the larynx is very familiar to most head and neck surgeons. Techniques to maximize the endoscopic exposure of this anatomy

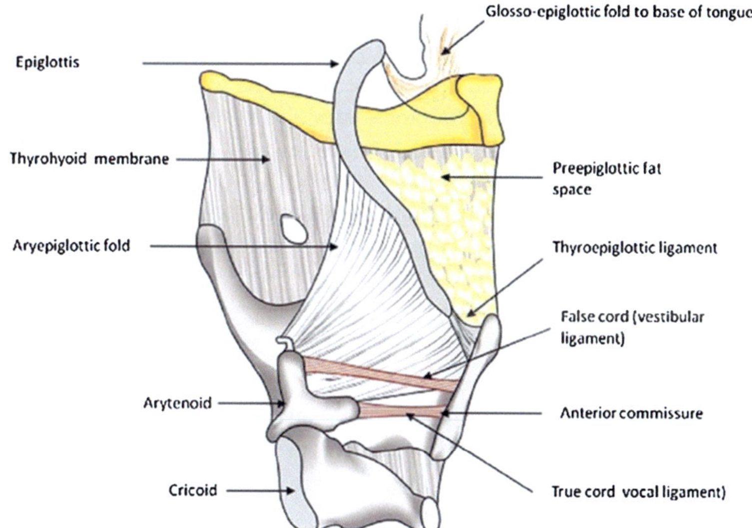

Fig. 9 A midline sagittal view which demonstrates the laryngeal framework, ligaments, and the pre-epiglottic space. From Joshi VM, et al. Imaging in laryngeal cancer. Indian J Radiol Imaging. 2012. Reprinted under Creative Commons license [24]

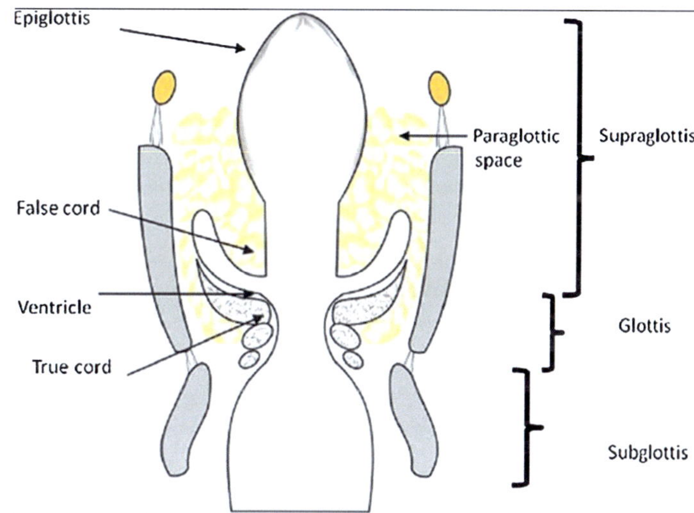

Fig. 10 Coronal section demonstrating the subdivisions, compartments, and barriers of the larynx. These are routes and barriers to tumor spread through the organ. From Joshi VM, et al. Imaging in laryngeal cancer. Indian J Radiol Imaging. 2012. Reprinted under Creative Commons license [24]

have been well described in the literature [23]. Cervical positioning and the choice of laryngoscope are critical elements of obtaining an appropriate view for surgery of the larynx. Knowledge of the structural and neurovascular anatomy of the larynx obtained from traditional endoscopic interventions form the basis of successful robotic surgeries of this region.

The larynx is divided into three main regions (Figs. 9 and 10). The supraglottic larynx extends from the level of the hyoid bone to the level of the laryngeal ventricle. Components of this region include the hyoid bone, epiglottis, arytenoid cartilages, aryepiglottic folds, false vocal folds, pre-epiglottic space, and the mucosa covering these structures. The glottic larynx extends from the laryngeal ventricles to 1 cm inferior to the level of the true vocal folds. The subglottic larynx extends from the inferior aspect of the glottic region to the inferior border of the cricoid cartilage and is mainly comprised of the cricoid cartilage and associated mucosa.

The laryngeal framework is comprised of the thyroid and cricoid cartilages and the hyoid bone.

The hyoid bone is the superior most structure and consists of a body and pairs of greater and lesser horns. It serves as an attachment point for the supra- and infra-hyoid strap muscles and the stylohyoid ligament. The thyroid cartilage forms most of the anterior and lateral walls of the larynx and is attached superiorly to the hyoid bone by the thyrohyoid membrane. The inferior horns articulate with the cricoid cartilage below. The cricoid is a signet shaped structure and is the only complete ring of the normal human airway. Anteriorly and laterally, the arch of the cartilage is relatively thin while the posterior lamina is 2–3 cm in height. The cricoid is attached to the first tracheal ring below by the cricotracheal ligament.

The endolaryngeal structures include the epiglottis, arytenoid cartilages, and the corniculate and cuneiform cartilages. The epiglottis is divided into three parts: the suprahyoid portion, the infrahyoid portion, and the petiole. The curved epiglottic cartilage contains numerous fenestrations which may act as a route of entry for carcinoma into the pre-epiglottic space. The arytenoid cartilages rest above and articulate with the cricoid cartilage. The paired cricoarytenoid units are the functional elements of the larynx involved in speech and swallowing. These units consist of the cricoid-arytenoid articulation, the corniculate and cuneiform cartilages, and the muscular attachments of the posterior cricoarytenoid, lateral cricoarytenoid, and interarytenoid muscles, and are innervated by branches of the superior laryngeal and recurrent laryngeal nerves. Generally, at least one of these units must be preserved when performing oncologic partial laryngeal resection in order to preserve meaningful function of the larynx.

The quadrangular membrane and conus elasticus are the paired fibroelastic sheets that also provide structure to the larynx and contain the laryngeal potential spaces. The quadrangular membrane extends from the sides of the epiglottis to the arytenoids, and is covered by mucosal folds on either side creating the aryepiglottic folds. The membrane extends inferiorly to form the vestibular folds, or false vocal folds. The conus elasticus is a more strongly developed layer. It originates from the superior aspect of the cricoid and sweeps upward and medially. Anteriorly the paired sheets of the conus elasticus attach to the inner surface of the thyroid cartilage near the midline. The superior edge of this sheet contributes to the vocal ligament and attaches to the vocal process of the arytenoid.

The portion of the pharynx most intimately involved with the larynx is the hypopharynx. The pyriform sinus is a subsite of the hypopharynx and sits just lateral to the endolarynx. The pyriforms are bounded laterally by the inner surface of the thyroid cartilage and medially by the pharyngoepiglottic folds. The pyriform sinuses funnel inferiorly into the esophageal inlet. The post-cricoid region and the posterior hypopharyngeal wall comprise the remainder of the hypopharynx. The mucosa of the hypopharynx is bounded by the muscle of the inferior constrictor muscle as it travels from one posterior border of the thyroid lamina to the other.

The larynx contains several adipose filled spaces that are formed by the above described structures (Figs. 9 and 10). These spaces must be considered when performing oncologic resections as they are routes of tumor spread. The pre-epiglottic space is anterior to the epiglottis and is bounded anteriorly by the thyrohyoid membrane, superiorly by the hyoid bone and hyoepiglottic ligament, inferiorly by the thyroepiglottic ligament, and laterally by the paraglottic spaces. The paired paraglottic spaces are bounded laterally by thyroid lamina, medially by the quadrangular membrane and conus elasticus, dorsally by the mucosa of the pyriform sinus, and are confluent anteriorly with the pre-epiglottic space [25].

TORS supraglottic laryngectomy has been described by Weinstein [26] and is an evolution of techniques using laryngoscopic exposures and laser-assisted supraglottic resections [27]. Though the steps of the procedure are explained elsewhere is this text, the operation includes the vertical transection of the epiglottis through the level of the vallecula. The dissection is carried anteriorly to the level of the hyoid bone and the contents of the pre-epiglottic space are dropped down and included in the resection. The surgeon dissects laterally and in a cranial-caudal direction.

In this manner, the pharyngoepiglottic fold is encountered which contains the neurovascular structures critical to the operation.

The neurovascular bundle pertinent to TORS supraglottic laryngectomy includes the superior laryngeal artery, superior laryngeal vein, and the internal branch of the superior laryngeal nerve. The superior laryngeal artery (SLA) provides the dominant blood supply to the supraglottic larynx. The SLA is most commonly a branch of the superior thyroid artery, but may arise directly from the external carotid artery as well. From its origin, it travels anteromedially, and along with the internal branch of the superior laryngeal nerve, pierces the thyrohyoid ligament at a point anterior to the superior horn of the thyroid cartilage to enter the larynx. Here it travels within the pharyngoepiglottic fold and divides into five branches to supply the supraglottic larynx [28]. The ascending branch is the most superficial when dissecting in a cranial-caudal direction, and courses across the upper aspect of the pyriform sinus to supply the epiglottis. The remainder of the branches includes the ventral branch supplying the laryngeal ventricle, the dorsal branch supplying the post-cricoid region, the medial branch supplying the false vocal folds, the dorsal branch supplying the post-cricoid region, and the descending branch supplying the thyroarytenoid muscle. For the purposes of TORS supraglottic laryngectomy, the ascending and ventral branches are most relevant.

Vascular control is obtained at the main trunk of the SLA. Goyal and colleagues describe identification of the main trunk at the level of the pharyngoepiglottic fold from a cranio-caudal approach (Figs. 11 and 12) [29]. Here, the main arterial trunk can be seen with blunt dissection of the pharyngoepiglottic fold immediately after it pierces the thyrohyoid membrane. Souvirón and colleagues describe a landmark-based approach to the main trunk of the SLA in which the neurovascular pedicle can be found in the superior (anterior) third of a triangle formed by the anterior commissure, the vocal process, and the attachment of the aryepiglottic fold to the epiglottis [30]. The spatial orientation of the pedicle

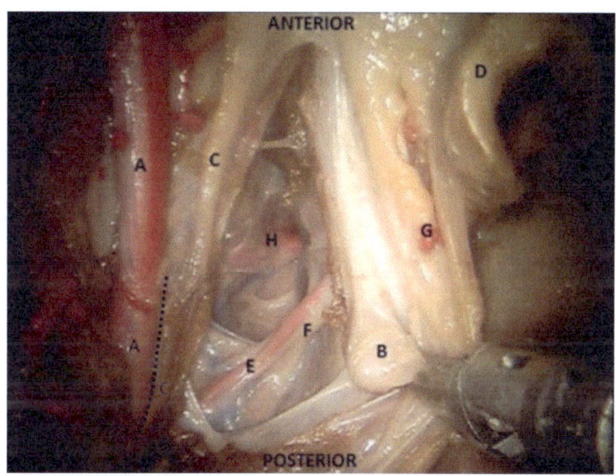

Fig. 11 Robotic dissection of the pharyngoepiglottic fold demonstrates the superior laryngeal neurovascular bundle. In this dissection the suprahyoid attachments were cut and the hyoid retracted medially. A—lingual artery, B—greater cornu of hyoid bone, C—digastric muscle and tendon, D—epiglottis, E—superior laryngeal artery (SLA), F—internal branch of superior laryngeal nerve, G—superior branch of the SLA, H—superior thyroid artery, *Dotted line*—lateral border of the digastric muscle as it comes over the lingual artery. From Goyal, N, et al. Surgical anatomy of the supraglottic larynx using the da Vinci robot. Head and Neck. 2013. Reprinted with permission [29]

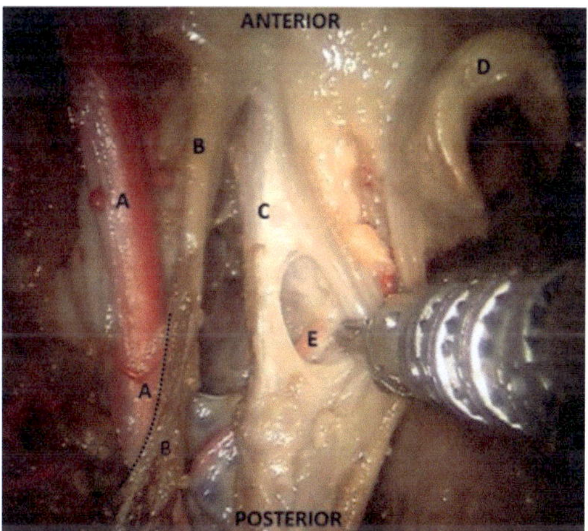

Fig. 12 The superior laryngeal bundle is seen on the medial aspect of the hyoid bone. A—lingual artery, B—digastric muscle and tendon, C—hyoid bone, D—epiglottis, E—superior laryngeal artery and internal branch of superior laryngeal nerve, *Dotted line*—lateral border of the digastric muscle. From Goyal, N, et al. Surgical anatomy of the supraglottic larynx using the da Vinci robot. Head and Neck. 2013. Reprinted with permission [29]

is such that either the superior laryngeal artery or superior laryngeal vein is found superficial to the internal branch of the superior laryngeal nerve in the majority (91 %) of specimens. In the minority, the nerve is the most superficial of the three. Regardless of the method used, control of the main SLA trunk with application of hemostatic clips is critical to avoid troublesome postoperative hemorrhage.

Multiple patterns of the intra-laryngeal branches of the SLA exist. In addition, there is a described aberrant SLA course in which the larynx is entered through a thyroid foramen posterior to the posterior border of the thyroid lamina [31]. In this variant, the main trunk is then found directly in the paraglottic space and can be controlled in this location, rather than within the pharyngoepiglottic fold. An additional consideration is the anastomoses between the ascending branch of the SLA and the suprahyoid branch of the lingual artery. This may lead to bleeding when the dissection includes tissues above the level of the hyoid bone.

The internal branch of the superior laryngeal nerve travels with the SLA through the thyrohyoid membrane and most commonly separates into two or three intra-laryngeal branches [32]. The upper one or two branches provide sensation to the mucosa of the epiglottis, vallecula, vestibule, and false vocal folds. The lower branch provides sensation to mucosa below the vestibule and the mucosa of the pyriform sinus, and motor innervation of the interarytenoid muscles. Much of the mucosal surface innervated by the upper branches is requisitely excised as a component of the oncologic resection, and preservation of these branches is thus superfluous. However, preserving the inferior branch may result in retained sensory innervation of mucosa of the hypopharynx and larynx below the vestibule, motor innervation of the inter-arytenoid musculature, and a preserved cough reflex, potentially improving outcomes postoperatively. With the knowledge of the spatial orientation of the neurovascular bundle within the pharyngoepiglottic fold, the magnification and visualization offered by the TORS approach may be exploited to prevent undue sacrifice of the innervation when placing clips on the vasculature.

Summary

As with traditional surgical approaches, successful and safe TORS procedures are predicated on a thorough understanding of the anatomy. Particular attention must be paid to the presence and course of the relevant neurovascular structures. Previous experience and knowledge of pharyngeal and laryngeal anatomy from a cervical perspective, as well as through traditional laryngoscopic exposures, must be integrated into considerations of the anatomic structures from the "inside-out" approach of experienced with TORS.

Each TORS procedure has its own pertinent vascular supply to consider. These neurovascular pedicles should be anticipated and handled accordingly. In addition, aberrations of the vascular anatomy due to congenital variations or mass effect of tumor must be considered. Preoperative evaluation with appropriate imaging is needed to avoid troublesome complications with hemorrhage and inadvertent neural damage. Particularly, the course of the ICA must be delineated to ensure that disastrous vascular trauma is avoided. Anatomic studies dedicated to the TORS perspective continue to build upon the body of knowledge and allow increasingly nuanced approaches.

References

1. Steiner W, Ambrosch P. Endoscopic laser surgery of the upper aerodigestive tract: with special emphasis on cancer surgery. New York: Theime Stuttgart; 2000.
2. Begum S, Cao D, Gillison M, Zahurak M, Westra WH. Tissue distribution of human papillomavirus 16 DNA in patients with tonsillar carcinoma. Clin Cancer Res. 2005;11(16):5694–9.
3. Janfaza P, Nadol JB, Galla RJ, Fabian RL, Montgomery WW, editors. Surgical anatomy of the head and neck. Philadelphia, PA: Lippincott Williams & Wilkins; 2011.
4. Ohtsuka K, Tomita H, Murakami G. Anatomy of the tonsillar bed: topographical relationship between the palatine tonsil and the lingual branch of the glossopharyngeal nerve. Acta Otolaryngol Suppl. 2002;546: 99–109.
5. Dallan I, Seccia V, Muscatello L, Lenzi R, Castelnuovo P, Bignami M, Montevecchi F, Tschabitscher M, Vicini C. Transoral endoscopic anatomy of the parapharyngeal space: a step-by-step logical approach with surgical considerations. Head Neck. 2011;33(4):557–61.

6. Holsinger FC, McWhorter AJ, Ménard M, Garcia D, Laccourreye O. Transoral lateral oropharyngectomy for squamous cell carcinoma of the tonsillar region: I. Technique, complications, and functional results. Arch Otolaryngol Head Neck Surg. 2005;131:583–91.
7. Weinstein GS, O'Malley BW, Snyder W, Sherman E, Quon H. Transoral robotic surgery: radical tonsillectomy. Arch Otolaryngol Head Neck Surg. 2007;133:1220–6.
8. Tubbs RS, Loukas M, Dixon J, Cohen-Gadol AA. Compression of the cervical internal carotid artery by the stylopharyngeus muscle: an anatomical study with potential clinical significance. Laboratory investigation. J Neuosurg. 2010;113:881–4.
9. Wang C, Kundaria S, Fernandez-Miranda J, Duvvuri U. A description of arterial variants in the transoral approach to the parapharyngeal space. Clin Anat. 2014;27(7):1016–22.
10. Goins MR, Pitovski DZ. Posttonsillectomy taste disturbance: a significant complication. Laryngoscope. 2004;114(7):1206–13.
11. Moore EJ, Janus J, Kasperbauer J. Transoral robotic surgery of the oropharynx: clinical and anatomic considerations. Clin Anat. 2012;25:135–41.
12. Lim CM, Mehta V, Chai R, Pinheiro CN, Rath T, Snyderman C, Duvvuri U. Transoral anatomy of the tonsillar fossa and lateral pharyngeal wall: anatomic dissection with radiographic and clinical correlation. Laryngoscope. 2013;123(12):3021–5.
13. Weinstein GS, O'malley BW. Transoral robotic surgery (TORS). San Diego: Plural; 2012.
14. Deutsch MD, Kriss VM, Willging JP. Distance between the tonsillar fossa and internal carotid artery in children. Arch Otolaryngol Head Neck Surg. 1995;121(12):1410–2.
15. Pfeiffer J, Ridder GJ. A clinical classification system for aberrant internal carotid arteries. Laryngoscope. 2008;118(11):1931–6.
16. Ozgur Z, Celik S, Govsa F, Aktug H, Ozgur T. A study of the course of the internal carotid artery in the parapharyngeal space and its clinical importance. Eur Arch Otorhinolaryngol. 2007;264(12):1483–9. Epub 19 July 2007.
17. Moore EJ, Ebrahimi A, Price DL, Olsen KD. Retropharyngeal lymph node dissection in oropharyngeal cancer treated with transoral robotic surgery. Laryngoscope. 2013;123:1676–81.
18. Byeon HK, Duvvuri U, Kim WS, Park YM, Hong HJ, Koh YW, Choi EC. Transoral robotic retropharyngeal lymph node dissection with or without lateral oropharyngectomy. J Craniofac Surg. 2013;24(4):1156–61.
19. Hollinshead WH. Anatomy for surgeons: the head and neck. 3rd ed. Philadelphia: Harper and Row Publishers; 1982.
20. Sanders I, Mu L. A three-dimensional atlas of human tongue muscles. Anat Rec. 2013;296(7):1102–14.
21. Dallan I, Seccia V, Faggioni L, Castelnuovo P, Montevecchi F, Casani AP, Tschabitscher M, Vicini C. Anatomical landmarks for transoral robotic tongue base surgery: comparison between endoscopic, external and radiological perspectives. Surg Radiol Anat. 2013;35(1):3–10.
22. Lauretano AM, Li KK, Caradonna DS, Khosta RK, Fried MP. Anatomic location of the tongue base neurovascular bundle. Laryngoscope. 1997;107(8):1057–9.
23. Vaughan CW. Vocal fold exposure in phonosurgery. J Voice. 1993;7(2):189–94.
24. Joshi VM, Wadhwa V, Mukherji SK. Imaging in laryngeal cancer. Indian J Radiol Imaging. 2012;22(3):209–26.
25. Reidenbach MM. The paraglottic space and transglottic cancer: anatomical considerations. Clin Anat. 1996;9(4):244–51.
26. Weinstein GS, O'Malley Jr BW, Snyder W, Hockstein NG. Transoral robotic surgery: supraglottic partial laryngectomy. Ann Otol Rhinol Laryngol. 2007;116(1):19–23.
27. Rudert HH, Werner JA. Endoscopic resections of glottic and supraglottic carcinomas with the CO_2 laser. Eur Arch Otorhinolaryngol. 1995;252(3):146–8.
28. Rusu MC, Nimigean V, Banu MA, Cergan R, Niculescu V. The morphology and topography of the superior laryngeal artery. Surg Radiol Anat. 2007;29(8):653–60.
29. Goyal N, Yoo F, Setabutr D, Goldenberg D. Surgical anatomy of the supraglottic larynx using the da Vinci robot. Head Neck. 2013;36:1126–31.
30. Souvirón R, Maranillo E, Vázquez T, Patel N, McHanwell S, Cobeta I, Scola B, Sañudo J. Proposal of landmarks for clamping neurovascular elements during endoscopic surgery of the supraglottic region. Head Neck. 2013;35:57–60.
31. Liu JL, Liang CY, Xiang T, Wang F, Wang LH, Liu SX, Yang HJ. Aberrant branch of the superior laryngeal artery passing through the thyroid foramen. Clin Anat. 2007;20:256–9.
32. Raikos A, Paraskevas GK. The thyroid foramen: a systematic review and surgical considerations. Clin Anat. 2013;26(6):700–8.

Establishing a Head and Neck Robotic Program at Your Institution

Scharukh Jalisi and Prachi Nene

History

Robotic technology has been slowly integrated into various fields of medicine with few complications. Advances in oncologic technology through robotic surgery have aimed to reduce patient mortality while maintaining similar surgical outcomes as other older techniques [1]. When robotic surgery was first explored, Intuitive Surgical® developed the da Vinci surgical robot for procedures originally in urology [2]. In recent years, robotic surgery has become smoothly incorporated into head and neck oncologic surgery.

Oropharyngeal squamous cell carcinoma (OPSCC) represents a significant problem in the head and neck cancer field, with 123,000 cases of malignancy each year [3]. Around the same time that OPSCC was recognized as a major burden in the field, a new technique of robotic surgery (TORS) was in the process of adaptation to the head and neck field by otolaryngologists at the University of Pennsylvania. Their aim was to facilitate transoral access to oropharyngeal cancers, in addition to other oral tumors. Since then much research has shown that TORS facilitates more rapid swallowing rehabilitation and a shorter hospital stay than other management techniques, essentially minimizing morbidity and mortality from the procedures [2].

Furthermore, numerous studies show TORS to be as safe as conventional non-robotic surgery methods (chemoradiation) with the same safety profile, and advances are constantly occurring to improve results [4, 5]. Due to the increasing demand for TORS in the head and neck field, it is necessary to increase the number of head and neck robotic programs in the country.

Training

Once the idea of a program for training surgeons in TORS is introduced, the next step shifts toward training. Adequate training of new surgeons is the crux of a flourishing robotics program at any hospital. In past studies evaluating the value of TORS programs in hospitals, surgeon training and experience is closely linked to the efficacy of a new program in robotic surgery [6]. Formal training in robotic surgery leads to better patient outcomes and shorter operative times. Furthermore, robotic surgery training has shown no negative impact on patient outcomes or learning curves [6].

S. Jalisi, M.D., M.A., F.A.C.S. (✉)
Department of Otolaryngology—Head and Neck Surgery, Division of Head and Neck Surgical Oncology and Skullbase Surgery, Boston University Medical Campus, Boston, MA, USA
e-mail: Scharukh.jalisi@bmc.org

P. Nene, B.A.
Division of Head and Neck Surgical Oncology and Skullbase Surgery, Department of Otolaryngology—Head and Neck Surgery, Boston University Medical Center, Boston, MA, USA
e-mail: pnene@bu.edu

G.A. Grillone and S. Jalisi (eds.), *Robotic Surgery of the Head and Neck: A Comprehensive Guide*,
DOI 10.1007/978-1-4939-1547-7_3,

The main disadvantage in the feasibility of establishing a robotic surgery program lies in training residents. To date, there are only 17 training centers in the United States [7]. Access to these training centers for their surgeons is the main challenge for many hospitals vying to establish a program. However, once this challenge is met, it is not difficult to train residents and surgeons in TORS.

Training requires considerable investment of money from surgeons and/or sponsoring hospitals. The initial training revolves around product training and animal labs. Thereafter the training is on actual patients. Currently this training can be performed by established proctors from the device manufacturer or in the hospital from another robotic trained surgeon.

The establishment of fellowships in TORS after residency in Otolaryngology has been proposed but to date has not been met with much enthusiasm. The main reason being that Head and Neck Oncology Fellowships already have a dearth of applicants and splintering them into further robotic fellowships would reduce the pool of necessary candidates. A successful study evaluating the proficiency of learning basic robotic skills showed that once a benchmark model for TORS trainings is established, it is very simple to teach residents fundamental tasks in robotic surgery [8]. However, the trend seems to show training programs slowly being added, as they were for robotic surgery in Urology [6, 8].

In addition, the current training for TORS that is in place consists of busy training centers filled with inanimate training tasks and proctored procedures. One group has developed a structured residency-based curriculum involving ex vivo tissue to help train residents in TORS. Their model has shown to yield very promising results in robotic surgery training [9]. The learning curve for TORS seems to be very promising, and its implementation is necessary for academic centers [10].

Ultimately, different effective models for training residents and surgeons in TORS through residency programs are necessary. As in Urology, trainees must attain the necessary knowledge and skills to provide safe patient care. In order to do this, a structured, competency-based curriculum, allowing the trainee to progress in a graduated manner, must be established, with proper credentialing [8].

Credentialing

Once a resident or surgeon has been trained via an approved TORS program, the issue at hand is to establish credentialing criteria. Currently there exist no nationally recognized credentialing criteria for TORS. Instead each academic medical center has its own criteria. At our institution the candidate seeking initial credentialing needs to demonstrate (a) board eligibility of certification in otolaryngology, (b) completion of the robotic manufacturer mandatory product and inanimate lab training, and (c) completion of three proctored TORS cases with a TORS credentialed surgeon in the institution.

Thereafter the candidate undergoes a Focused Provider Practice Evaluation for 6 months for monitoring of any complications. Once they pass this then they will have an Ongoing Provider Practice Evaluation annually. Ideally each institution should establish a "minimum" number of cases required annually to maintain credentialing.

Proctoring

As in robotic surgery in the field of Urology, no standardized credentialing system is established to evaluate surgical ability and training in TORS. Proctoring, as in Urology, may be an effective modality used to appraise robotic surgical skill in head and neck surgery [11]. Rather than preceptor involvement in which surgeons are actively involved in the surgeries done, proctoring will ensure safety while training new residents and surgeons while allowing independence for the trainees. Currently proctoring is an added expense to any new program since the proctor has to be hired via the robot manufacturer unless there are trained TORS surgeons within the academic medical center.

Feasibility

Robotic surgery advances have transformed the standard of care for head and neck surgery. Patient interest has grown immensely since the introduction of robotic surgery in head and neck surgery, and improvements in TORS have made establishing programs more realistic [6].

Establishing a robotic surgery program at an institution comes with both advantages and disadvantages. One hindrance to this is the high costs associated with the equipment and training associated with robotic surgery in any field. However, as in other fields, formally trained robotic surgeons have better patient outcomes, and given an efficient system, robotic-assisted procedures have cost-comparable statistics to open surgical alternatives [6]. In addition lower length of stay can improve hospital resource utilization. Additionally, the high cost associated with purchase of the equipment and maintenance can be counterbalanced by high surgical volume using robotic surgery. This cost can be counter balanced in institutions where multiple surgical specialties can utilize the robot. In our institutions the robot is used by Thoracic Surgery, Urology, Gynecology and Otolaryngology allowing for economies of scale to counter the high cost of equipment.

On the other hand this places "specialty hospitals" in a conundrum since the cost of the robot outweighs efficiencies due to lack of non-otolaryngology utilization. Some specialty hospitals have worked out arrangements with other hospitals to utilize their robot. We do not feel this is a safe practice unless the otolaryngologist can manage complications directly in an off-site institution.

Moreover, the cost for training can be extremely high per surgeon. It is estimated by one institution that the cost for training one trainee lies close to $9,500 [7]. This does not include other staff training that may be necessary. The question remains of how many patients are needed to justify such a high cost for a hospital. However, such costs can be offset again by high surgical volume and industry of the trained surgeons, once they are independent in operating with TORS.

A guideline may be to establish a robotic surgery committee at each institution, which may evaluate the needs of each department appropriately to allocate resources for TORS. This committee should establish a coordinator for the Robotic Program whose function should be to orient and train residents, nursing staff, and new surgeons and aim to maximize the robot utilization by managing a central robot schedule. We have also worked with Robotic "block time" to allow different surgical groups access to the robot on certain days of the week.

Additional research may be necessary to evaluate establishing TORS center programs at institutions, as doing so may be daunting at first [12]. With careful planning, care to safety, and efficiency, establishment of a robotic surgery program in Otolaryngology is possible and can be integral to the success of any Head and Neck surgery department.

References

1. Bhayani MK, Holsinger FC, Lai SY. A shifting paradigm for patients with head and neck cancer: transoral robotic surgery (TORS). Oncology (Williston Park). 2010;24(11):1010–5.
2. Hans S et al. Transoral robotic surgery in head and neck cancer. Eur Ann Otorhinolaryngol Head Neck Dis. 2012;129(1):32–7.
3. Parkin DM et al. Global cancer statistics, 2002. CA Cancer J Clin. 2005;55(2):74–108.
4. Hockstein NG, O'Malley Jr BW, Weinstein GS. Assessment of intraoperative safety in transoral robotic surgery. Laryngoscope. 2006;116(2):165–8.
5. Lui VW, Grandis JR. Primary chemotherapy and radiation as a treatment strategy for HPV-positive oropharyngeal cancer. Head Neck Pathol. 2012;6 Suppl 1:S91–7.
6. Luthringer T et al. Developing a successful robotics program. Curr Opin Urol. 2012;22(1):40–6.
7. Kokot N. Pathways and pitfalls for establishing a TORS program in an academic practice. http://www.globalroboticsinstitute.com/sites/default/files/wrs/presentations/ENT%20%20Pathways%20and%20Pitfalls%20for%20establishing%20a%20TORS%20Program%20in%20an%20Academic%20Practice.pdf. Accessed 1 April 2014.

8. Lee JY et al. Best practices for robotic surgery training and credentialing. J Urol. 2011;185(4):1191–7.
9. Curry M et al. Objective assessment in residency-based training for transoral robotic surgery. Laryngoscope. 2012;122(10):2184–92.
10. White HN et al. Learning curve for transoral robotic surgery: a 4-year analysis. JAMA Otolaryngol Head Neck Surg. 2013;139(6):564–7.
11. Zorn KC et al. Training, credentialing, proctoring and medicolegal risks of robotic urological surgery: recommendations of the society of urologic robotic surgeons. J Urol. 2009;182(3):1126–32.
12. Richmon JD, Agrawal N, Pattani KM. Implementation of a TORS program in an academic medical center. Laryngoscope. 2011;121(11):2344–8.

Costs Versus Outcomes of Robotic Surgery of the Head and Neck

Scharukh Jalisi and Shaheer Piracha

Introduction

Advances in oncologic technology through robotic surgery have aimed to reduce patient mortality while maintaining similar surgical outcomes as other older techniques [1]. When robotic surgery was first explored, Intuitive Surgical® developed the da Vinci surgical robot for procedures originally in urology [2]. In recent years, robotic surgery has become smoothly incorporated into head and neck oncologic surgery.

Oropharyngeal squamous cell carcinoma (OPSCC) represents a significant problem in the head and neck cancer field, with 123,000 cases of malignancy each year [3]. Around the same time that OPSCC was recognized as a major burden in the field, a new technique of robotic surgery (TORS) was in the process of adaptation to the head and neck field by otolaryngologists at the University of Pennsylvania. Their aim was to facilitate transoral access to oropharyngeal cancers, in addition to other oral tumors. Since then much research has shown that TORS facilitates more rapid swallowing rehabilitation and a shorter hospital stay than other management techniques, essentially minimizing morbidity and mortality from the procedures [2].

Furthermore, numerous studies show TORS to be as safe as conventional non-robotic surgery methods (chemoradiation) with the same safety profile, and advances are constantly occurring to improve results [4, 5]. In order to be able to deploy this wonderful new technology, institutions do have to look at the cost vs benefit ratio of this technology. The literature has mixed data on the cost benefits of robotic surgery.

Costs

It is imperative for organizations to understand what the cost of performing robotic surgery is as compared to traditional surgery. Armed with this data organizations can evaluate resource allocation and utilization in the enterprise. Unfortunately most of these studies are published in the non-head and neck surgery literature, but the costing can be pertinent to our specialty.

Recently an article evaluating 24,312 radical nephrectomies of which 7,787 were performed robotically was published comparing the costs between laparoscopic and robotic surgery [1]. This study showed median total hospital costs for robotic assisted surgery were $15,149 compared

S. Jalisi, M.D., M.A., F.A.C.S. (✉)
Department of Otolaryngology—Head and Neck Surgery, Division of Head and Neck Surgical Oncology and Skullbase Surgery, Boston University Medical Campus, Boston, MA, USA
e-mail: Scharukh.jalisi@bmc.org

S. Piracha, M.D.
Department of Otolaryngology, Boston University, Boston, MA, USA
e-mail: shaheer@bu.edu

G.A. Grillone and S. Jalisi (eds.), *Robotic Surgery of the Head and Neck: A Comprehensive Guide*, DOI 10.1007/978-1-4939-1547-7_4, © Springer Science+Business Media New York 2015

to $11,735 for laparoscopic surgery ($p<0.001$). There was no difference in perioperative complications or the incidence of death. Another study [2] has shown that robotic surgery is safer than laparoscopic surgery. In this study Yu et al. showed that robotic assisted laparoscopic surgery and laparoscopic surgery versus open surgery were associated with shorter length of stay for all procedures, with robotic assisted laparoscopic surgery being the shortest for radical prostatectomy and partial nephrectomy (all $p<0.001$). For most procedures robotic assisted laparoscopic surgery and laparoscopic surgery versus open surgery resulted in fewer deaths, complications, transfusions, and more routine discharges. Safety of a procedure does play into overall costs in an institution. Lower number of blood transfusions may lead to fewer ICU stays and hence reduce the overall cost of admission.

Robotic applications in Gynecology have also been reviewed. A study by Barnett et al. on management of endometrial cancers [3] showed that laparoscopy is the least expensive surgical approach for the treatment of endometrial cancer. Robotic surgery is less costly than abdominal hysterectomy when the societal costs associated with recovery time are accounted for and is most economically attractive if disposable equipment costs can be minimized to less than $1,496 per case.

Since robotic surgery can have a cost burden to the healthcare system it has been studied by national health care systems. One such study using data from the Japanese National Health Insurance System (JNHIS) showed that only institutions which perform more than 300 robotic operations per year would obtain a positive cost benefit performance and avoid financial deficit with the projected JNHIS reimbursement [4]. The hope is that a reduction in price of robotic equipment by the manufacturer would result in a decrease in the cost per procedure.

Recently a European study looked at costing data comparing total laryngectomy with transoral laser microsurgery (TLM) and transoral robotic surgery (TORS) [5]. This study showed that the total cost for supraglottic open (135–203 min), TLM (110–210 min), and TORS (35–130 min) approaches were 3,349€ (3,193–3,499€), 3,461€ (3,207–3,664€), and 5,650€ (4,297–5,974€), respectively. For total laryngectomy, the overall costs were 3,581€ (3,215–3,846€) for open and 6,767€ (6,418–7,389€) for TORS. TORS cost is mostly influenced by equipment (54 %) where the other procedures are predominantly determined by personnel cost (about 45 %). The authors concluded that TORS is more expensive than standard approaches and mainly influenced by purchase and maintenance costs and the use of proprietary instruments.

Kang et al used the da Vinci to treat 338 patients with thyroid cancer with total ($n=104$) and subtotal ($n=234$) thyroidectomies using endoscopic thyroid surgery with a gasless transaxillary approach. They reported a mean operating time of 144 min with a mean postoperative hospital stay of 3.3 days [6]. In contrast, another Korean study presented a series of 52 patients who underwent non-robotic endoscopic hemithyroidectomy with a gasless transaxillary approach. They reported a mean operating time of 154 ± 68 min with a mean postoperative hospital stay of 6.37 ± 2.83 days [7]. Thereby reducing the OR and inpatient cost manifold. Emerging evidence suggests that the longer operating times attributable to a steep learning curve will reduce with experience in the use of the robot.

Breitenstein et al. reported the amortization for the robotic system per case as $1,275 based on an amortization period of 5 years and 300 cases per year. The higher costs of robotic surgery are mainly due to the high purchase and maintenance costs [8].

Byrd et al. [9] evaluated the cost-effectiveness of transoral robotic surgery (TORS) for the diagnosis and treatment of cervical unknown primary squamous cell carcinoma (CUP). The incremental cost-effectiveness ratio for sequential and simultaneous examination under anesthesia with tonsillectomy (EUA) and TORS base of tongue resection was $8,619 and $5,774 per additional primary identified, respectively. The TORS was able to identify the primary tumor in 19 of 22 patients (86.4 %).

Even in the case of robotic thyroidectomy (RT) institution specific data showed that even in a high-volume institution, the cost of the robot was estimated at $1.5 million bringing the cost of robot to $1,703 per case. Using these values, the relative costs of RT were $5,742 for a short case and $5,848 for a long case. Additionally the up-front cost of training for the surgeon and the operative staff involved in the thyroid cases is high. Certainly, many institutions will have support staff already trained and competent in using the robotic system, which means that adding RT does not add personnel costs. However, the surgeon must pay approximately $3,000 to undergo training, exclusive of travel, accommodations, and lost clinical revenue during that time, and many surgeons choose to pursue further training or mentorship before implementing the procedure [10].

In our prior chapter it has been shown that for the cost of Robotic Surgery of the head and neck to be truly worthwhile for an institution, it is essential that the robotic instrumentation is used by multiple departments to dilute out the costs. In our institution the Robot is used by Urology, Thoracic Surgery, Gynecology, General Surgery, and Otolaryngology- Head and Neck Surgery. It is interesting that most studies note that the most common deterrent to achieving economies of scale in institutions is the cost of disposables and the robotic equipment. This new technology will likely be further embraced if the cost of robotic technology is reduced.

Outcomes

There is an increasing amount of data on robotic surgery outcomes. This is the most important parameter to consider given the costs surrounding robotic surgery. Kelly et al. [5] recently did a systematic literature review assessing for outcomes of TORS with early (T1-2) oropharyngeal squamous cell cancer (OPSCC). A total of 206 papers were identified, with 11 meeting the inclusion criteria (190 patients). For T1-2 OPSCC, the aggregate local control rate was 96.3 % with an overall survival rate of 95.0 %. Rates of prolonged (>12 month) tracheostomy tube and gastrostomy tube dependence were 0.0 % and 5.0 % respectively. This indicated that TORS was a viable alternative for early stage OPSCC.

In another study [11] the authors compared the efficacy of robotic thyroidectomy via a gasless, axillary approach with conventional cervical and endoscopic techniques by meta-analysis. Those who underwent robotic surgery reported greater cosmetic satisfaction, with a pooled net mean difference of −1.35 (95 % confidence interval (CI): −1.69, −1.09). Robotic approach operative time was longer than that of the conventional approach (95 % CI: 29.23, 54.87), with a trend to be shorter than the endoscopic approaches. Robotic surgery had similar risks to open and endoscopic approaches.

Local control and margin status have been a topic of debate around robotic surgery. There has been discussion about whether or not there is adequate margin control with robotic surgery. Weinstein et al. [12] reported their study in which 30 patients were enrolled with previously untreated OPSCC and no prior head and neck radiation therapy. Follow-up duration was at least 18 months. At the time of diagnosis, 9 tumors were T1 (30 %); 16 were T2 (53 %); 4 were T3 (13 %); and 1 was T4a (3 %). The anatomic sites of these primary tumors were tonsil in 14 (47 %), tongue base in 9 (30 %), glossotonsillar sulcus in 3 (10 %), soft palate in 3 (10 %), and oropharyngeal wall in 1 (3 %). There was only 1 patient (3 %) who had a positive margin after primary resection; further resection achieved a final negative margin. Perineural invasion was noted in 3 tumors (10 %). No patient received postoperative adjuvant therapy. At a mean follow-up of 2.7 years (range, 1.5–5.1 years), there was 1 patient with local failure (3 %). This indicates a very high local control rate potentially saving the patient adjuvant therapy in OPSCC.

TORS is a modality that purports that quality of life is preserved by obviating the need for typical external and transcervical approaches to access OPSCC. Another study looked at patient's quality of life at 6 months and 12 months after TORS and adjuvant radiation therapy. Combination TORS and adjuvant therapy caused a temporary decrease in several domains at 6 months, returning to baseline including swallowing function in all patients [13].

Another study reported on 47 patients with stages III and IV advanced oropharyngeal carcinoma and mean follow-up was 26.6 months. There was no intraoperative or postoperative mortality. Resection margins were positive in 1 patient (2 %). At last follow-up, local recurrence was identified in 1 patient (2 %), regional recurrence in 2 (4 %), and distant recurrence in 4 (9 %). Disease-specific survival was 98 % (45 of 46 patients) at 1 year and 90 % (27 of 30 patients) at 2 years. Based on pathologic risk stratification, 18 of 47 patients (38 %) avoided chemotherapy, and 5 patients (11 %) did not receive adjuvant radiotherapy and concurrent chemotherapy in their treatment regimen. At minimum follow-up of 1 year, only 1 patient required a gastrostomy tube. The authors concluded that transoral robotic surgery treatment regimen offers disease control, survival, and safety commensurate with standard treatments and an unexpected beneficial outcome of gastrostomy dependency rates that are markedly lower than those reported with standard nonsurgical therapies [14].

Conclusions

In this chapter we have shown that there is sparse but upcoming data on outcomes of Robotic head and neck surgery. TORS has been shown to be at least equivalent to traditional surgery in terms of safety, margin, and local control in early and late stage oropharyngeal squamous cell cancers. Moreover there is a reduction in gastrostomy tube dependence rates. On the other hand this improved safety and quality of life for patients comes at a cost. It seems that the main driver of costs is the maintenance and purchase of disposables and the system. In order to achieve economies of scale and justify institutional expenditure on purchase of a robotic system, it seems TORS should be performed in institutions where multiple services can utilize the robot and perform at least 300 robotic cases per year. Overall robotic surgery is here to stay and healthcare systems need to embrace this new technology with creative economic investments and collaborations.

References

1. Yang DY, Monn MF, Bahler CD, Sundaram CP. Does robotic assistance confer an economic benefit during laparoscopic radical nephrectomy? J Urol. 2014; 192:671–6. doi:10.1016/j.juro.2014.04.018.
2. Yu HY, Hevelone ND, Lipsitz SR, Kowalczyk KJ, Hu JC. Use, costs and comparative effectiveness of robotic assisted, laparoscopic and open urological surgery. J Urol. 2012;187(4):1392–8. doi:10.1016/j.juro.2011.11.089. Epub 16 Feb 2012.
3. Barnett JC, Judd JP, Wu JM, Scales Jr CD, Myers ER, Havrilesky LJ. Cost comparison among robotic, laparoscopic, and open hysterectomy for endometrial cancer. Obstet Gynecol. 2010;116(3):685–93. doi:10.1097/AOG.
4. Kajiwara N, Patrick Barron J, Kato Y, Kakihana M, Ohira T, Kawate N, Ikeda N.Cost-Benefit Performance of Robotic Surgery Compared with Video-Assisted Thoracoscopic Surgery under the Japanese National Health Insurance System. Ann Thorac Cardiovasc Surg. 2014. doi:10.5761/atcs.oa.14-00076. Epub 16 May 2014.
5. Dombrée M, Crott R, Lawson G, Janne P, Castiaux A, Krug B. Cost comparison of open approach, transoral laser microsurgery and transoral robotic surgery for partial and total laryngectomies. Eur Arch Otorhinolaryngol. 2014;271:2852–34.
6. Kang SW, Lee SC, Lee SH, Lee KY, Jeong JJ, Lee YS, Nam KH, Chang HS, Chung WY, Park CS. Robotic thyroid surgery using a gasless, transaxillary approach and the da Vinci S system: the operative outcomes of 338 consecutive patients. Surgery. 2009; 146(6):1048–55.
7. Koh YW, Kim JW, Lee SW, Choi EC. Endoscopic thyroidectomy via a unilateral axillo-breast approach without gas insufflation for unilateral benign thyroid lesions. Surg Endosc. 2009;23(9):2053–60. doi:10.1007/s00464-008-9963-3. Epub 5 June 2008.
8. Breitenstein S, Nocito A, Puhan M, Held U, Weber M, Clavien PA. Robotic-assisted versus laparoscopic cholecystectomy: outcome and cost analyses of a case-matched control study. Ann Surg. 2008;247(6):987–93.
9. Byrd JK, Smith KJ, de Almeida JR, Albergotti WG, Davis KS, Kim SW, Johnson JT, Ferris RL, Duvvuri U. Transoral robotic surgery and the unknown primary: a cost-effectiveness analysis. Otolaryngol Head Neck Surg. 2014;150(6):976–82.
10. Broome JT, Pomeroy S, Solorzano CC. Expense of robotic thyroidectomy: a cost analysis at a single institution. Arch Surg. 2012;147(12):1102–6.

11. Jackson NR, Yao L, Tufano RP, Kandil EH. Safety of robotic thyroidectomy approaches: meta-analysis and systematic review. Head Neck. 2014;36(1): 137–43.
12. Weinstein GS, Quon H, Newman HJ, Chalian JA, Malloy K, Lin A, Desai A, Livolsi VA, Montone KT, Cohen KR, O'Malley BW. Transoral robotic surgery alone for oropharyngeal cancer: an analysis of local control. Arch Otolaryngol Head Neck Surg. 2012;138(7):628–34.
13. Leonhardt FD, Quon H, Abrahão M, O'Malley Jr BW, Weinstein GS. Transoral robotic surgery for oropharyngeal carcinoma and its impact on patient-reported quality of life and function. Head Neck. 2012;34(2): 146–54.
14. Weinstein GS, O'Malley Jr BW, Cohen MA, Quon H. Transoral robotic surgery for advanced oropharyngeal carcinoma. Arch Otolaryngol Head Neck Surg. 2010;136(11):1079–85.

Operating Room Setup, Instrumentation, and Safety Considerations in Transoral Robotic Surgery

Jeffrey S. Jumaily, Lance Maggiacomo, and Gregory A. Grillone

Introduction

Safe and efficient management of patients undergoing transoral robotic surgery (TORS) starts with a highly functioning team and effective communication. Communication, which should begin when the TORS procedure is first scheduled and conclude when the patient is safely in the post-anesthesia care unit, is important to ensure availability of all team members, proper equipment and instrumentation setup, and safe and efficient completion of the procedure. A highly functioning team requires proper training of all team members. Surgeon training for TORS is discussed elsewhere in this book but it should be emphasized here that, while many operating rooms have personnel trained in the use of the da Vinci® Robotic System for other specialties, appropriate TORS specific training is necessary for all members of the team who will participate in the planning and execution of TORS procedures.

J.S. Jumaily, M.D. • G.A. Grillone, M.D.
Department of Otolaryngology Head and Neck Surgery, Boston Medical Center, Boston University School of Medicine, Boston, MA, USA
e-mail: Jeffrey.jumaily@bmc.org

L. Maggiacomo, R.N., B.S.N. (✉)
Department of Surgery, Boston Medical Center, 88 East Newton Street, Boston, MA 02118, USA
e-mail: lance.maggiacomo@bmc.org

Equipment and Instrumentation

A well written surgeon's preference card is an effective tool in efficient preparation of the surgical suite for a TORS procedure. This tool will communicate to the staff the important equipment and instrumentation needed for a safe procedure and should include details of safe handling and positioning of the equipment. The night before surgery the team assigned to the case should review the TORS procedure manual and the physician's preference card. The size of the operating room used for TORS procedures should be large enough to accommodate the considerable amount of equipment required.

Primary equipment required for TORS:

1. da Vinci® Robot (which consists of patient-side cart, surgeon consoles, and vision cart)
2. Laryngoscopy and airway carts
3. Secondary video tower
4. Procedural case cart (contains all the needed instrumentation)
5. Flexible waveguide-based CO_2 laser (if needed).

Other equipment and instrumentation required for TORS:

1. Surgical high-magnification camera head (45 FOV)
2. Surgical wide-angle camera head (60 FOV)
3. High-definition 3D imaging system
4. Thirty (30) degree surgical endoscope
5. Zero (0) degree surgical endoscope

G.A. Grillone and S. Jalisi (eds.), *Robotic Surgery of the Head and Neck: A Comprehensive Guide*, DOI 10.1007/978-1-4939-1547-7_5, © Springer Science+Business Media New York 2015

6. Robotic instruments (selected by surgeon in advance)
7. Patient surgical bed with gel pads and mattress and warming blanket
8. Three sterile surgical tables
9. Two Mayo stands
10. Sequential compression device
11. Cautery unit with Bovie pedal and bipolar pedal (for assistant at bedside), two Bovie pads, and reusable bipolar cord
12. Four chairs with height adjustment capability—two at bedside (for the nurse and the bedside surgical assistant), one for the teaching console (if applicable), and one at surgeon console.
13. Three rectangular OR instrument carts and one small square OR instrument cart.

The da Vinci® Robotic System can be equipped with various instruments and camera-endoscope units that attach to the arms of the robot. The manufacturer's manual and catalogue contains a list of available attachments and should be referred to for the most up-to-date information.

TORS cases also require surgical instruments in addition to the da Vinci® Robotic System and its components. These instruments are used by the surgical assistant at the bedside. Many of these instruments are found in a standard tonsil kit and should include:

1. Surgical headlight
2. Lip and tongue retractors
3. Needle holders
4. Debakey forceps
5. Metzenbaum or tonsil scissors
6. Hemostats
7. Suction cautery
8. Yankauer suction
9. Small and medium vascular clips

Room Setup (Fig. 1)

The room setup should provide adequate space for surgical personnel to move around the room. Extraneous equipment should be removed from the room to maximize available space. The procedural case cart, surgeon consoles, and ancillary equipment should be positioned at the periphery of the room. The rest of the needed equipment should also be placed and set up at the periphery of the room and positioned so that there is a clear pathway to the patient surgical bed once the patient is in the room. The patient surgical bed should be set up for efficient patient transfer from the stretcher and assembled appropriately for a TORS procedure. The head attachment of the patient surgical bed should be placed at the foot of the bed, and the base of the bed should be turned 180° so that the patient's head will rest on the repositioned head attachment. This bed arrangement allows space for the base of the patient-side cart to fit under the bed. The sterile surgical tables should be set up at the periphery of the room at the foot of the patient's surgical bed, with a clear pathway to move at the beginning of the procedure. The patient-side cart is then draped and the camera-endoscope units are calibrated. Before the patient is brought into the room it should be confirmed that all appropriate equipment is present, turned on, and functioning properly including all three components of the da Vinci® Robotic System.

Patient Positioning

Once the patient enters the room the entire surgical team should be focused on the patient's comfort and safety. When the patient is safely transferred and secured on the surgical bed, a universal protocol is performed and general endotracheal anesthesia is induced.

The bed is turned 180° with the patient's feet towards anesthesia. An extended breathing circuit is used to reach the endotracheal tube. All intravenous lines and monitoring lines are positioned for easy access by the anesthesiologist and cushioned with gauze to prevent undue pressure on the patient. Both of the patient's arms are wrapped in gel arm wraps. Arms are then tucked at the patient's side. The patient's head is placed on a low profile "gel donut." The vertex of the patient's head should be at the very edge of the OR table. Other equipment needed for TORS procedures may include a foam or gel mattress and warming blanket. Once the head of the

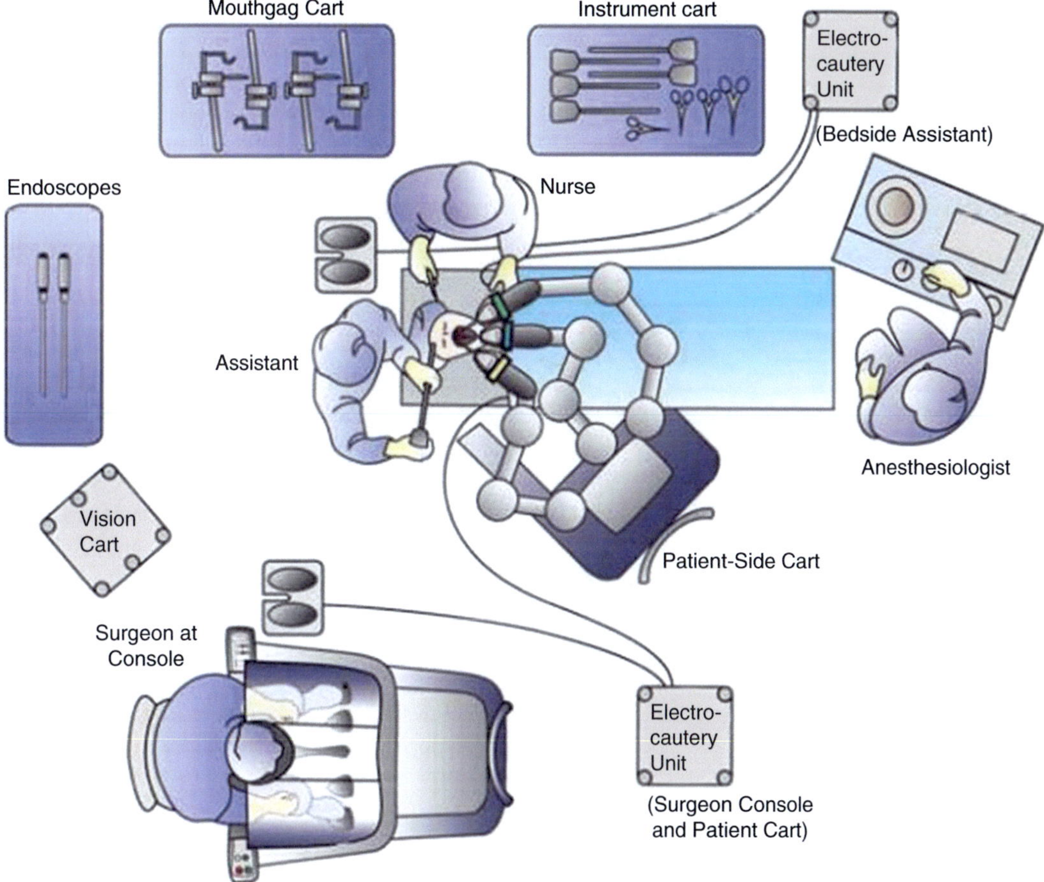

Fig. 1 Diagram showing typical OR setup for TORS case. Da Vinci® Transoral surgery procedure guide. PN 871671 Rev. D 3/11 [2]

patient surgical bed is turned 180° from the anesthesia machine, the suction machine, electrocautery machine, sequential compression device, blanket warmer, and other equipment should be placed near the patient's feet, beside or behind the anesthesia machine to avoid interference with the robotic equipment.

Equipment Tables

Tables that hold the endoscopes, robotic instruments, various mouth gags, and other instruments used are placed behind the surgical assistant and scrub nurse for easy access and interchange during the procedure (Figs. 1, 2, and 3).

Surgical Assistant Positioning

The assistant to the surgeon positioned at the patient's head attends to the surgical site with handheld instruments. The assistant observes the surgical site directly and well on one of the video monitors and performs tasks such as suctioning, cautery, applying vascular clips, and ensuring that robotic arms do not cause injury to patient.

Anesthesia Considerations

The patient should be intubated with a single lumen reinforced tube for oropharynx cases. If the laser is used or the hypopharynx or larynx will be instrumented close to the endotracheal tube, then a laser safe tube should be employed to minimize airway fire risk. The route of intubation (nasal or oral) and the position of the

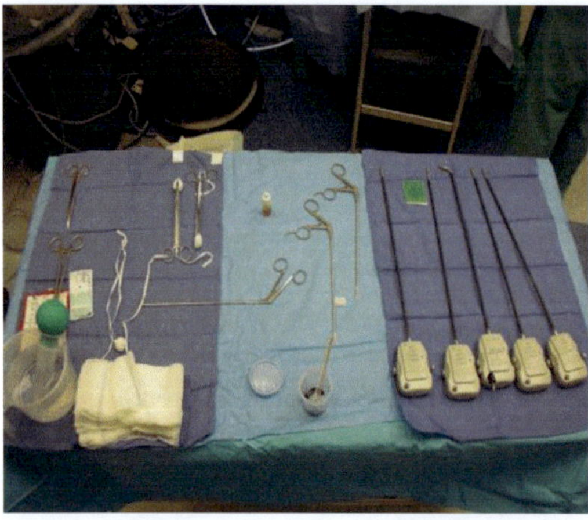

Fig. 2 Setup of the camera cart. Da Vinci® Transoral surgery procedure guide. PN 871671 Rev. D 3/11 [2]

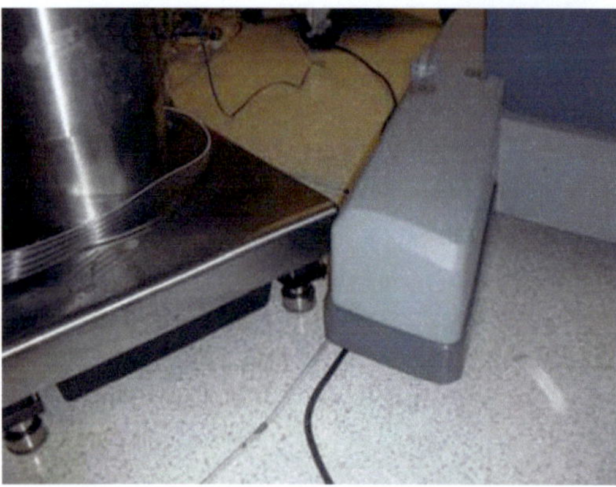

Fig. 3 Positioning of the OR table and patient-side cart. Da Vinci® transoral surgery procedure guide. PN 871671 Rev. D 3/11 [2]

endotracheal tube depend on the specific type of TORS procedure being performed and on surgeon preference.

Da Vinci® Robot Patient-Side Cart Setup

(a) Docking

The patient-side cart is moved to the edge of the patient bed and aligned at a 30° angle from the long axis of the patient surgical bed. It is important to note that some surgical beds have a wider base that limits proximity of patient-side cart base to the patient. In those instances an alternative position may be needed or the surgical bed may need to be changed. The relationship of the surgical bed base and the base of the patient-side cart is the same for every case; therefore, it may facilitate faster room setup if permanent marks are placed on the OR floor to allow staff to position the equipment appropriately each time (Fig. 3).

(b) Mouth gags and retractors

There are several types of mouth gags and retractors that are useful in TORS procedures depending on the type of procedure and patient anatomy.

The most commonly used retractors are the Feyh–Kastenbauer (FK) retractor, Crow-Davis (or Boyle Davis), McIvor and Dingman mouth gags, and the Jennings mouth gag. The Feyh–Kastenbauer (FK) retractor from Gyrus ACMI (Tuttlingen, Germany) is equipped with various tongue blades that allow enhanced exposure of the vallecula, hypopharynx, and supraglottic larynx (Fig. 4). The Crow-Davis (or Boyle-Davis) mouth gag is useful for exposure of the lateral wall of the oropharynx (Fig. 5). The McIvor and Dingman mouth gags are also useful for exposure of the lateral oropharynx. These mouth gags come with two types of tongue blades. Blades with a groove for the endotracheal tube allow the tube to be fixed in the midline. These are the blades typically used for routine (non-TORS) tonsillectomy but the hump formed by the groove projects into the oral cavity and may limit placement or movement of the robotic instruments. Flat blades have a lower profile and allow more space in the oral cavity for movement of the robotic instruments but require that the endotracheal tube be fixed to the contralateral (from the surgical site) side of the oral cavity. Flats blades also have a suction port which can be used for smoke evacuation.

The Jennings mouth gag has no tongue blade and is designed primarily to maintain the upper and lower jaws open. It is useful for TORS procedures on the base of the tongue when combined with anterior retraction of

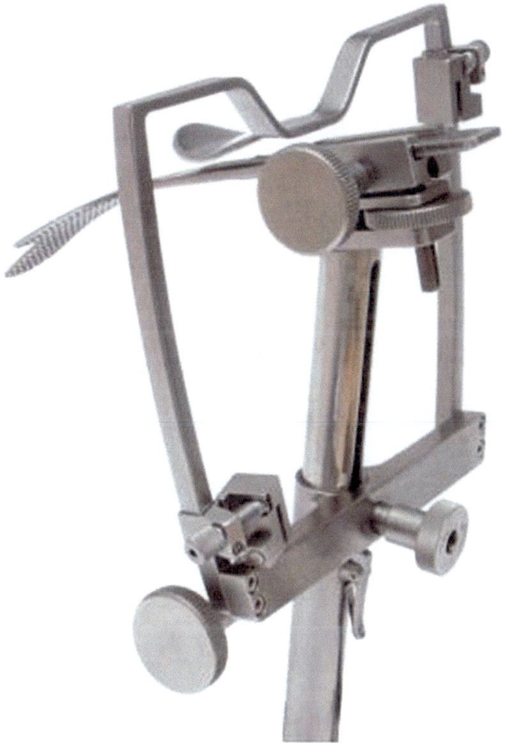

Fig. 4 FK-WO retractor. Da Vinci® transoral surgery procedure guide. PN 871671 Rev. D 3/11 [2]

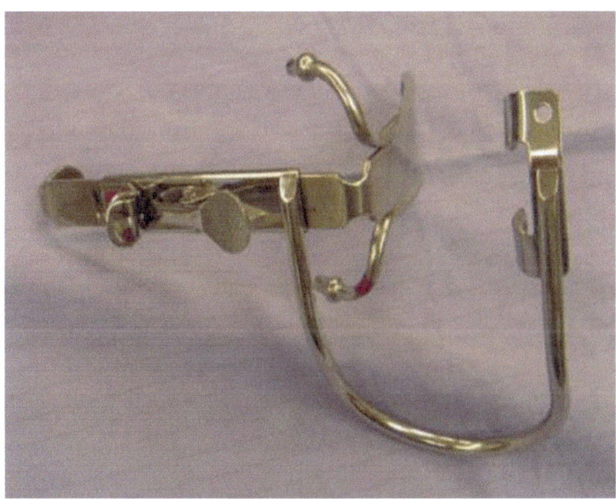

Fig. 5 Crow-Davis Retractor. Da Vinci® transoral surgery procedure guide. PN 871671 Rev. D 3/11 [2]

the tongue. Figure 6 shows a typical setup of the mouth gag table.

The surgeon should place the desired mouth gag before final positioning of the patient-side cart. Once the mouth gag is placed, it should be suspended using a low profile suspension device to avoid interference from the robotic arms. The suspension device should be fixed to the patient surgical bed on the side opposite the patient-side cart.

(c) Camera-endoscope and instrument arm setup
After the mouth gag is in place, the robotic arms are moved and positioned over the patient's chest so that the distal portion of the robotic trocar holders is hovering a few centimeters above the patient's mouth. The trocars are then placed in the trocar holders, and camera-endoscope arm is positioned with trocar in the center of the patient's mouth. The right and left instrument arms are placed just inside the corners of the mouth taking care not to put pressure on the lips or teeth.

Once the arms are in the patient's mouth, the patient surgical bed should not be moved and this should be clearly communicated to all staff in the room.

Step-by-step guide to placement of instrument and camera-endoscope arms:

- The camera-endoscope arm is positioned vertically over the chest and inserted midline through open jaws of the mouth gag.
- Initially the camera arm should be as high as possible on pedestal to visualize the target structures. This minimizes collisions with the other arms. After the camera-endoscope is placed, the pedestal arm is lowered gradually until desired structures are seen.
- The camera-endoscope arm should not come into contact with the upper teeth or gingiva.
- The right and left instrument arms are positioned in place such that cannula remote center (thick black line) is at the level of the mouth gag (outside the mouth). The arms should be kept as far as possible from the camera to minimize collisions.
- The angle of the instruments is adjusted so that only the tip of the instrument is seen by the camera view (Fig. 7). A clear plastic lip protector is recommended to prevent injury to the lips by the instruments.

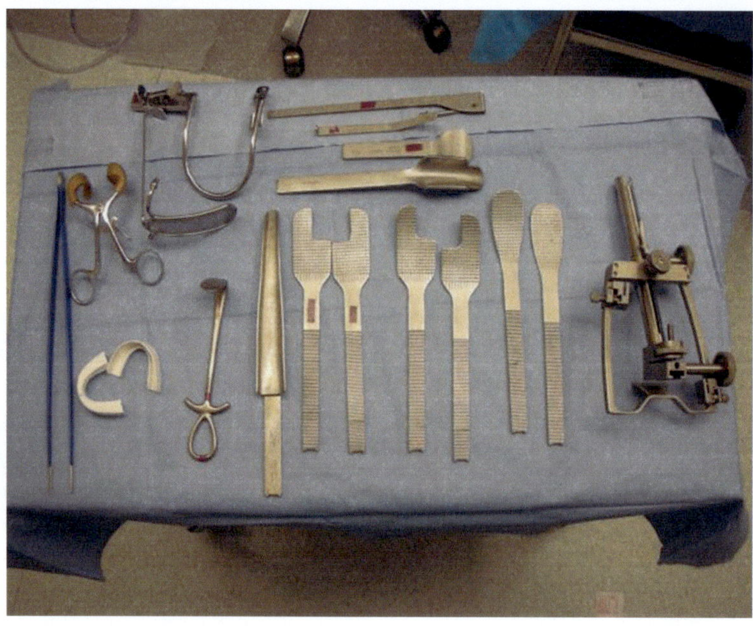

Fig. 6 Mouth gag table setup. Da Vinci® transoral surgery procedure guide. PN 871671 Rev. D 3/1 [2]

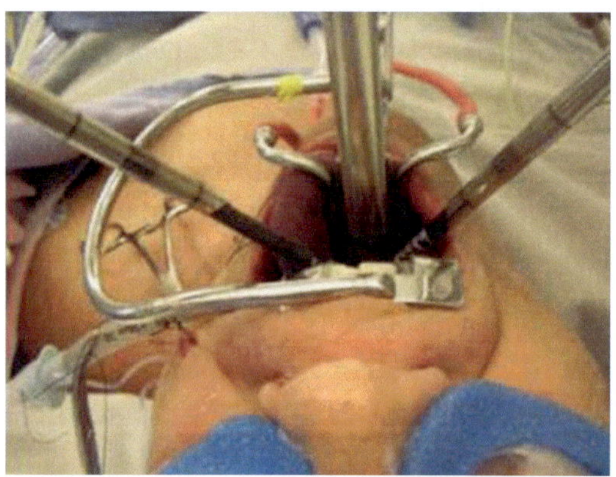

Fig. 7 A view of the patient's face with all instruments in place. Clear plastic lip protector should be used to protect lips (not shown in this picture). Da Vinci® transoral surgery procedure guide. PN 871671 Rev. D 3/11 [2]

Safety Considerations

(a) Airway fire

If a laser is to be used during TORS, a metal lined or other laser safe endotracheal tube should be used, and the patients head, eyes, and upper chest should be covered with wet towels. All other laser safety procedure should be followed to prevent fires and laser injuries to the patient and staff. The algorithm for the management of airway fires published by the American Society of Anesthesia is shown in Fig. 8.

The risk of fire is also present when using the cautery arm of the da Vinci® Robot. The fire precautions for TORS are the same as for other transoral procedures such as tonsillectomy. All staff in the room must be aware of the fire risk and of their role in the event of an airway fire. The anesthesia team should use appropriately low FiO_2 levels to minimize risk of fire.

The first steps when a fire is noted are to turn off the oxygen and remove the endotracheal tube. The mouth gag or retractor may need to be released first before the endotracheal tube can be removed completely. There should be 1 L of saline in an open container available to be poured in the mouth. If the fire is extinguished, ventilation should be reestablished. The endotracheal tube should be inspected for missing parts that may be still be in the airway. A bronchoscopy can be performed to evaluate the airway for remaining foreign bodies and retrieve them if present.

(b) Eye protection

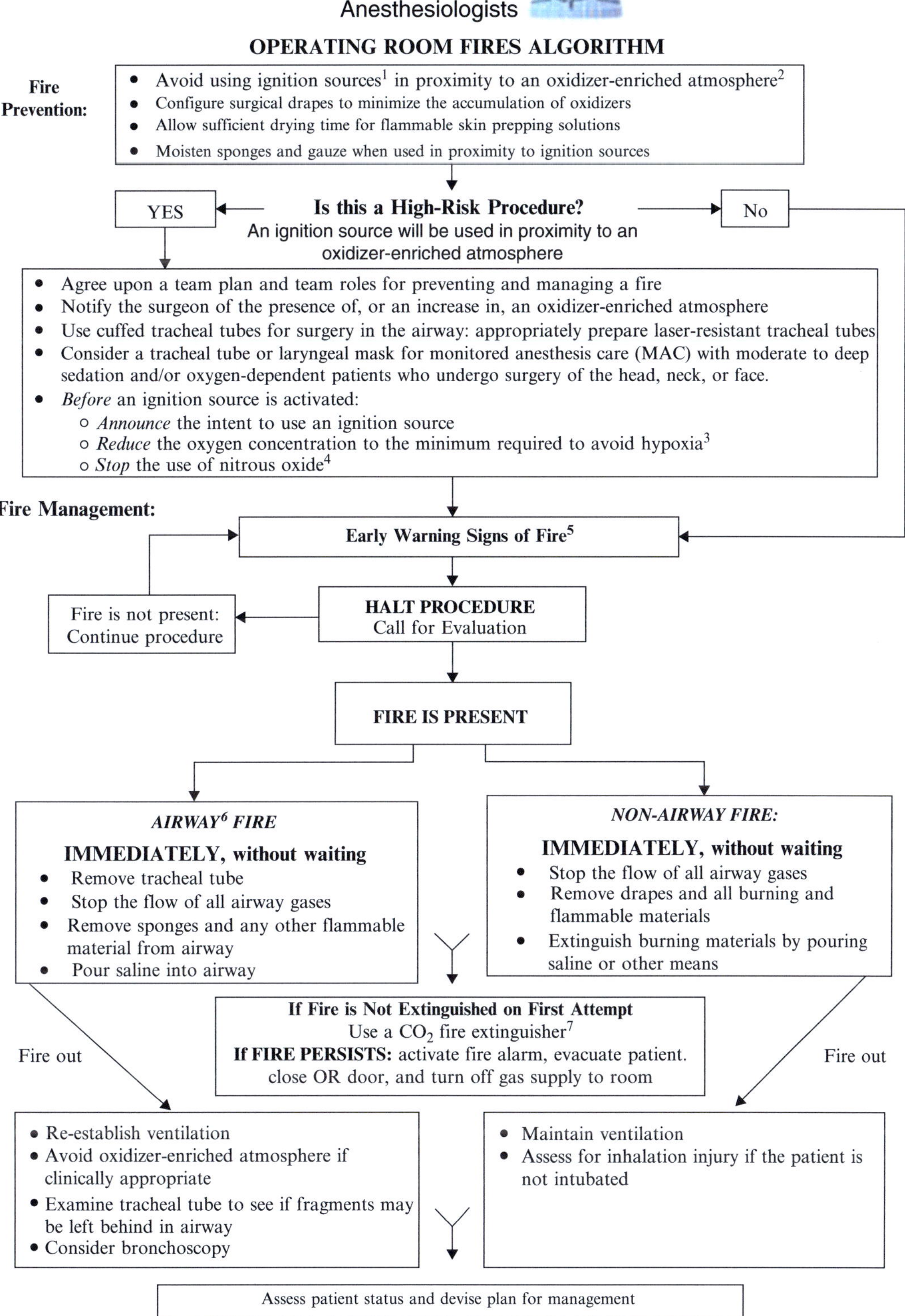

Fig. 8 American Society of Anesthesia (ASA) OR fire algorithm [1]

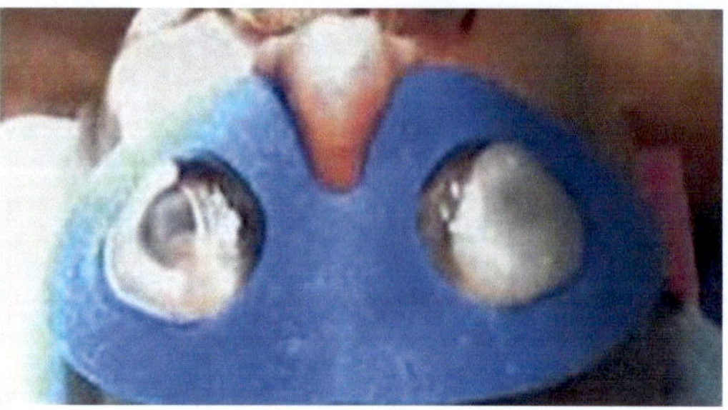

Fig. 9 Optigard eye protection

"Optigard eye protection" should be used for all TORS procedures. They are adhesive backed, foam goggles with hard plastic lenses that are placed over the patient's eyes to protect them from any possible pressure from any of the robotic or surgical instruments (Fig. 9).

(c) Lip/mouth injury

A white latex free silicone tooth guard is placed over the teeth to provide a level of protection. A clear plastic "lip retractor" should be used to protect the lips from injury by the instrument arms of the robot (Fig. 10). This can be placed before or after placement of the mouth gag.

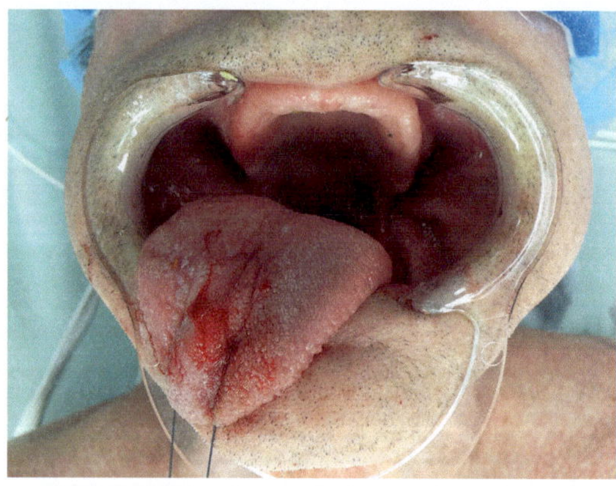

Fig. 10 Clear plastic lip protector in place

References

1. American Society for Anesthesiologist. Practice Advisory for the Prevention and Management of Operating Room Fires. An Updated Report by the American Society of Anesthesiologists Task Force on Operating Room Fires. Anesthesiology. 2013; 118:271–90.
2. da Vinci® Transoral Surgery Procedure Guide. PN 871671 Rev. D 3/11.

Robotic Surgery in Pediatric Otolaryngology

Elam Adil, Bao Anh Le, Hiep T. Nguyen, and Reza Rahbar

Introduction

Advances in technology have led to a paradigm shift from traditional open procedures to minimally invasive surgery (MIS). Robotic assisted surgery (RAS) is a form of MIS, which already has widespread applications in urology, gynecology, cardiothoracic surgery, and neurosurgery. RAS has been associated with a more rapid recovery, better cosmetic results, decreased pain, and lower rate of postoperative infection [1–3]. In addition, this emerging technology has been proven to be safe, produce comparable results, and can be cost-effective when compared with other surgical approaches.

The use of RAS in Otolaryngology—Head and Neck Surgery was first described in 2005 [4–6]. Transoral robotic surgery (TORS) was determined to be feasible using mannequin head, cadaver, and canine models. Intraoperative safety was next established using a cadaveric head [7]. It was found that dental, cervical spine, and mandible fractures could not be achieved despite applying maximal torque and pressure through the robotic arms. Once feasibility and safety were established, the first human applications were described including transoral radical tonsillectomy and supraglottic laryngectomy [8, 9]. The use of TORS has since expanded and numerous case series have been reported.

In pediatric otolaryngology, RAS is still in its infancy. Size of the robotic surgical instruments initially limited access to pediatric oropharyngeal structures. However, miniaturization of instrumentation has dramatically expanded the scope of surgical options. Clinical applications in pediatric otolaryngology that have been reported include laryngeal cleft repair, lingual tonsillectomy, and thyroglossal duct cyst excision [10–12].

History

There are three types of surgical robots: active, semiactive, and passive. An active robot system can complete an entire procedure without any surgeon input. A semiactive robot requires some surgeon input to carry out directed movements, while a passive robot is under complete control of the surgeon. Puma 560 was the first passive robotic surgical system. It was developed in 1985 with 6° of freedom, which allowed for increased precision of

E. Adil, M.D., M.B.A. (✉) • R. Rahbar, D.M.D., M.D.
Department of Otology and Laryngology,
Harvard Medical School, Boston, MA, USA

Department of Otolaryngology and Communication Enhancement, Boston Children's Hospital,
Boston, MA, USA

B.A. Le, B.S.
Tufts University Dental School of Medicine,
Boston, MA, USA

H.T. Nguyen, M.D.
Department of Urology, Boston Children's Hospital,
Boston, MA, USA

G.A. Grillone and S. Jalisi (eds.), *Robotic Surgery of the Head and Neck: A Comprehensive Guide*,
DOI 10.1007/978-1-4939-1547-7_6, © Springer Science+Business Media New York 2015

neurosurgical biopsies. A number of surgical robots have been introduced since then, but the only FDA approved system for Transoral Robotic Surgery (TORS) is the da Vinci Robot (Intuitive Surgical Inc., Sunnyvale, CA, USA) [13]. The origin of the da Vinci Surgical Robot stems from the National Aeronautics and Space Administration's (NASA) need to offer surgical care for astronauts while away on space missions [14, 15]. Both the Stanford Research Institute and the US Army saw promise in this technology. The US Army needed a way to provide surgical care to a wounded soldier as soon as possible, without putting the surgeon in harm's way. Intuitive Surgical Corporation was developed in 1995, 10 years after the introduction of the Puma system, to produce telerobotic systems for commercial public use [16]. In 2005, the first robot assisted otolaryngic procedure was described by Mac Leod and Melder who excised a vallecular cyst [17].

A review of the last 10 years of robotic surgery in pediatrics was published recently [18]. A total of 2,393 procedures in 1,840 patients were identified. Most cases were derived from the North American literature, with only 14 % of cases from Europe, 4 % from the Middle East, and 3 % from Asia. Genitourinary procedures were most commonly reported ($n = 1{,}434$) with pyeloplasty ($n = 672$) as the most commonly cited procedure. Gastrointestinal procedures accounted for 882 reported procedures and there were 77 reported pediatric thoracic cases. The authors note that the number of reported cases has increased dramatically since 2010 with six reports including over 100 cases each. Also of note, there are no randomized clinical trials of RAS in pediatrics to date.

Advantages and Disadvantages

There are both advantages and disadvantages to RAS. One of the biggest advantages of RAS when compared to traditional open techniques is the EndoWrist instruments have 90° of articulation and 7° of freedom. This translates into greater range of motion when compared to the human wrist, which allows for increased dexterity. Fatigue reduction is another advantage to RAS. During open head and neck procedures, most surgeons stand for the duration of the case. While using the robot, the surgeon is seated with his/her forearms resting on a pad and the head resting against the console, which results in less body fatigue. In addition, the surgeon avoids the need to physically twist and turn to move instruments and see the operative field. With improved comfort and view of the operative field, suturing is technically easier. Studies suggest that robotic surgery is less stressful for surgeons during complex tasks [19]. Furthermore, the robotic system's 3-dimensional endoscopes with tenfold magnification improve visualization of the surgical field allowing for more precise dissection and suture placement.

When compared to endoscopic techniques, there are several advantages of RAS. First, the robotic system has the ability to eliminate tremor. Through hardware and software filters, a surgeon's movements can be scaled down. Because of this ability, large hand movements are transformed into micromovements, which allows for more precision [1]. There is also improved hand eye coordination given that there is no fulcrum effect as is seen with endoscopic surgery [20].

Aside from the advantages compared to open and endoscopic techniques, there are several unique advantages of RAS. The robotic system provides a new vehicle for teaching. Trainees and surgeons can sit next to each other at different consoles and practice tissue holding and suturing techniques [21]. The daVinci Skill Simulator is a training tool made specifically for the robot. It can be attached to the console to allow virtual skills training using the same robotic interface [22]. There are currently no standardized residency curriculums that formally support the teaching of robotic surgical skills, but with the increase in RAS, this is likely to change.

Another unique advantage to RAS is the ability to perform telesurgery in which a surgeon performs a procedure on a patient from a remote location [23]. Marescaux and colleagues first described the feasibility and safety of a robot assisted telesurgery. They performed a laparoscopic cholecystectomy from a surgical console in New York on a patient in Strasbourg, France using a high-speed connection. They successfully completed the procedure in less than an hour with no complications.

There are some known disadvantages associated with RAS. As with any new technology, there is a learning curve for surgeons. The lack of haptic feedback can be a significant problem. Because of the lack of hands-on tissue manipulation, the early robotic surgeon can have issues with tearing tissue or suture. However, with time, evaluation of adjacent tissue can give the surgeon feedback about the amount of pressure being applied. Cost is also a downside to this technology with the average system costing $1.5–2.5 million. In addition, maintenance fees are $100,000 per year and instrument heads cost approximately $2,000 each and have limited life spans. The physical size of the unit also can be cumbersome with most hospitals requiring a dedicated robotic surgery room to accommodate the surgeon's console, patient side cart, and instruments. The operating room staff also require additional training to become familiar with the instrumentation and to reduce surgical set-up time. Finally, as mentioned previously, there have not been any randomized controlled studies comparing RAS to endoscopic or open procedures to evaluate its effectiveness.

Current Technology

The 5 mm EndoWrist instruments are currently the smallest instruments available. All of the EndoWrist needle holders and tissue graspers can open their jaws from 0 to 30°. They differ in their intended application and the amount of force applied at their jaws. The 5 mm needle driver has medium jaw opening and closing force at its tip. There are no suture cut 5 mm needle drivers available. Round tip scissors have medium force during closing and opening. Curved scissors have low jaw closing force, but medium jaw opening force. The Schertel grasper is used for fine tissue handling and has low jaw opening and closing force. The Maryland dissector has similar tissue handling forces. DeBakey forceps have low jaw closing force, but medium jaw opening force. The needle driver and tissue graspers all have 20 uses per instrument, while the scissors have 12 uses.

For tissue cautery, there are 5 mm hooktip and spatula tip EndoWrist cautery heads available. These both have 18 uses. There is also a 5 French laser fiber introducer with 20 uses. Finally, there are Harmonic ACE ultrasonic shears which use mechanical energy to coagulate and cut tissue. This instrument has 20 uses.

Current Literature in Pediatric Otolaryngology

Peer reviewed literature on the use of RAS in pediatric otolaryngology is limited. The first study published in this area examined the feasibility and safety of RAS in the pediatric airway [10]. The da Vinci Surgical Robot (Intuitive Surgical Inc., Sunnyvale, CA, USA) was initially trialed on 4 cadaver larynxes placed in a larynx holder. It was found that the surgeon had great dexterity and suturing within the endolarynx was successful using 5-0 and 6-0 Vicryl sutures (Ethicon Inc, Somerville, NJ). 3D depth perception was possible with the 12-mm, 3-dimensional endoscope, but not the 8-mm, 2-dimensional endoscope. Next, RAS was attempted in five pediatric patients with laryngeal clefts. In the patients, the procedure could not be completed due to limited transoral access. RAS was successful in 1 patient with a type 1 laryngeal cleft and another with a type 2 cleft. The procedure was performed using spontaneous ventilation and exposure was provided using a Crowe-David mouth gag. The best view was obtained using the 30° endoscope. Use of the robot increased surgical time by an average of 40 min when compared to an endoscopic repair. There were no complications.

Robot assisted pediatric lingual tonsillectomy was recently reported [11]. Sixteen patients with a mean age of 12 years (range 5–19 years) underwent lingual tonsillectomy for obstructive sleep apnea ($n=11$), dysphagia ($n=2$), upper airway obstruction ($n=1$), exercised induced breathing difficulty ($n=1$), and recurrent tonsillitis ($n=1$).

All patients in this study were orally or nasotracheally intubated, which did not impede surgical access. Either the Feyh–Kastenbauer, Dingman, or McIvor retractor was used for access. The 12-mm 3-dimensional endoscope was used for visualization in all cases. The 5-mm Maryland blade and 5-mm spatula cautery were used to perform the lingual tonsillectomies. Robot docking time, estimated blood loss, and mean operative time were compared between the first five cases, next five cases, and last six cases to establish a learning curve. Mean docking time was significantly lower between the first five cases (9 min) and the next five cases (3 min). Estimated blood loss and mean operative time was not significantly different between groups; however, there was a trend such that blood loss decreased with increased case number. All patients were extubated in the operating room at the conclusion of the procedure. Ten patients were admitted to the intensive care unit following surgery and ten patients were discharged on postoperative day one. Median hospitalization was 1 day with a range of 1–13 days. Two patients had a postoperative bleed which required admission and monitoring without a secondary surgical procedure. Two patients also developed pneumonia. One patient had fever of unclear etiology and 4 patients had poor pain control. No patients required tracheostomy or gastrostomy tube placement.

Robot assisted marsupialization of a lingual thyroglossal duct cyst was also recently described [12]. In this case report, a 2 month female presented with stridor, respiratory distress, cyanotic episodes, and dysphagia since birth. A red-purple mass originating from the tongue base and obstructing a view of the larynx was seen on examination. Computed tomography (CT) scan revealed a 1.5 cm homogenous midline tongue mass and normal thyroid gland. The patient was orally intubated and exposure was provided using a Farabeuf retractor. The 0°, 3-dimensional endoscope was used in addition to the 5 mm Maryland blade and 5 mm cautery. The mass was marsupialized and the patient was successfully extubated in the intensive care unit 2 hours after surgery. She resumed breastfeeding that day without difficulty and was discharged home on postoperative day 3 in stable condition. There was no recurrence based on a follow-up magnetic resonance imaging (MRI) performed at her 10 month visit. This is the youngest reported patient to undergo TORS, which indicates that there is potential to use this technology in very small patients.

Conclusion

Robotic surgery naturally found its way into some specialties, such as urology, because of the large incisions required for traditional open approaches and the tissue handling limitations (specifically suture placement) of endoscopic techniques. Robotic surgery in otolaryngology has been slow to develop because many head and neck structures can be easily accessed through existing orifices such as the mouth. In addition, surgical incisions within the head and neck heal well because of its abundant blood supply. In pediatric otolaryngology, instrument size limitations were initially a limiting factor. However, the advent of 5 mm instrumentation has made RAS a potential alternative to endoscopic airway surgery. Robot assisted laryngeal cleft repair, lingual tonsillectomy, and lingual thyroglossal duct cyst excision have already been described. As RAS technology continues to improve, larger studies with expanded use are on the horizon.

References

1. Kim VB, Chapman WHH, Albrecht RJ, et al. Early experience with telemanipulative robot-assisted laparoscopic cholecystectomy using da Vinci. Surg Laparosc Endosc Percutan Tech. 2002;12(1):33–40.
2. Fuchs KH. Minimally invasive surgery. Endoscopy. 2002;34(2):154–9.
3. Allendorf JDF, Bessler M, Whelanetal RL. Postoperative immune function varies inversely with the degree of surgical trauma in a murine model. Surg Endosc. 1997;11(5):427–30.
4. Hockstein NG, Nolan JP, O'Malley Jr BW, Woo YJ. Robotic microlaryngeal surgery: a technical feasibility study using the da Vinci surgical robot and an airway mannequin. Laryngoscope. 2005;115(5):780–5.
5. Hockstein NG, Nolan JP, O'Malley Jr BW, Woo YJ. Robot-assisted pharyngeal and laryngeal microsurgery: results of robotic cadaver dissections. Laryngoscope. 2005;115(6):1003–8.

6. Weinstein GS, O'Malley Jr BW, Hockstein NG. Transoral robotic surgery: supraglottic laryngectomy in a canine model. Laryngoscope. 2005; 115(7):1315–9.
7. Hockstein NG, O'Malley Jr BW, Weinstein GS. Assessment of intraoperative safety in transoral robotic surgery. Laryngoscope. 2006;116(2):165–8.
8. Weinstein GS, O'Malley Jr BW, Snyder W, Sherman E, Quon H. Transoral robotic surgery: radical tonsillectomy. Arch Otolaryngol Head Neck Surg. 2007;133(12):1220–6.
9. Solares CA, Strome M. Transoral robot-assisted CO_2 laser supraglottic laryngectomy: experimental and clinical data. Laryngoscope. 2007;117(5):817–20.
10. Rahbar R, Ferrari LR, Borer JG, Peters CA. Robotic surgery in the pediatric airway: application and safety. Arch Otolaryngol Head Neck Surg. 2007;133(1): 46–50.
11. Leonardis RL, Duvvuri U, Mehta D. Transoral robotic-assisted lingual tonsillectomy in the pediatric population. JAMA Otolaryngol Head Neck Surg. 2013;139(10):1032–6.
12. Kayhan FT, Kaya KH, Koc AK, Altintas A, Erdur O. Transoral surgery for an infant thyroglossal duct cyst. Int J Pediatr Otorhinolaryngol. 2013;77(9): 1620–3.
13. Moore EJ, Olsen KD, Kasperbauer JL. Transoral robotic surgery for oropharyngeal squamous cell carcinoma: a prospective study of feasibility and functional outcomes. Laryngoscope. 2009;119(11): 2156–64.
14. Lanfranco AR, Castellanos AE, Desai JP, Meyers WC. Robotic surgery: a current perspective. Ann Surg. 2004;239(1):14–21.
15. Satava RM. Surgical robotics: the early chronicles: a personal historical perspective. Surg Laparosc Endosc Percutan Tech. 2002;12(1):6–16.
16. Cadiere GB, Himpens J, Vertruyen M, Bruyns J, Fourtanier G. Nissen fundoplication done by remotely controlled robotic technique. Ann Chir. 1999;53(2): 137–41.
17. McLeod IK, Melder PC. Da Vinci robot-assisted excision of a vallecular cyst: a case report. Ear Nose Throat J. 2005;84(3):170–2.
18. Cundy TP, Shetty K, Clark J, et al. The first decade of robotic surgery in children. J Pediatr Surg. 2013;48: 858–65.
19. Berguer R, Smith W. An ergonomic comparison of robotic and laparoscopic technique: the influence of surgeon experience and task complexity. J Surg Res. 2006;134(1):87–92.
20. Prasad SM, Ducko CT, Stephenson ER, Chambers CE, Damiano Jr RJ. Prospective clinical trial of robotically assisted endoscopic coronary grafting with 1-year follow-up. Ann Surg. 2001;233(6):725–32.
21. Feifer A, Al-Ammari A, Kovac E, Delisle J, Carrier S, Anidjar M. Randomized controlled trial of virtual reality and hybrid simulation for robotic surgical training. BJU Int. 2011;108(10):1652–7.
22. Blavier A, Cadière GB, Gaudissart Q, Nyssen AS. Comparison of learning curves and skill transfer between classical and robotic laparoscopy according to the viewing conditions: implications for training. Am J Surg. 2007;194(1):115–21.
23. Marescaux J, Leroy J, Rubino F, et al. Transcontinental robot-assisted remote telesurgery: feasibility and potential applications. Ann Surg. 2002;235(4): 487–92.

Transorbal Robotic Surgery for Sleep Apnea

Claudio Vicini, Filippo Montevecchi, Mohamed Eesa, and Iacopo Dallan

Introduction

Da Vinci tongue base reduction (TBR) and supraglottoplasty (SGP) are devised in order to provide similar functional outcomes of the classic open approach described by Chabolle and Coll. (1999) [1] as well as all the potential benefits of a completely transoral approach (TORS) [2–4]. The da Vinci System 3D HD visualization, wristed instrumentations and intuitive movement help to provide the ultimate, precise and endoscopic approach for TBR&SGP. A really reduced invasiveness, a significant efficacy and relatively limited surgical time are the keys of this procedure.

C. Vicini, M.D. (✉) • F. Montevecchi, M.D.
Department of Special Surgery, Otolaryngology—Head & Neck Surgery Division, Oral Surgery Unit, University of Pavia in Forlì, G.B. Morgagni L. Pierantoni Hospital, Viale C. Forlanini 34, 47121 Forlì, Italy
e-mail: claudio@claudiovicini.com

M. Eesa, M.D.
Department of Otolaryngology—Head & Neck Surgery, University of Zagazig, Zagazig, Egypt

I. Dallan, M.D.
Ear Nose and Throat Unit, Azienda Ospedaliero-Universitaria Pisana, Pisa, Italy

Indications

Mild to severe OSAHS patients (Apnoea Hypopnea Index > 20) usually with Excessive Daytime Sleepiness (Epworth Sleepiness Scale > 10), significant obstruction at tongue base (Fig. 1) (Cormak and Lehane Grading > 2) and/or supraglottic area prolapse endoscopically demonstrated are the ideal application for TORS procedure, provided that a sufficient oropharyngeal exposure is possible (interincisive distance >2.5 cm). UARS and mild OSAH as well may be approached if prominent tongue base and/or supraglottic instability is the main concern.

The preoperative diagnostic approach is basically the same for all potential surgeries of sleep related breathing disorders: history, conventional ENT examination, awake fiberendoscopy (Naso Pharyngo Laryngoscopy), biometrics (Body Mass Index [BMI], Neck Circumference, Tonsils Grading 0 to IV, Mallampati–Friedman Scoring I to IV, Cormack and Lehane Scoring), psychometrics (Epworth Sleepiness Scale, Cognitive Functions Test Battery, Anxiety and Depression Scales, Electronic Reactometry), Imaging (basically Panorex® & Lateral Cephalogram), Quality of Life SF36 questionnaire. In this particular group of patients Sleep Endoscopy and Neck CT or MRI proved to be a very useful additional set of investigations for better defining soft tissue collapsing pattern during sleep and relative obstructing mass composition (lymphatic tissue vs. muscle) in base of tongue (BOT) bulging (Fig. 2).

G.A. Grillone and S. Jalisi (eds.), *Robotic Surgery of the Head and Neck: A Comprehensive Guide*, DOI 10.1007/978-1-4939-1547-7_7, © Springer Science+Business Media New York 2015

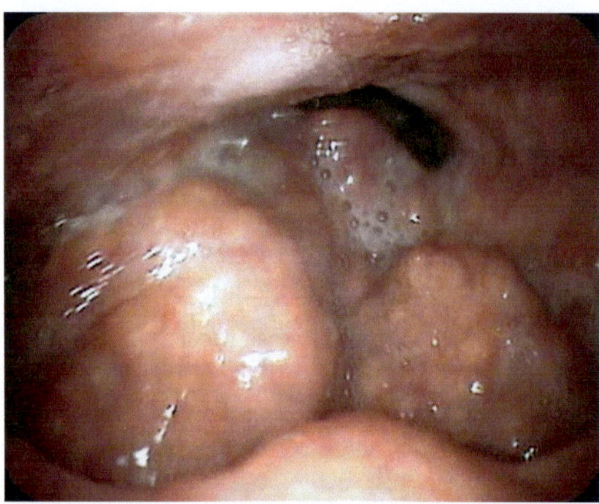

Fig. 1 Lymphatic tongue base obstruction (endoscopic view)

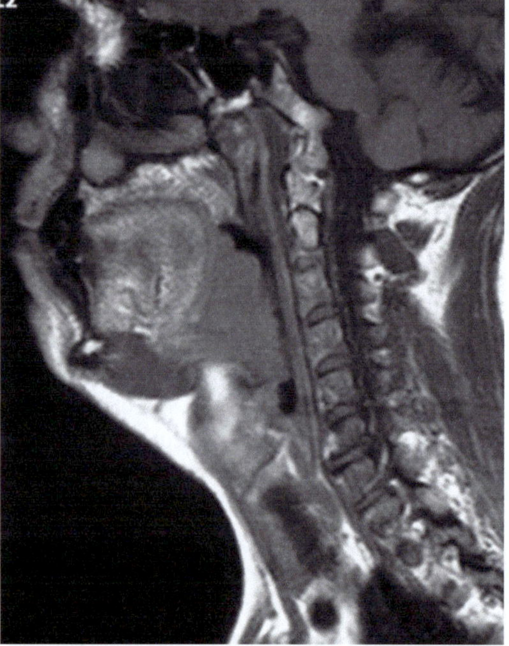

Fig. 2 Lymphatic tongue base obstruction (MRI pre-op)

In many cases patients are referred to surgery after continuous positive airway pressure (CPAP) not acceptance or drop-out. In a significant number of patients TORS is proposed as a revision procedure after previous surgery failure. Additional complaints commonly reported by most of the patients are related to BOT enlargement; foreign body sensation in the throat, swallowing difficultics and chronic cough.

Associated nasal obstructive problems as well as palate and tonsil disproportionate anatomy may be treated in the same time of TORS with additional surgical steps in the same operation (multilevel surgery including nose reconstruction and Expansion Sphincter Pharyngoplasty according to Pang & Tucker Woodson, that replaced in our experience the more classical but less effective uvulopalatopharyngoplasty).

Cardiovascular and neuropsychological comorbidities usually related to OSAHS must be accurately evaluated by the anaesthesiological team, in order to rule out too high risk patients or properly managing the more complex cases. Obesity is the most common dysmetabolic condition encountered as well as arterial hypertension and metabolic syndrome. It is worth to mention that TORS for OSAHS is a BMI sensitive procedure. In patients with BMI>30 the expected success rate decreases along with the BMI increasing. Specific technical features of TORS for OSAHS must be pointed out. Airway problems are very probable in induction as well as in post-op survey for OSAHS patients.

1. Difficult intubation facilities are always at disposal, and endoscopic assisted intubation was necessary in 80 % of our cases, not different from Literature figures.
2. Especially for most severe OSAHS cases a safety tracheostomy is strongly recommended for post-op ventilation assistance, moreover if nose and oropharynx are operated in the same time. One more key point for tracheostomy is the degree of difficulty in case of reintubation for airway problems or post-op bleeding. The present policy of our group is to discuss any single case with the anaesthesiological team and share the final decision about a planned tracheostomy, that is no more adopted in mild to moderate cases, without significant comorbidities, scheduled for a limited surgical treatment (tongue base and supraglottis without nose and/or palate) and expected to be easily reintubated if necessary. If required, tracheostomy is the first step of TORS. A specific study comparing conventional/incisional with dilatiative/percoutaneous is still running in our Institution. Preliminary unpublished

data seem to favour the dilatative, more expensive but less aggressive and easy to perform out of the operating room in the patients' preparation area. An additional advantage of tracheostomy to be stressed is a completely tube free surgical field during robotic procedure, very useful in case of very narrow pharynx. In our Institution post-op Protocols for severe OSAHS patients require routine tracheostomy. A prolonged post-op intubation inside the recovery room may be an alternative solution. We use to check the airway by fiberoptics in order to optimize the timing of tube removal, usually about few hours after the surgery, and in order to avoid the intubation induced edema, sometimes more prominent than postsurgical one.

Technique

Tongue base exposure is achieved in the standard TORS approach with a combination of tongue body traction with strong sutures and tongue body displacement by Storz® Davis Meyer Mouth Gag. A complete set of tongue blades of different sizes with integrated suction tubes (for smoke and blood) is of paramount importance. FK® Mouth Gag is available on the table but usually is not necessary for TBR in most cases but sometimes may be useful for SGP. A small size blade proved to be the most suitable tool in most cases, especially in the first steps of BOT approach. Cheek retraction by means of disposable auto-retaining retractors (Leone Orthodontics and Implantology®, Florence, Italy) is possible in order to gain more space laterally, especially for a better view of the 2nd surgeon for his manoeuvres. 12 mm 30° 3D scope (upward facing) is our preferred choice. If available 8 mm scope may be very interesting in particular cases (small interincisive distance, extreme macroglossia, etc.).

Only two robotic 5 mm Endo Wrist® arms are used for each patient: a Maryland Dissector 400143/420143 for grasping and dissection of tissues and a Monopolar Cautery with Spatula Tip 400142/400160 for dissection and coagulation. No clip placement is usually required, but in few special cases large vessel clipping proved to be very helpful. Sometimes additional haemostasis is provided by an insulated ball-end coagulation-suction tube Storz® Cat. 12067R at disposal. An insulated long blunt angled-tip bipolar forceps Storz® Cat. 842219 is of paramount importance for safe coagulation in the peripheral aspects of the surgical field. A bipolar Dessi's coagulating device originally designed for FESS may be helpful as well. Two additional hands with a suction device type mini-Yankauer are offered by the assistant surgeon at the head of the patient. Tissue displacement for better surgical exposure, blood and smoke suctioning are the basic jobs of the assistant surgeon.

Some special remarks about specificity of OSAHS TORS may be discussed into detail:

The patient's so-called supine "sniffing position" is preferred in order to achieve the best compromise for basic good exposure and possibility to apply all possibly required external manoeuvres of neck compression/ lateral displacement in order to enhance the exposure of different areas during the dissection.

1. A single case customized combination of tongue base traction and properly selected mouth-gag blade length is the key for a really good exposure. It requires a correct amount of tongue base bulging into the surgical field for the best manipulation.
2. In extremely huge tongue situations, the smallest Storz blade may allow a lateral inrolling of the tongue body margins. In this situation the operative arms introduction may be difficult. The use of a longer and wider blade is possible in order to sustain the lateral tongue body profiles, provided that a lower degree of tension of the tongue suture is set in order to allow a more posterior tongue base bulging.
3. Repositioning of tongue blade may be rarely necessary and in our experience it would be considered as the last choice. Usually the shortest blade or the medium blades are very effective for completing tongue base as well as epiglottis procedures. If a second blade is to be inserted after first resection step, the new position must be checked in a very precise way in order to avoid losing the orientation.

4. Only in few cases FK mouth gag proved to be crucial, especially for supraglottic exposure; it's usually not necessary in tongue base exposure.

TORS approach in OSAHS surgery includes two different surgical procedures usually combined in the same patient [5–9]:

1. Tongue Base Reduction (TBR)
2. Supra Glotto Plasty (SGP)

Tongue base reduction (TBR): It's basically a different application and a proper modification of the tongue base resection described by O'Malley and Coll. in 2006 [10]. The goal of TBR is to enlarge the oropharyngeal section in the anterior wall area as well as classically palatine tonsils removal and lateral pharyngoplasty address the more common lateral oropharyngeal wall obstruction. As in the lateral oropharyngeal wall, in tongue base area, there is surgically safe superficial layer composed of lymphoid tissue easy to remove and surgically dangerous deep muscular layer composed of muscles covering great vessels (lingual artery and its dorsal branches) and functionally crucial nerves (hypoglossus nerve and lingual nerve).

The end point of TBR may be probably achieved when the obtained surgical view shifts from a Cormack & Lehane Grade IV to a Grade II, or far less commonly, to a Grade I. In all but few cases lymphoid tissue as well as tongue base muscle must be removed in order to clear the so called Retrolingual Space or Posterior Airway Space (PAS).

The more lymphatic hyperplasia, the less muscular tissue violation. Conversely, if lingual tonsil is no more than a thin layer, a more aggressive muscular resection is required in order to get the Cormack & Lehane Grade II goal. The mean volume of removed tissue is of about 15 cc, but sometimes the overall volume may be over 50 cc. Surgical steps are quite standardized in a precise and may be logic sequence, and may be sequentially applied in most of the approached cases [11]:

1. Midline split of the two lingual tonsils from foramen caecum down to identify epiglottic tip and vallecula. The section is carried out by Monopolar Cautery and get in depth the junction between tonsil and muscle. Sometimes difficult to identify in extreme lingual tonsil hyperplasia, foramen caecum is the key point for starting the dissection. This point must be stressed because it locates the upper limit of the resection, helping the surgeon to spare circumvallate papillae area and taste function, and in the same time giving to the surgeon a reasonable location of the midline. Approaching this step of the dissection with the scope tip relatively far from the surgical field (low magnification and a wide angle view of the surgical field) is strongly recommended in order to enhance the 3D awareness of the surgical anatomy. At the end of this first step lingual tonsil is completely split in midline, and a deep groove joining foramen caecum to midline glosso-epiglottic area at the lymphoid-muscle junction in depth is our goal.
2. Superior (sulcus terminalis), lateral (amigdalo-glossus sulcus) and inferior (glosso-epiglottic sulcus) borders of the right lingual tonsil are identified and possibly marked by cautery. This sequence is possible only in case of moderate to mild lingual tonsil hyperplasia. In extreme lingual tonsil hyperplasia after midline splitting, the subsequent step is a central tongue base debulking in order to allow better lateral manipulation and limits identification. After central debulking the following steps are basically the same.
3. In case of moderate to mild lingual tonsil hyperplasia the right lingual tonsillectomy is performed "en block" up to down keeping the section close to the muscular plane (Fig. 3); during this step the scope is kept closer to the surgical field (greater magnification) for better identification of vessels and, by far less commonly, nerves.
4. Left lingual tonsillectomy is completed in the same way after side inversion of the robotic tools
5. The surgical field is now inspected in order to evaluate the residual degree of obstruction. If Cormack and Lehane Grade > 2 is measured, additional resection in true muscle area is required.
6. The key of this step is to remove a sufficient amount of muscle in order to open the posterior airway space as well as to avoid any

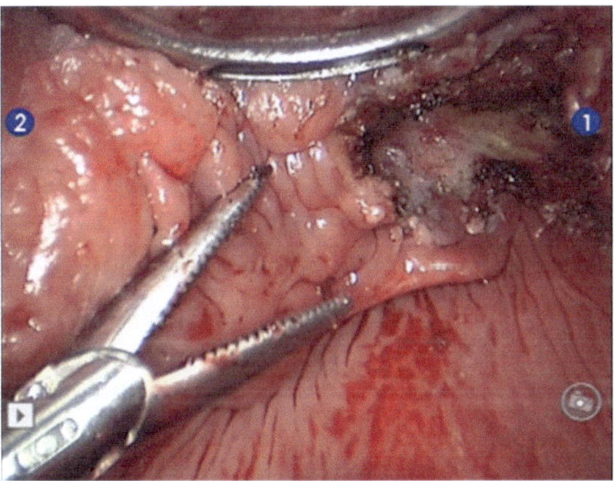

Fig. 3 Intraoperative surgical view after right-side tongue base reduction

possible injury to XII cranial nerve, lingual nerve and lingual artery. Sequert and Coll. [12], Lauretano and Caradonna [13] and O'Malley and Coll [10] published very interesting cadaveric dissections with practical landmarks for the main structures. Our group collected a 2 days full-time dissection experience in fresh cadaver in Vienna with a robotic-like endoscopic setting (data in press). Tuker Woodson [14] stresses the importance of intraoperative tongue mapping with ultrasound if available. All the authors admit that a reliable pre-location of all these structures is virtually impossible due to the enormous inter-individual anatomical variations and to the extreme mobility of active tongue, and, last but not least, due to the important shape modification produced by the surgical setting (traction sutures, mouth gag blades, head and mandible position). In our experience two points must be remarked:

(a) Basically a muscle layer thinner than 10 mm may be removed without real problems inside the entire BOT limits.
(b) In midline area an additional strip of 5 mm at each side of midline and 5 mm in depth may be resected without major additional risks.
(c) The paramount importance of 3D da Vinci® close view with magnification is the key for the identification of the crucial structures to avoid damaging them, working carefully step by step with a mix of blunt and sharp dissection with robotic instruments.
(d) One more simple rule is based upon the normal anatomical relationship between main trunk of the lingual artery and hyoid bone greater cornu. Irrespective of tissue manipulation by the blades for the exposure, the course of lingual artery trunk runs parallel to the hyoid greater cornu within 10 mm from the hyoid bone itself. Any dissection, if necessary, within this area should be really careful.

SUPRA GLOTTO PLASTY (SGP) it's very often carried out after TBR in the same patient and during the same operation. The key of SGP is to fix the inward inspiratory collapse of floppy and/or redundant tissue in epiglottis, ary-epiglottic folds and arytenoids area. In Literature four different surgical actions are described and suggested, separately or in different combination:

1. Resection of excessive amount of tissue (-ectomy or -plasty)
2. Mucosal removal in order to promote scarring and retraction (-scar-pexy)
3. Suturing in order to stabilize too mobile structures (-suture-pexy)
4. Section and release of too short ligaments. (-release)

Robotic laryngeal supraglottic resection was described by Weinstein and Coll [15] in cadaver, Hockstein and Coll [16] introduced different robotic procedures in the same area in a similar cadaver model, and more recently Solares and Strome [17] proposed in cadaver and dog model a Robot-Laser coupling for supraglottic laryngectomy. All these surgical manipulations are made extremely easy by TORS approach, with particular regard to intrapharyngeal suturing otherwise really demanding. The extra time required for laryngeal step after TBR is usually less than 15 min. The most common choice in supraglottic area includes the following basic steps:

1. Vertical midline splitting of supra-hyoid epiglottis; the section is carried out along the midline, following the medial glosso-epiglottic fold, from the tip down to spare at

least 5 mm over the deep vallecular plane (a sufficient strip of cartilage is left for preventing aspiration)

2. An horizontal section on both sides is done in a plane joining the vertical section in midline and running laterally immediately over the pharyngo-epiglottic fold, in order to leave a lateral fold preventing aspiration, and in order to avoid possible bleeding from the superior laryngeal vessels.
3. During the post-op scarring of the vallecular and peri-vallecular area, a progressive adhesion and stabilization of the residual epiglottis to the tongue base is observed.

After the robotic assisted step, if necessary, palate and/or nose may be addressed in a conventional way inside a single step multi-site procedure. Our group could demonstrate that expansion sphincter pharyngoplasty (ESP) proved to be the most effective associated procedure in palate area. Coupling ESP instead of uvulopalatopharyngoplasty (UPPP) in a series of multilevel procedure, the final post-op AHI could drop to 9 instead of 19 as in the group of UPPP palate associated surgery [18].

Postoperative

After 1-h stay in the recovery room, the patient is transferred directly to the ear, nose and throat ward. Morphine in sustained release form is used for analgesia for the first 3–5 days. Pain intensity within the first week is about 3.5 in a visual analog scale of 0–10. A liquid diet is permitted on the second day and solid diet is resumed after a week. Average hospital stay is about 5 days.

In our experience, complications were rare and transient. No conversion to open technique was needed. No complications related to robot instrumentation occurred. A few cases of self-limiting delayed bleeding in the first 1–3 weeks were treated by simple observation. Transient hypogeusia occurred in some patients, but this resolved within a few weeks. Average level of dysphagia was fairly low, as measured by MDADI, a dysphagia-specific quality-of-life questionnaire. In Fig. 4 are summarized our results in a pilot group of 107 patients out of our overall series of 160 TORS for OSAHS.

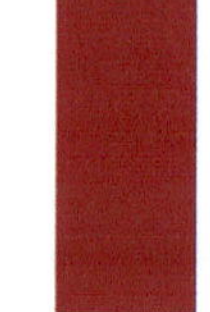
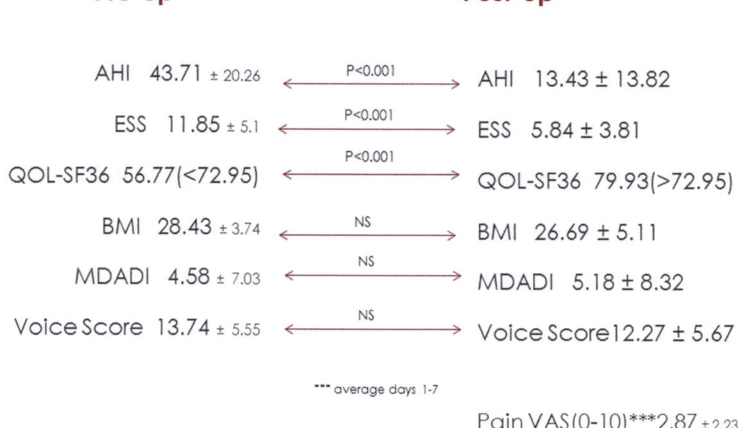

Fig. 4 Outcomes

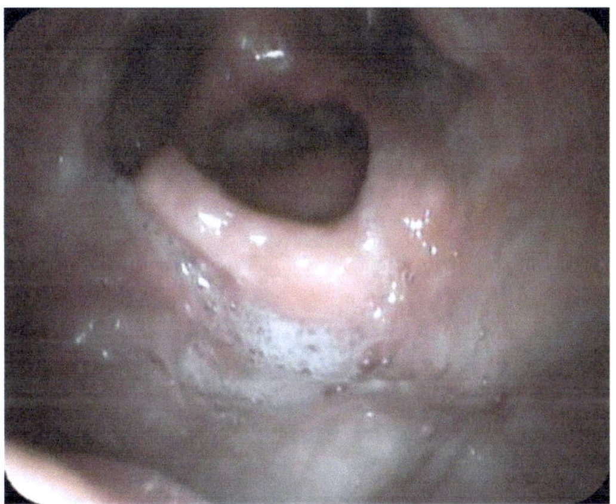

Fig. 5 Endoscopic view 3 months after surgery

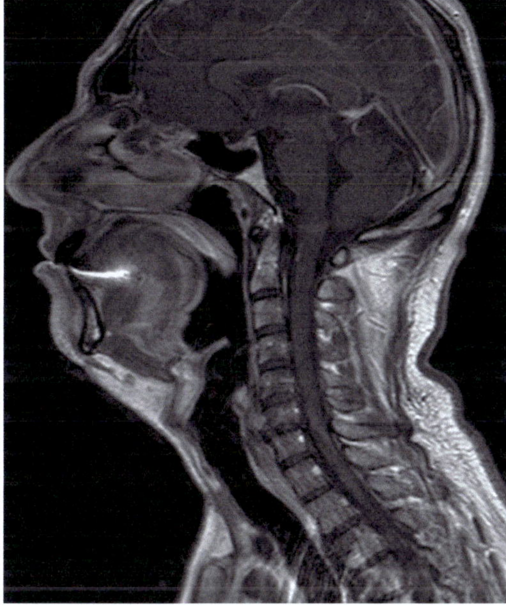

Fig. 6 MRI post-op 3 months after surgery

A significant reduction of AHI and ESS was achieved as well as a statistical improvement of Lower Oxygen Saturation and Quality of Life (SF36 score), without any significant reduction of BMI. Usually post-op follow-up by means of endoscopy and sleep study is performed between 3rd and 6th month (Figs. 5 and 6).

Some key points for selecting the best patients and for performing the best job as possible may be listed.

The most suitable candidates for TORS are:

- Subjects with BMI lower than 30, irrespective to pre-op AHI
- With tongue base obstruction related to low, lymphatic and ball-like overgrowth of tissue in supra vallecular area
- With no additional nose or palate obstruc tion or with well-known nose and or palate obstruction eligible for a specific corrective surgery with a reasonable expected success rate

The less suitable candidates for TORS are:

- Subjects with BMI higher than 30,
- With tongue base obstruction related to very high tongue base, with not limited but diffusely reduced posterior airway, or with tendency of the tongue base borders to roll in during inspiration
- With additional nose or palate obstruction or with well-known nose and or palate obstruction eligible for a specific corrective surgery with a low expected success rate
- The single surgical key point worth to be stressed is the success dependency upon the removed tissue volume. A resection of less than 7 cc proved to be ineffective in most of the cases.

Conclusions

TORS would be considered an additional option for treating OSAHS related to obstruction in both the tongue base and supraglottic larynx. Further studies are needed to elucidate long-term outcomes of TORS for OSAHS. Other areas in need of further investigation include optimizing patient selection criteria, surgical instrumentation and improvements in both short-term and long-term functional outcomes.

References

1. Chabolle F, Wagner I, Blumen MB, Séquert C, Fleury B, De Dieuleveult T. Tongue base reduction with hyoepiglottoplasty: a treatment for severe obstructive sleep apnea. Laryngoscope. 1999;109: 1273–80.

2. Friedman M, Hamilton C, Samuelson CG, Kelley K, Taylor D, Pearson-Chauhan K, Maley A, Taylor R, Venkatesan TK. Transoral robotic glossectomy for the treatment of obstructive sleep apnea-hypopnea syndrome. Otolaryngol Head Neck Surg. 2012;146(5):854–62.
3. Lee JM, Weinstein GS, O'Malley Jr BW, Thaler ER. Transoral robot-assisted lingual tonsillectomy and uvulopalatopharyngoplasty for obstructive sleep apnea. Ann Otol Rhinol Laryngol. 2012;121(10):635–9.
4. Lin HS, Rowley JA, Badr MS, Folbe AJ, Yoo GH, Victor L, Mathog RH, Chen W. Transoral robotic surgery for treatment of obstructive sleep apnea-hypopnea syndrome. Laryngoscope. 2013;123(7):1811–6.
5. Vicini C, Dallan I, Canzi P, Frassineti S, La Pietra MG, Montevecchi F. Transoral robotic tongue base resection in obstructive sleep apnoea-hypopnoea syndrome: a preliminary report. ORL J Otorhinolaryngol Relat Spec. 2010;72(1):22–7.
6. Vicini C, Montevecchi F, Dallan I, Canzi P, Tenti G. Transoral robotic geniohyoidpexy as an additional step of transoral robotic tongue base reduction and supraglottoplasty: feasibility in a cadaver model. ORL J Otorhinolaryngol Relat Spec. 2011;73(3):147–50.
7. Vicini C, Dallan I, Canzi P, Frassineti S, Nacci A, Seccia V, Panicucci E, La Pietra MG, Montevecchi F, Tschabitscher M. Transoral robotic surgery of the tongue base in obstructive sleep Apnea-Hypopnea syndrome: anatomic considerations and clinical experience. Head Neck. 2012;34(1):15–22.
8. Vicini C, Montevecchi F, Tenti G, Canzi P, Dallan I, Huntley TC. Transoral robotic surgery: tongue base reduction and supraglottoplasty for obstructive sleep apnea (Original Research Article). Oper Tech Otolaryngol Head Neck Surg. 2012;23(1):45–7.
9. Vicini C, Montevecchi F, Scott MJ. Robotic surgery for obstructive sleep apnea. Curr Otorhinolaryngol Rep. 2013;1:130–6.
10. O'Malley Jr BW, Weinstein GS, Snyder W, Hockstein NG. Transoral robotic surgery (TORS) for base of tongue neoplasms. Laryngoscope. 2006;116:1465–72.
11. Dallan I, Seccia V, Faggioni L, Castelnuovo P, Montevecchi F, Casani AP, Tschabitscher M, Vicini C. Anatomical landmarks for transoral robotic tongue base surgery: comparison between endoscopic, external and radiological perspectives. Surg Radiol Anat. 2013;35(1):3–10.
12. Sequert C, Lestang P, Baglin AC, Wagner I, Ferron JM, Chabolle F. Hypoglossal nerve in its intralingual trajectory: anatomy and clinical implications. Ann Otolaryngol Chir Cervicofac. 1999;116:207–17.
13. Lauretano AM, Li KK, Caradonna DS, Khosta RK, Fried MP. Anatomic location of the tongue base neurovascular bundle. Laryngoscope. 1997;107:1057–9.
14. Woodson BT. Innovative technique for lingual tonsillectomy and midline posterior glossectomy for obstructive sleep apnea. Oper Tech Otolaryngol Head Neck Surg. 2007;18:20–8.
15. Weinstein GS, O'Malley Jr BW, Hockstein NG. Transoral robotic surgery: supraglottic laryngectomy in a canine model. Laryngoscope. 2005;115:1315–9.
16. Hockstein NG, Nolan JP, O'Malley Jr BW, Woo YJ. Robot-assisted pharyngeal and laryngeal microsurgery: results of robotic cadaver dissections. Laryngoscope. 2005;115:1003–8.
17. Solares CA, Strome M. Transoral robot-assisted CO_2 laser supraglottic laryngectomy: experimental and clinical data. Laryngoscope. 2007;117:817–20.
18. Vicini C, Montevecchi F, Pang K, Bahgat A, Dallan I, Frassineti S, Campanini A. Combined transoral robotic tongue base surgery and palate surgery in obstructive sleep apnea-hypopnea syndrome: expansion sphincter pharyngoplasty versus uvulopalatopharyngoplasty. Head Neck. 2014;36(1):77–83.

Robotic Surgery for the Management of Oropharyngeal Malignancies

Eric J. Moore

Introduction

Oropharynx Cancer

The oropharynx encompasses the soft palate, the palatine tonsils, the base of tongue, and a portion of the posterior and lateral pharyngeal wall between the nasopharynx and hypopharynx. The oropharynx is lined by squamous epithelium, and it contains numerous salivary glands and lymphoid tissue. Squamous cell carcinoma comprises the majority of cancers in the oropharynx. Oropharynx squamous cell carcinoma (OP SCCA) comprises approximately 12 % of all head and neck cancers, with an increasing incidence each year [1]. Historically, OP SCCa has been a disease associated strongly with heavy tobacco and alcohol use. While these two carcinogens continue to play a role in the development of OP SCCa, human papilloma virus (HPV, particularly type 16) has been recognized as the most common factor associated with oropharynx cancer in the United States and other developed cancers. HPV 16 is also the most common factor in the development of cervical cancer in women, and the incidence of OP SCCa related to HPV 16 is expected to eclipse the incidence of cervical cancer by 2020 [2].

Like nearly every cancer, OP SCCa can be treated by surgical removal, radiation therapy, chemotherapy, or combinations of these treatments. Historically OP SCCa has been treated by surgery and postoperative radiation therapy. But the OP is a difficult area in which to obtain adequate surgical exposure. Traditional surgical exposure of the OP has been obtained by mandibulotomy and pharyngotomy. These "open approaches" require tracheostomy and reconstruction and have been criticized for their surgical morbidity and prolonged healing time. With the rising popularity of concomitant chemotherapy and radiation therapy for head and neck carcinoma, the treatment of OP SCCA shifted predominantly to nonoperative treatment throughout the early 2000s [3]. But advances in surgical technology, an alteration in the patient age and prognosis related to the rising incidence of HPV-related OP SCCa, and a realization of the long-term morbidity of chemoradiation therapy have led to a resurgence in interest in transoral surgery for these cancers [4, 5].

This chapter will describe the patient candidacy, indications, technique, postoperative care, additional treatment, and complications of transoral robotic surgery (TORS) for cancers of the tonsil and base of tongue.

E.J. Moore, M.D. (✉)
Professor-Otolaryngology/Head and Neck Surgery, Mayo Clinic-Rochester, MN, USA
e-mail: moore.eric@mayo.edu

G.A. Grillone and S. Jalisi (eds.), *Robotic Surgery of the Head and Neck: A Comprehensive Guide*,
DOI 10.1007/978-1-4939-1547-7_8, © Springer Science+Business Media New York 2015

Transoral Surgery

Minimally invasive surgery takes advantage of either small "ports" or natural body orifices for access of instrumentation. The oropharynx is ideally positioned next to the mouth which provides a wide natural body orifice. The first descriptions of transoral surgery of the oropharynx came from Huet in France and utilized electrocautery to remove the tonsil and superior pharyngeal constrictor muscle for carcinoma of the tonsillar fossae [6]. Going deeper into the oropharynx than the tonsillar fossae has posed challenges for procedures performed with a handheld electrorcautery and other rigid instruments. After the development of transoral laser microsurgery (TLM) by Jako and Strong, some surgeons began to utilize carbon dioxide laser applied through a micromanipulator and tubular laryngoscopes to gain access to and remove tumors from the oropharynx. This use of TLM for oropharynx neoplasms was pioneered by Steiner of Goettingen, Germany [7]. Because many of the tumors in the oropharynx could not be circumferentially visualized or removed completely through the laryngoscope, Steiner advocated "piecemeal" resection of the tumor and careful assessment of the interface between the tumor and the surrounding normal tissue at its borders. This technique violated the traditional concept of en bloc removal that was revered by oncologic surgeons since Halsted's original description early in the twentieth century. Steiner's landmark paper demonstrating 85 % local control in T1 and T2 tumors and overall control of 80 % in T3 and T4 tumors established a basis for the value of transoral surgery in oropharynx cancer treatment [8].

Even with its growing acceptance as a treatment option for oropharyngeal malignancies, TLM is not without its limitations. The inability to utilize two hands for dissection and manipulation of the tumor, the need to alternate between the laser and an electrocautery when vessels and bleeding are encountered, and the inability to work around the "corners" of the oropharynx create challenges. Limitations in visualization of the entire tumor and inability to manipulate the tumor with more than one hand can make TLM technically difficult, and training and experience is necessary to achieve an acceptable level of competence.

The desire to take advantage of transoral access while avoiding the limitations of TLM has led some oncologic surgeons to adopt the da Vinci Surgical System (Intuitive Surgical, Sunnyvale, CA) for OP surgery [9–11]. Transoral Robotic Surgery (TORS) provides visualization with a 0° or 30° binocular telescope and surgical manipulation of tissue with 540° wristed instrumentation. The instrumentation was ushered into the Otolaryngology literature by Neil Hockstein while he was a resident at the University of Pennsylvania in 2005 [12]. Hockstein authored the original studies on feasibility and safety of TORS in cadavers and patients [13]. Further studies culminated on the Food and Drug Administration approval of TORS for selected tumors of the head and neck [14]. Since that time, a number of studies have documented local control rates, overall survival rates, and safety and complication rates of TORS for OP SCCa that are at least as favorable as other transoral modalities [9, 15]. Surgical advantages of TORS include 540° wristed instrumentation, angled high definition telescopic optics, tremor reduction, and two-handed tissue manipulation. Multiple studies have shown that with proper patient selection, TORS of OP SCCa can result in better swallowing function, decreased gastrostomy tube and tracheostomy tube dependence, shorter hospitalization and recovery time, and decreased overall morbidity compared to open surgical techniques and nonoperative therapy.

Disadvantages of TORS relate to the size of the instrument and the orientation of the arms that can make access and exposure of tumors difficult or impossible in some patients. Other disadvantages include the expense of the instrumentation, the lack of tactile feedback, and the training and experience necessary to use and maintain the instrument properly.

Transoral Robotic Surgery

Candidacy

The first step in TORS is appropriate patient selection: who is an ideal candidate and who is an unfavorable candidate for this technique. This decision making is vital for success and is dependent on operator experience and judgment. This candidacy selection begins with patient history paying careful attention to the symptoms and length of their presence, comorbidities, prior treatment, current speech and swallowing function, weight loss, social status and support, and patient concerns and anxiety. Following that, a careful physical exam should assess mouth opening and dentition. The tumor should be carefully palpated with a gloved index finger and the induration, friability, submucosal spread, and mobility should be assessed. Flexible nasopharyngoscopy looks at the medial and inferior extent of the tumor, the involvement of the epiglottis and lateral pharyngeal wall, the status of the glottic mobility, and the ability to clear secretions with swallow. Recording the endoscopy can help with review of the operative plan, discussion of the tumor with the patient and colleagues, and discussion of the airway management with the anesthesiologist. The neck is carefully assessed for size and mobility of adenopathy. Imaging with computerized tomography CT) with contrast can help with metastatic workup and assessment of the primary tumor and lymph node relationship to the great vessels, skull base, and mandible.

Patient candidacy can be divided into three major categories: patient comorbidities, anatomic constraints, and tumor characteristics [16].

Patient Comorbidities

Transoral surgery results in an oropharyngeal wound that heals by secondary intention. During this time, the patient is at risk for bleeding, aspiration, wound infection, dehydration, airway compromise, poor nutritional support, and sleep deprivation. The successful outcome balances on a race between rapid remucosalization and the occurrence of these complications. Therefore, the ideal patient must not only be able to tolerate some of these insults, but they must also be able to rapidly contract and heal the wound. Patient comorbidities that tip this balance toward an unfavorable outcome include:

- Immune suppression
- Advanced age
- Dementia
- Coagulopathy
- Congestive Heart Failure
- COPD
- Severe malnutrition
- Diabetes
- Prior treatment causing microvascular compromise

The presence of one or a few of these factors may not completely disqualify the patient from TORS, but the surgeon should counsel the patient appropriately and tread cautiously when these factors are present or severe.

Anatomic Constraints

Transoral surgery uses the mouth as the access point, and it requires the placement of an oral retractor to gain access. Experience of the surgeon can often help predict after office exam alone which patients can be exposed and which ones will pose difficulties. In the absence of experience, or when the access is in doubt, and operative exam under anesthesia may help decide candidacy. Specific anatomic constraints that pose challenges include:

- Trismus: mouth opening <1.5 cm—this can be caused by pain, previous treatment, tumor invasion of the pterygoid muscles
- Mandibular transverse dimensions: the mandibular width needs to be wide enough to accommodate the blade of the retractor and allow the tongue to spill around its sides rather than displacing it posteriorly into the operating field
- Retrognathia: a posteriorly positioned mandible and displace the tongue posteriorly and inferiorly into the operating field
- Macroglossia
- Cervical spine inflexibility
- Prominent incisor teeth
- Mandibular tori
- Medial internal carotid arteries

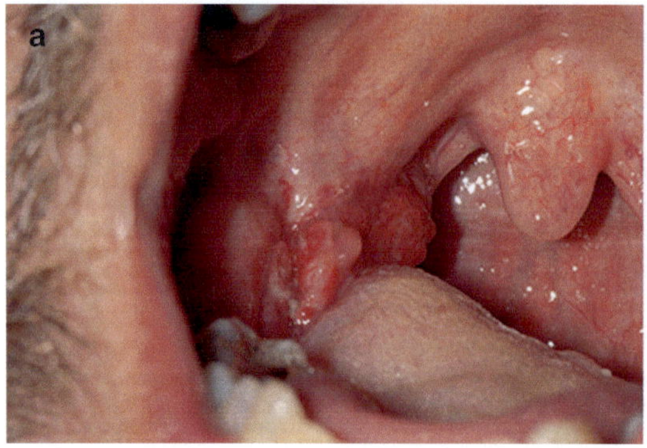

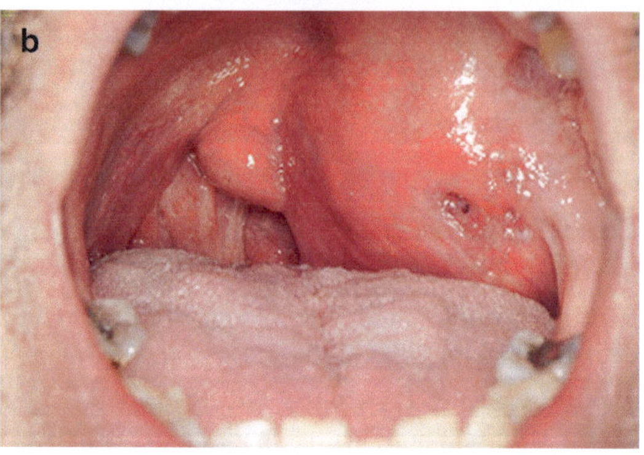

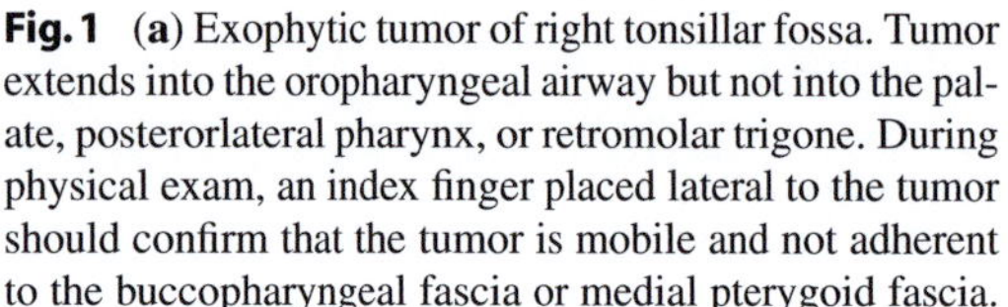
Fig. 1 (**a**) Exophytic tumor of right tonsillar fossa. Tumor extends into the oropharyngeal airway but not into the palate, posterorlateral pharynx, or retromolar trigone. During physical exam, an index finger placed lateral to the tumor should confirm that the tumor is mobile and not adherent to the buccopharyngeal fascia or medial pterygoid fascia. (**b**) A left tonsil tumor showing endophytic growth pattern and submucosal invasion into soft palate. These tumors are often fixed and immobile. Palpation and imaging can help the surgeon discern the lateral boundaries of the tumor, but fixed tumor are not ideal tumors to approach transorally

Tumor Characteristics

The primary goal of all OP SCCa surgery is complete removal of the entire tumor with clear microscopic margins. As Jesse stated decades ago, "the primary cause of failure of treatment of oral cancer is the inability to completely resect the tumor." Proper assessment of the tumor boundaries and its relationship with normal tissue and structures is a vital step in assessing surgical candidacy. This is done through careful history and physical examination, palpation of the tumor and its lateral borders, flexible nasolaryngopharyngoscopy, and careful review of a CT with contrast to appreciate the relationship of the primary tumor and metastases with the internal and external carotid arteries, skull base, and mandible. The ideal tumor for transoral resection is easily accessible, is mobile to palpation, and demonstrates an exophytic growth pattern [17] (Fig. 1). Particular tumor characteristics that make a patient a candidate for TORS include:

- Fixation of the tumor to the lateral or posterior pharyngeal wall, including deep extension to the parapharyngeal space
- Significant involvement of the internal carotid artery as it passes through the parapharynx and retropharynx
- Mandibular invasion
- Skull base invasion

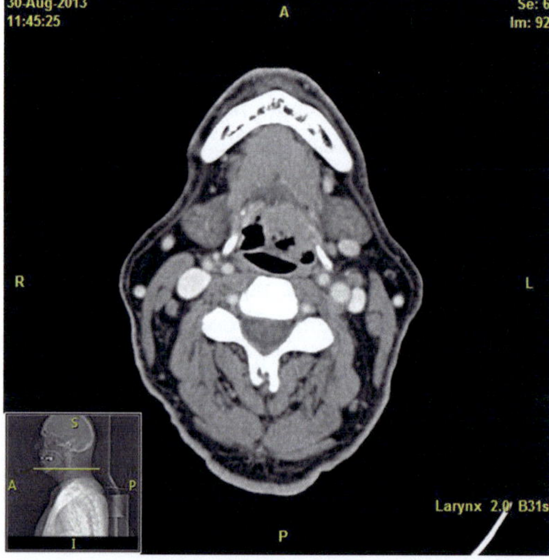

Fig. 2 Axial CT scan with contrast demonstrating a base of tongue tumor on the left side of the patient that extends lateral to the hyoid bone. Tumors in this area often involve the lingual artery, dorsal lingual artery, and hypoglossal nerve. If the surgeon is going to approach these tumors transorally, then dissection should proceed very cautiously in this area to avoid bleeding. Alternative approaches include transhyoid pharyngotomy or neck dissection prior to transoral tumor removal

- Distal extension down the lateral pharyngeal wall toward the parapharynx
- Anterior extension from the tongue base toward the root of tongue
- Extension lateral to the hyoid bone to involve the lingual artery and hypoglossal nerve (Fig. 2).

Patient selection is vital for successful completion of TORS. If a patient would benefit from complete surgical removal of the tumor but is not a good candidate for TORS, the surgeon should also possess the ability to perform TLMS and open surgery through pharyngotomy or mandibulectomy in order to individualize the procedure to the patient and tumor and maximize the outcome.

Anesthesia

After proper patient selection and counseling, the patient arrives in the operating room and the airway needs to be secured. The tumor can impact the anesthesiologist's access to the glottis and trachea. Communication with the anesthesiologist needs to be thorough and lucid, and it can be aided by a video of the nasopharyngoscopy of the airway. The communication includes a discussion of the choice of intubation technique and the tube, as well as the perioperative anesthesia issues of paralysis, pain control, blood pressure control, anticipated blood loss, length of procedure, and oxygen content of the anesthetic. The preoperative anesthesia briefing should include not only the preferred airway, but also a backup plan in the event of complications.

Approaches to securing the airway include intubation under general anesthesia or awake versus sedated intubation. Using either of these approaches, tracheal intubation can be achieved via a transoral, transnasal, or tracheostomy route. Our preferred intubation is a transoral route with the use of traditional laryngoscope or Glide scope (Verathon, Bothell, WA). The tube is secured to the lower lip on the side opposite the tumor with tape. Fiberoptic intubation can also be useful.

Deciding on the proper endotracheal tube entails choosing a tube that will not kink, is not readily flammable, and is of appropriate size and position to deliver anesthesia but not obstruct the surgeon's view of the tumor. We typically use a wire-reinforced laser-safe endotracheal tube.

Taping the tube to the contralateral lower lip or suturing it to the contralateral lower dentition or labial mucosa can secure the tube. Airway fire is a risk in transoral surgery, and an airway fire can occur in the presence of the fire triad: a fuel source (the tube), an ignition source (cautery, laser), and an oxidizer (oxygen). Before beginning the procedure, the surgeon should communicate with the anesthesiologist that the FiO_2 should be kept below 30 % throughout the transoral surgery to decrease the chance of a fire [18]. A suction placed in the mouth can remove excess plume and also decrease the accumulation of oxygen in the event of a cuff leak around the endotracheal tube. The patient should be paralyzed during the transoral portion of the case to allow maximal exposure. Prophylactic antibiotics should be given prior to the start of the operation.

Transoral Surgical Equipment

After securing the airway, and administering endotracheal anesthesia, the surgeon should take advantage of the relaxed patient to perform a last thorough oropharyngeal exam. The tumor should be thoroughly palpated to confirm its mobility, and the surgeon should make a mental map of the confines of the tumor and their relationship to visual landmarks. Proper exposure of the tumor requires an oral retractor. This is most commonly done with a Feyh–Kastenbauer (FK) laryngeal retractor (Gyrus ACMI, Southborough, Massachusetts), or a Crowe-Davis retractor.

The most commonly used robotic instruments are the 5 mm EndoWrist Shertel grasper, the 5 mm Maryland dissector, and the 5 mm monopolar cautery (Intuitive Surgical). The assistant at the head of the table commonly uses a laryngeal suction, a suction cautery, endoscopic graspers, and endoscopic lip appliers. The assistant has a vital role in maintaining a smoke-free, dry, and clean working field, and can also assist in retraction and tumor exposure.

TORS Approach

Once intubation is complete, with the patient lying supine, the operating table is positioned so that the head is turned 90° from the anesthesia team [19] (Fig. 3). The teeth are protected with

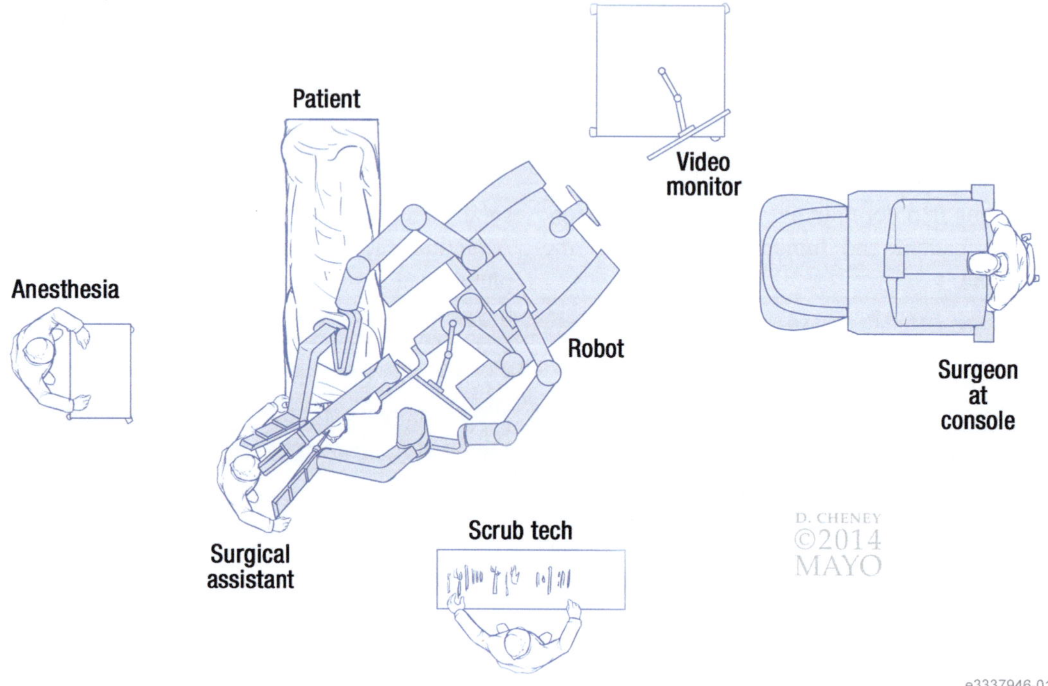

Fig. 3 Bird's-eye view of the TORS setup in the operating room. Note the relationship of the TORS side cart to the edge of the bed, which allows proper positioning of the robotic arms. The surgical assistant sits at the head of the bed, while the surgeon sits at the console

moldable thermoplastic sheeting (WFR/Aquaplast Corp., Wyckoff, NJ). The oral retractor is placed, and sometimes a trial of several blades and multiple angles is attempted to obtain the absolute best exposure of the tumor possible. The surgeon uses a headlight during retractor placement, and care is taken not to injure the teeth and lips during opening of the retractor. The retractor is then suspended to the left side of the bed using a Storz Laryngoscope holder (Karl Storz, Tuttlingen, Germany). The robot is now docked on the right of the patient with the base even with the head and slightly angulated away from the operating table. Three robotic arms are used for TORS: the camera is placed with the middle arm, the left arm is used to hold a dissector/grasper, and the right arm is used to hold the monopolar cautery. A 0° camera is mounted for lateral oropharyngectomy, and the 30° binocular camera is used pointing up for base of tongue resection. The arms are positioned so that the pivot point is at the level of the oral commissures, and the arms are placed so that they have the least chance of colliding. A red rubber catheter is placed transnasally and hooked to suction for smoke evacuation. A surgical assistant with experience in transoral surgery sits at the head with access to a variety of instruments including suction cautery, suction cannulas of various sizes, laryngeal graspers, bipolar cautery which is long enough to reach the base of tongue, and endoscopic vascular clip appliers. The monitors should be placed so that the surgical assistant and/or nurse/tech has easy visualization of the robotic surgical field. The assistant should have the ability to audibly communicate during the procedure so that repositioning of the robotic arms or retractor, manipulation of the tissue, clearance of blood and hemostasis, and other appropriate collaboration can occur.

Lateral Oropharyngectomy

Lateral oropharyngectomy can be performed with a headlight and electrocautery as has been

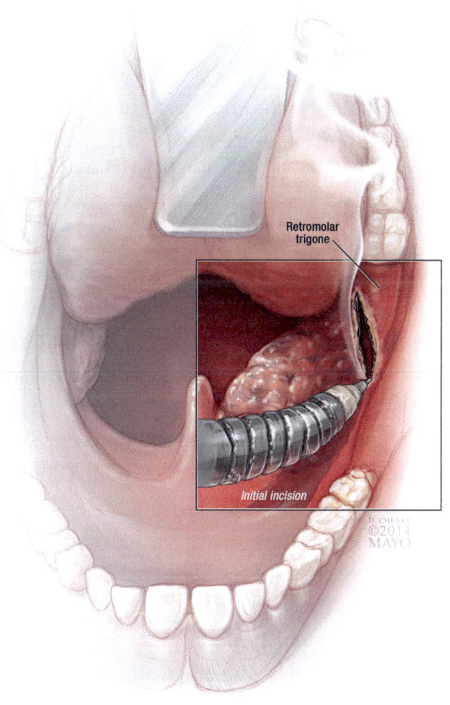

Fig. 4 Initial transoral oropharyngectomy cut performed lateral to tumor allows dissection down to the medial pterygoid fascia and allows proper plane of dissection onto buccopharyngeal fascia

described for decades, but it is enhanced by TORS by improved detail in the visualization and improved dexterity at the inferior extent of the tumor which often involves the base of tongue at the glossotonsillar sulcus [6]. With the tumor exposed and the robot docked, the procedure begins with a cut in the oral mucosa lateral and superior to the tumor near the retromolar trigone (Fig. 4). The incision is carried to the pterygomandibular raphe which serves as an anatomic landmark for the surgeon to develop the correct lateral dissection plane. Dissection is carried along the medial pterygoid fascia while retracting the tumor and the tonsil laterally. This action leads the surgeon into the plane between the superior pharyngeal constrictor, which will be taken with the specimen as a deep margin, and the buccopharyngeal fascia which will remain and separate the oral cavity from the parapharynx [16, 17, 20] (Fig. 5). Recall that the pterygomandibular raphe separates the superior pharyngeal constrictor from the buccinators muscle as it runs from the hamulus of the medial pterygoid plate and the mandible. At this point, it is helpful to make a medial incision through the palate mucosa and musculature and continue this incision inferiorly through the palatopharyngeus muscle (posterior tonsillar pillar)

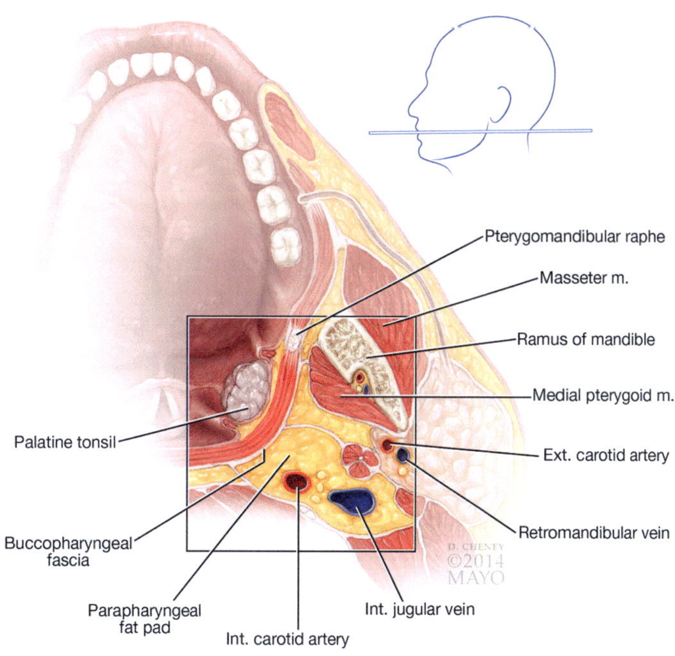

Fig. 5 Axial cut showing the important anatomical relationships the head and neck surgeon needs to be aware of as he or she begins to dissect out the tumor. Special attention should be paid to the relationship of the buccopharyngeal fascia, the parapharyngeal fat, and the internal carotid artery

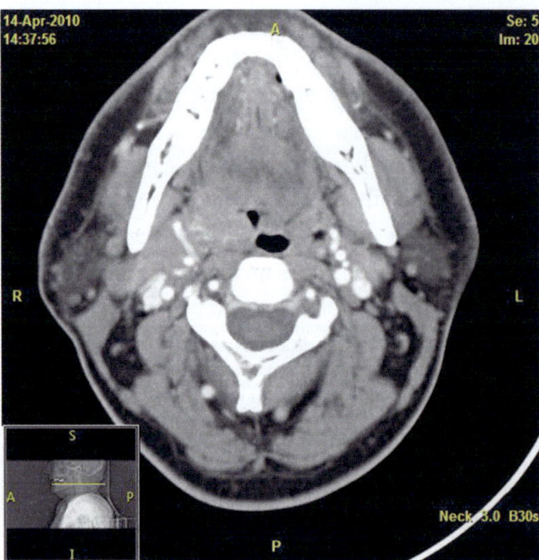

Fig. 6 Axial CT scan with contrast demonstrating a right-sided tonsillar carcinoma and the adjacent facial artery with multiple vascular feeders lateral to the tumor. The surgeon will encounter the most robust vascular supply to the tumor at its lateral borders, and these vessels usually come from the ipsilateral facial and lingual artery

and pharyngeal mucosa and superior pharyngeal constrictor medially. Making these medial defining incisions at this point prevents the surgeon from continuing the dissection and excision too far medially as the tumor is rolled from lateral to medial during the final stages of removal. Inferior cuts can be made inferior to the tumor border and including the glossotonsillar sulcus and lingual tonsil as necessary for adequate tumor removal.

The most critical portion of tumor removal is the lateral dissection, as this is where the majority of the vascular supply to the tonsil from the lingual and facial arteries enters the specimen [16] (Fig. 6). The correct plane of dissection is critical at this portion of the operation. After establishing the lateral border of dissection as the buccopharyngeal fascia and the medial specimen with the palatoglossus, palatopharyngeus, and superior pharyngeal constrictor muscles, the surgeon dissects along the buccopharyngeal fascia, often bluntly with the spatula of the cautery. Dissection continues inferiorly with some medial tension on the specimen provided by the grasping instrument. Often this instrument is used gently as a retractor, as grasping a friable tumor multiple times will just lead to more bleeding and fragmentation of the specimen. Proceeding inferiorly the obliquely oriented styloglossus muscle and the vertically oriented stylopharyngeus muscle are encountered. The glossopharyngeal nerve may be visualized anterolaterally between these muscles. Numerous vascular contributions from the lingual, facial, and ascending pharyngeal vessels of various diameter may be encountered at this location and can be controlled by vascular clips applied by the assistant. If the facial or lingual arteries are encountered, they should be managed by multiple vascular clips. If bleeding is encountered that obscures vision, the surgeon can grasp the vessel with the robotic grasper to tamponade the vessel, and the assistant can apply pressure to the external neck at the level of the greater cornu of the hyoid bone. The styloglossus and stylopharyngeus muscles superiorly provide a medial barrier between the surgeon and internal carotid artery, and its pulsations and that of the external carotid artery can be seen transmitted through these structures and the parapharyngeal fat deep to the buccopharyngeal fascia. Inferiorly, the styloglossus and stylopharyngeus muscles can be transected t where they travel between the superior and middle pharyngeal constrictor to free the specimen. Blunt dissection at this level to free the muscles can prevent injury to the lingual artery. As the specimen is freed by final inferior cuts at the base of tongue and medial cuts at the medial superior pharyngeal constrictor, the surgeon and assistant should confirm orientation of the specimen that is not lost when removing the tumor through the mouth. It should be recognized that oncologic effectiveness is not necessarily improved by intact removal of the specimen. If at any time the volume of tumor prevents proper exposure of the operative area, the tumor can be transected and removed in sections, as is common in TLMS. The assistant grasps the tumor and the surgeon releases it. The tumor is then removed with orientation intact and placed on a towel and marked appropriately to prepare it for examination by the pathologist. The surgeon should visually inspect and palpate the specimen to confirm complete tumor removal and recognize any areas where the margins of resection may not be complete. The oropharynx is then carefully inspected for bleeding vessels, communication with the neck through the buccopharyngeal fascia,

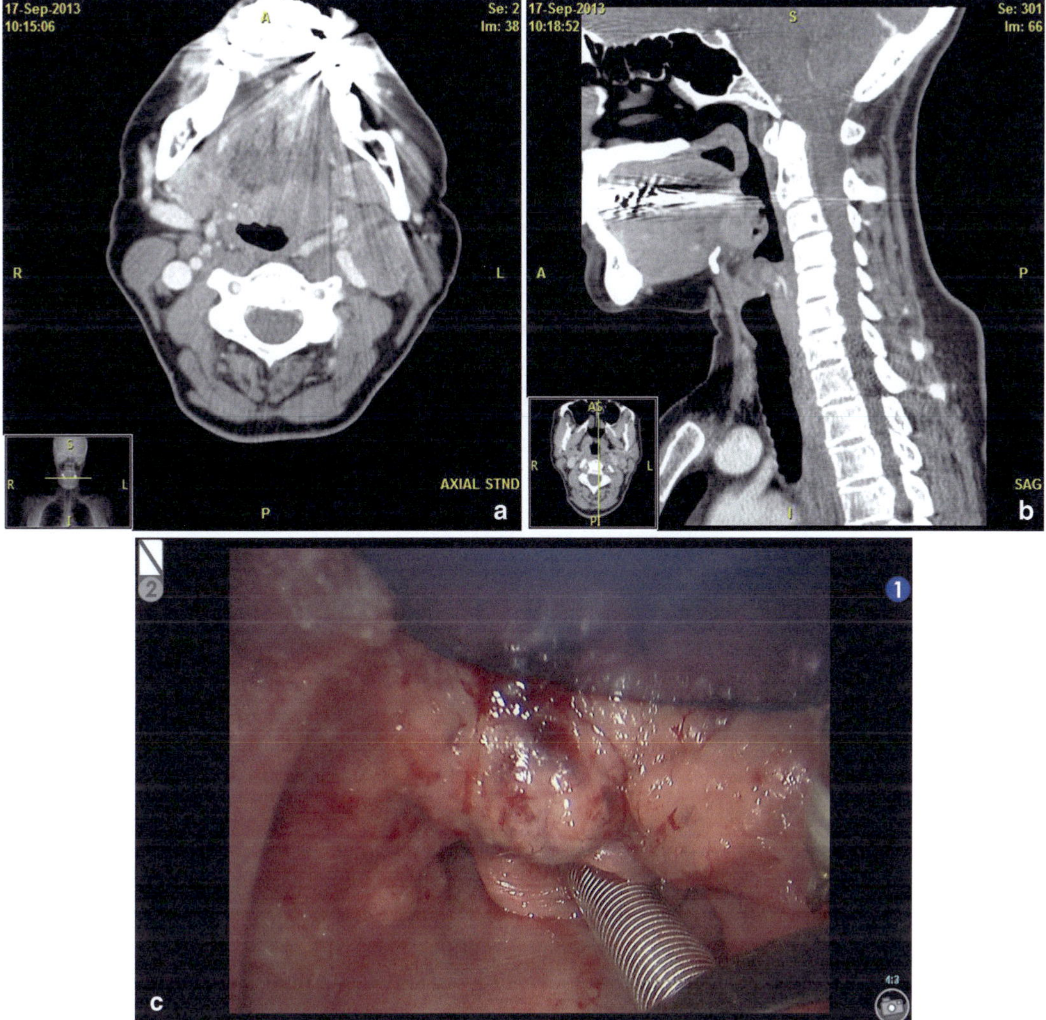

Fig. 7 The surgeon can use both physical exam and imaging to help create a mental image of the tumor to aid with operative planning. (**a**) Axial CT scan with contrast showing a left well-encapsulated lingual mass abutting the facial artery. (**b**) Sagittal CT scan showing that the tumor does not extend beyond the hyoid bone, making it a good TORS candidate. (**c**) Intraoperative view of the tumor

and any suspicious areas that might contain residual tumor. The robot arms are removed and the oral retractor is completely released to relieve venous congestion of the tongue while the tumor is being inspected by the pathologist.

Base of Tongue Resection

It is important for the surgeon to perform a careful physical examination of the BOT tumor prior to transoral excision, as it allows the surgeon to create a 3D image of the tumor and correlate it with preoperative imaging if available, as well as assess the tumor for mobility. This should be done before the retractor is placed, as the anatomy of the oropharynx can become distorted. With retractor placement, one should try to provide the widest tumor exposure, as this step is crucial for successful tumor removal (Fig. 7). The placement of a tongue stitch or applying tongue retraction with a sponge before mouth gag or laryngoscope insertion can help the surgeon with tongue retraction in order to obtain deeper access.

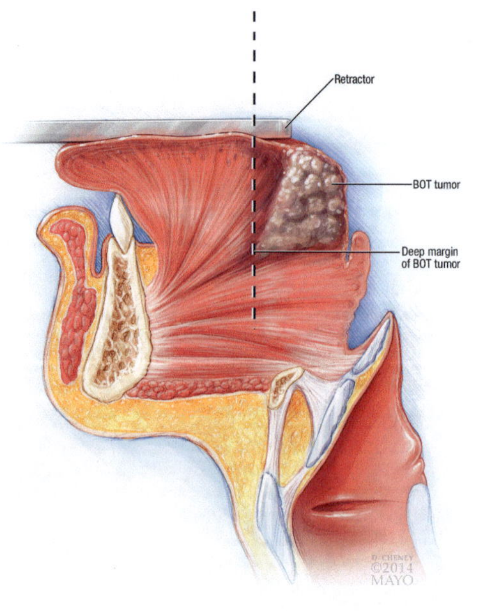

Fig. 8 The initial mucosal cut is made anteriorly in BOT lesions, allowing the tumor to fall posteriorly. This provides proper visualization throughout the procedure. It is important to palpate the deepest extent of the BOT tumor before removal. The placement of the retractor can limit tumor excision depending on the tumor's extent, and if this is the case, an open surgical technique may be required over a transoral one

Both the anterior edge and most of the inferior extent of the tumor should be visualized, and adjustments may need to be performed throughout the procedure to maintain maximum exposure [11].

With exposure maximized, the surgeon can make a vertical cut through the tumor, exposing its greatest depth. This is useful since tangential cuts (to the tumor) across the BOT can fail to include the full tumor depth and unintentionally leave tumor within the deep intrinsic tongue musculature (Fig. 8). For the first step, the initial mucosal cuts are made anteriorly, allowing the tumor to fall posteriorly into the operative field. In order to recognize the inferior extent of the tumor throughout dissection, the first inferior cut should be made at the level of the vallecula. For counter-traction along the plane of dissection, the surgeon can retract along the healthy mucosa of the anterior margin. Tumor extent helps to guide the placement of both the medial and lateral cuts.

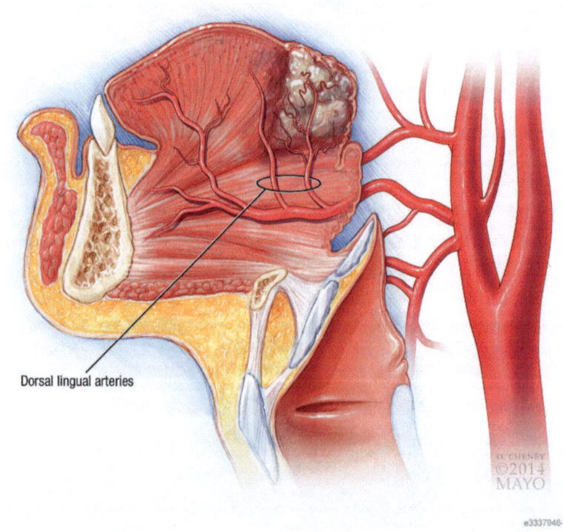

Fig. 9 Sagittal view showing the important vasculature that the head and neck surgeon can encounter during the excision of a BOT lesion, with the dorsal lingual artery and its branches being the most relevant

Again, if the tumor is too large to see the borders for these cuts, transection of the tumor and removal in sections can be performed. Dissection is then carried out either in an anterior to posterior, or superior to inferior direction through the mucosa, lymphoid tissue, and tongue musculature, while making sure to preserve a cuff of normal tissue encircling the tumor. Once the tumor is freed, it is grasped by the surgical assistant, oriented, and passed along to pathology for frozen section analysis. The surgeon should again inspect the defect for bleeding and suspicious tissue, and then release the retractor while the specimen is being evaluated.

During the procedure, the surgeon should be aware of the dorsal lingual artery laterally along with contributions of the lingual artery. This is especially true for tumors that extend deeply and laterally beyond the hyoid bone, reaching the hyoglossus muscle, where both the lingual artery and hypoglossal nerve are in close proximity (Fig. 9). For adequate hemostasis, these vessels should be clipped with two to three clips on the patient's side, and one clip on the tumor side. As described above for bleeding from the lingual artery during lateral oropharyngectomy, external pressure in the area of the greater cornu of the hyoid bone can be applied to slow blood flow until a clip can be applied. For tumors with this type of lateral extent, it may be safer to proceed with an external approach and allow for more confident resection of margins.

Margin Analysis

The entire oncologic goal of TORS for OP SCCa is complete microscopic margin clear resection of the cancer. As has been affirmed for decades, the most common cause of patient mortality from cancer is the failure to completely eradicate the tumor at its primary source [21]. The best opportunity to accomplish this momentously important task is at the primary source. If the surgeon waits for final pathology confirmation and finds that the permanent margins are positive, it can be difficult, if not impossible, to correlate that positive margin with its original location in the oropharynx. Consequently, it is mandatory that an experienced frozen section pathologist is available as a member of the operative team. Equally important is the ability to communicate with that pathologist directly. The frozen section pathology result is only as good as the weakest length in that communication chain. The specimen needs to be removed, oriented, transported to the pathology lab with no loss of orientation, inked at the appropriate border, cut, placed on the chuck, cut with a microtome, placed on the slide, stained, and then examined by the pathologist for tumor at the cut margin. This multistep process needs to be performed for the medial, lateral, superior, inferior, and deep edges of the specimen (Fig. 10). Any of these specimens that have tumor at the margin need to be correlated to the appropriate location in the operative bed, and a new resection margin needs to be excised and the process repeated. Obviously there are multiple hazards in this process including loss of orientation, failures in communication, and errors in inking and cutting that could result in a false positive or negative margin. In our institution, the surgeon who removes the specimen examines it grossly and transports it to the pathologist directly and has a face-to-face communication with the pathology team to ensure that the communication link is as strong as possible. In this manner, we have been able to achieve a 99 % correlation with frozen and final pathology and a 99 % local control rate for OP SCCa resected by transoral surgery. The surgeon should continue to clear margins by repeated resection until all margins are microscopically clear of tumor, or a structure is encountered that cannot be safely resected.

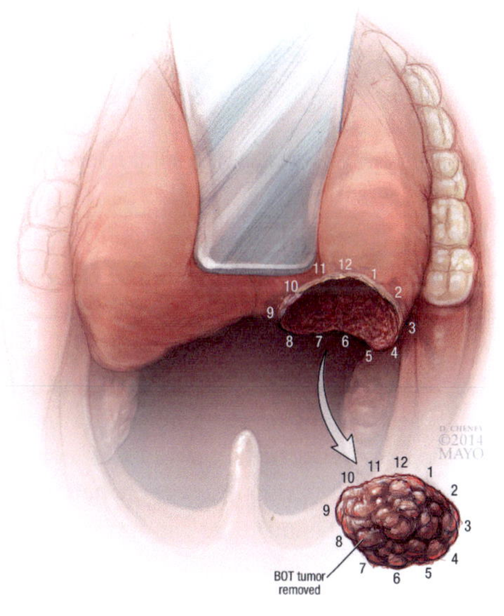

Fig. 10 For both tonsillar and BOT tumors, it is important that the surgeon maintain proper orientation of the specimen as it is passed on to pathology for frozen section. This ensures that any margins that are positive can be accurately re-excised

It has been a point of contention as to how much normal tissue should be excised along with the primary tumor, with suggested margins ranging from 1 mm to up to 10 mm of normal tissue [22]. Although in theory these values may ring true, practically they are less plausible. Oropharyngeal tissue contracts as much as 50 % after being removed and thus a 5 mm margin can become only a 2 mm margin once it reaches the pathologist. If one were to take a deep margin any greater than 2.4 mm in the tonsillar fossa, one would sacrifice the major vessels within the parapharyngeal space. Hinni analyzed 128 tonsillar carcinomas that were treated transorally where the average deep margin was only 1.98 mm, but he still found the 5-year local control rate to be 99 % [21]. We agree with Hinni that a clear microscopic margin is the goal, and that this goal holds up to equal oncologic effectiveness for transoral resection of OP SCCa whether the margin is 1 mm or 10 mm.

Revision Surgery

The decision to use TORS as a treatment option goes back to the initial description of patient candidacy. In the author's experience the issue with TORS as salvage therapy is twofold:

1. One needs to be able to obtain margins for adequate resection. One can imagine the primary previously untreated tumor as being contained in a box. Thus during resection, when negative margins are obtained, one can be fairly certain the tumor in its entirety has been removed. Once a patient has had chemoradiation, the tumor is no longer confined to a "box," instead there are now islands of tumor leading to the possibility of obtaining negative margins around one island, but leaving residual tumor behind. A similar issue is seen when tumors begin to invade lymphatics or neurovascular structures and begin to spread outside of its "box."
2. The majority of TORS defects are left to heal by secondary intention. Some authors advocate vascularized flaps in patients who have been chemoradiated, but again this somewhat defeats the purpose of the minimally invasive approach. Patients with a history of prior chemoradiation have an increased risk of developing non-healing wounds and wound infections. In patients with TORS as the primary treatment, the chance of a cure approaches 90 % (14), whereas in patients where TORS is a salvage treatment, the chance of a cure without significant morbidities drops to 70 % [15].

Neck Dissection

Neck dissections are often part of the management for oropharyngeal malignancies, and either ipsilateral or bilateral neck dissections can be performed. If the patient has N0-N2b or N3 disease, they typically undergo an ipsilateral select neck dissection (levels II–IV). The submandibular gland can be retained without any loss of oncologic effectiveness in the neck disease, and this structure can be very helpful in reinforcing the thin tissue between the oropharyngeal dissection and the neck dissection to reduce fistula [23]. The retropharyngeal nodes can be involved in oropharyngeal SCCa if there is significant invasion of the tumor into the soft palate or posterior pharyngeal wall. If these areas are involved, then careful review of the radiographs and palpation of this area should ensue. In the presence of radiographic or clinical evidence of retropharyngeal nodal adenopathy, then the retropharyngeal nodes should be removed. These nodes lie just medial to the internal carotid artery and are often in contact with its medial border. They usually number between 1 and 3 [24]. The nodes can be removed directly through the transoral defect where they are often readily accessible, or the surgeon can dissect up through the neck dissection along the medial surface of the internal carotid artery while retracting the hypoglossal nerve and digastric muscle superiorly. Dissection of the retropharyngeal nodes can lead to a communication between the neck and oropharynx that may need to be closed by suturing the retropharyngeal fascia to the edge of the remaining superior pharyngeal constrictor muscle.

The timing of the neck dissection if done concomitantly with primary transoral resection is also important, and is based on tumor involvement with vascular structures and the possible development of an orocervical communication or pharyngocutaneous fistula [25]. Delayed neck dissection can be performed several weeks after transoral tumor removal, allowing time for healing. Advantages of waiting include the surgeon having a chance to review any delayed positive margins, possibly lowering the need for tracheostomy with less laryngopharyngeal swelling, and decreasing the risk of creating an orocutaneous communication [17].

Simultaneous neck dissection is what is performed at our institution. Advantages of performing the neck dissection at the time of the transoral procedure include exposing the patient to only a single anesthetic, requiring only one hospitalization, and providing the surgeon with immediate feedback regarding staging information that can be used to initiate adjuvant therapy, which usually begins 3–4 weeks following surgery. There is some concern that there is a higher risk of creating an orocutaneous fistula with simultaneous neck dissection, but even so, the rate of persistent pharyngocutaneous fistula is rare [20, 26]. This was emphasized in a retrospective study of patients undergoing TORS with simultaneous neck dissection which showed that although 29 % of patients (42/148) were found to have an orocervical communication intraoperatively, only 4 % (6/148) resulted in a pharyngocutaneous fistula [25]. To identify any orocervical communication, the nares are plugged and then sterile saline used to irrigate the oropharynx vigorously. One should be able to see the pharynx swell into the neck without a fluid leak. Any leak that is identified should be repaired intraoperatively. If the communication is less than 1 cm, primary closure followed by Tisseel (Baxter Bioscience, Deerfield IL) application on the cervical side can be performed. A suction drain needs to be placed in the neck. This can be removed once output is less than 10 cc over 24 h and a clear liquid diet started on postoperative day one. In the case that the communication is greater than 1 cm, Moore et al. recommend suturing the constrictor muscle, closing part of the digastric muscle to the sternocleidomastoid muscle lateral to the defect, and then applying Tisseel over the repair. In these patients a suction drain with the same removal protocol is placed, as well as keeping the patient strictly NPO for the initial 24–48 h with a nasogastric feeding tube in place. This is followed by slowly advancing to a clear liquid diet, and then eventually to a regular diet as long as no leak is observed. With this method of vigilant observation for any orocutaneous fistula intraoperatively and its immediate repair, along with aggressive management of any developing orocutaneous fistulas postoperatively, simultaneous neck dissections can be safe and effective.

The timing of the neck dissection, before or after transoral resection, can be decided based on any concern of extension of disease around the great vessels. If this is the case, an ipsilateral neck dissection should be performed first with a cotton patty placed over the carotid for isolation and protection during transoral dissection. Even though complications associated with transoral surgery are reduced compared to open approaches, bleeding postoperatively can be life threatening if serious. With this in mind, Salassa et al. recommend tying off the entire external carotid system when pharyngeal defects are large enough to expose named arteries [27]. If the pharyngeal defects are only moderate, ligation of the lingual, facial, and superior laryngeal arteries can be considered depending on their involvement.

Defect Management

In appropriately selected patients, the resultant defect from TORS for OP SCCa can be left to heal by secondary intention. The environment is typically ideal for this type of wound healing: warm, moist, well vascularized, and bathed in a solution with antibacterial properties [28]. The advantages of secondary intention healing are multiple, as the resultant healed wound is mucosalized, contracted, and sensate, and mimics the surrounding environment better than a reconstructed defect could [19] (Fig. 11a, b). Occasionally, the resultant wound requires some type of reconstruction, and some authors are more enthusiastic about placing flaps into the transoral defect than others. Most of the time, the defects that warrant consideration of reconstruction encompass more than 50 % of the soft palate, leave bone exposed at the medial mandible, or involve a significant communication with the mouth and the neck and its vasculature. Reconstruction can be necessary in these defects, and options include skin grafts or local mucosal flaps, local/regional pedicle flaps, or ultimately large regional pedicle or free flaps. We will focus our attention on local/regional pedicle flaps as this is the most advanced option that is feasible when transoral resection is performed via TORS as the robot can be used to sew in these flaps. Although robotic surgery has been described for both the harvest and inset of pedicled and microvascular

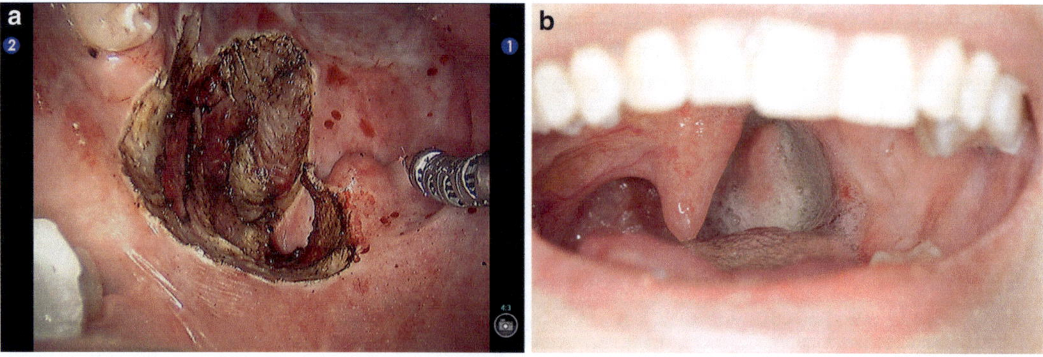

Fig. 11 A left tonsil defect shown immediately after clearance of margins during transoral surgery (**a**), and 10 days after surgery showing early mucosalization and healing of the lateral pharynx (**b**)

flaps, once the defect requires a larger pedicled flap or a free flap, the surgeon should reconsider if TORS is a suitable option, or if instead the resection should be done in an open fashion that makes exposure and inset easier. Factors that can affect the choice of reconstruction include fistulization risk, bleeding, wound breakdown, and functional outcomes such as speech, deglutition, and phonation.

Any defects of the soft palate or tonsillar fossa that are small enough can be allowed to heal by secondary intention or even closed primarily. Any defects that involve more than 50 % of the soft palate or communicate with the neck require more extensive reconstruction; otherwise the patient risks developing rhinolalia and nasal regurgitation. Three local pedicled flaps that have the ability to be sewn in using the robot include the buccal fat pad flap, the inferiorly based facial artery musculomucosal (FAMM) flap, and the anterograde or retrograde submental artery island flap (Fig. 12). All three of these flaps offer excellent reconstructive options for patients with intermediate oropharyngeal defects, while at the same time avoiding the complexity of having a separate donor site with its own morbidities in a more distant part of the body.

Things to keep in mind in order to successfully use a local pedicled flap include using a Doppler intraoperatively, especially when the patient has a history of a prior neck dissection or a neck dissection is being performed concomitantly. Both of these scenarios can interrupt the facial artery blood supply proximally and distally in the case of the submental flap, and only proximally in the FAMM flap. When performing a neck dissection with plans to use the submental flap, it is important to preserve the blood supply of the submental artery as well as its venous runoff. Nodal dissection can be done effectively, even in area I, and still preserve the blood supply to the submental flap, but it requires modification in standard technique, sometimes some individual nodal removal from the fat overlying the digastric and mylohyoid muscles, and careful management of the facial artery and vein and meticulous clipping and division of the branches around the submandibular gland.

Postoperative Care

Postoperative care of the transoral surgery patient begins immediately at the end of the operation prior to extubation. The airway is examined with the aid of a laryngoscope for hematoma or blood, and supraglottic or glottis edema. If the airway is questionable, a tracheostomy is placed. Special caution should be observed in patients with prior neck dissection and radiation, as they can present with delayed upper airway edema. In most patients, a tracheostomy is not necessary, and the patient can be extubated and observed in the post-anesthesia recovery unit prior to sending the

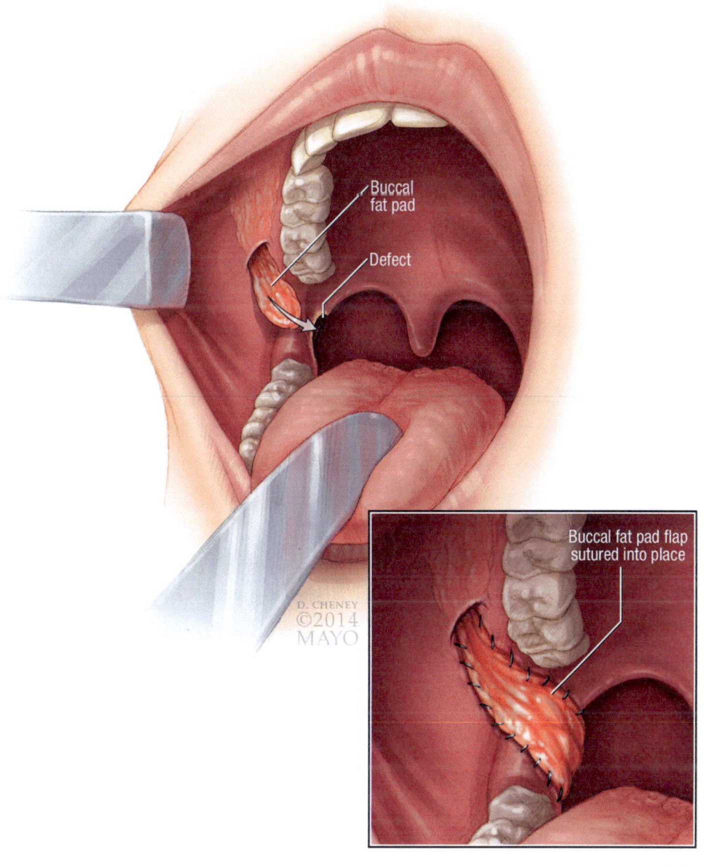

Fig. 12 Use of the buccal fat pad flap for oral defects following transoral removal of an oropharyngeal malignancy

patient to the general floor. In the first 48 h, pain management, pulmonary toilet, oral hygiene, and ambulation are critical for avoidance of complications.

Proper wound care, including adequate drain care, is important to help monitor for any signs of fistula development. If the development of a fistula is a concern, the drain should be kept in place until there are less than 10 cc output over 24 h, otherwise the drain can be removed when there are less than 30 cc of output over 24 h. In any patient where an orocervical communication was observed intraoperatively, a 5-day minimum course of antibiotics should be prescribed. Oral hygiene, such as sponge brushes dipped in saline, chlorhexidine gluconate 0.12 % (Peridex, 3 M ESPE), or 1.5 % sodium bicarbonate, helps keep the mouth moist and make it easier for the patient to swallow and begin oral intake.

In many cases following transoral surgery, the patients are able to resume swallowing immediately postoperatively and can be started on a clear diet with the goal eventually being a mechanical soft diet. An NGT is placed in patients who are predicted to have pain, dysphagia, or an increased risk of aspiration postoperatively, as well as in patients where an orocervical communication occurred during the procedure. If pain is the only concern, the patient can be started on a clear diet immediately, but if dysphagia or aspiration is a concern, it may be prudent to obtain a speech therapy consultation while in the hospital along with a bedside swallow evaluation. For most patients with an NGT, the feeding tube can be removed once sufficient caloric intake is achieved. If the NGT was placed because of concerns for a pharyngocutaneous fistula developing, the feeding tube is left in place for 10–14 days until they are evaluated as an outpatient for speech and swallow abilities as well as their risk of aspiration.

Another key aspect to postoperative care is adequate pain control. Transoral surgery is almost always a very painful operation. At our institution, we start the patient on IV narcotics until oral or enteral access is available after which the patient can be changed over to oral narcotics along with scheduled acetaminophen if necessary. Due to a large majority of transoral defects being left to granulate in, the use of NSAIDs or any anticoagulation medications is not recommended. By controlling a patient's pain, it encourages earlier ambulation, which in turn helps with pulmonary toilet and gastrointestinal ileus. Ambulation is encouraged to begin on postoperative day one, along with sitting in a chair when not sleeping or resting.

Adjuvant Therapy

Traditionally, adjuvant therapy has been prescribed in the form of radiation therapy or chemoradiation therapy based upon the presence of nodal metastasis, extracapsular extension of the nodal metastasis, and extent of primary resection and clearance of margins [29, 30]. The extent of adjuvant therapy necessary to achieve the highest oncologic control is controversial in oropharyngeal squamous cell carcinoma treatment owing to the paucity of controlled clinical trials investigating this topic. Further complicating matters is the heterogeneity of outcomes between HPV-mediated disease and HPV-negative tumors [31]. Clinical reports exist of single modality being sufficient in patients with completely resected primary tumors and single nodal metastasis or N0 necks [32, 33]. In smokers, patients with N2b or greater neck disease, and in patients with extracapsular extension or HPV-negative tumors, radiation therapy is given at our institution to the necks at risk for metastasis.

Complications

Bleeding

Although rare, with only an incidence of 3–8 %, postoperative hemorrhage after oropharyngeal surgery can be life threatening [27, 34]. Prevention of postoperative bleeding can already begin at the time of surgery by carefully placing 2–3 clips on the patient side of any vessel greater than 2 mm in diameter, and also by identifying any vessels that may be in spasm and then retract into the soft tissue, and subsequently cauterizing them. As discussed previously, the lingual, facial, and superior thyroid arteries or even the entire external carotid artery system for large pharyngeal defects should be ligated during the neck dissection. Following surgery, in the immediate postoperative period, bleeding can also be prevented by performing a cautious extubation, controlling a patient's hypertension, keeping the patient NPO for 7–10 days (with placement of NGT), having the patient avoid Valsalva maneuvers or vigorous activities, and finally telling the patient not to take any anticoagulants for 3 weeks.

Postoperative bleeding can be divided into major and minor bleeds. Minor bleeds usually occur at around 9–14 days after surgery, with the patient noticing blood tinged sputum that occurs for minutes to hours. Conservative management tends to be the mainstay of treatment for minor mucosal bleeds and includes the use of ice water, stopping any anticoagulants, observation, or bedside cautery.

Major bleeding is attributed to erosion into already controlled vessels or vasodilation of vessels that were previously in vasospasm during surgery and thus not clipped. There are two reasons why major bleeding can quickly progress to catastrophic bleeding: first, large named vessels are frequently clipped during surgery and then simply left within the open wound bed as it slowly granulates in over a period of 3–4 weeks, and second, most patients undergoing transoral resection have compromised swallowing ability and cannot protect their airway properly in the event of a major bleed [34].

It is not hypotension or exsanguination that is so dangerous with oropharyngeal bleeding, but rather the risk of asphyxiation and airway compromise. With most bleeding occurring within 7 days of the surgery, it is important for both the surgical team and the patient with their family to have a plan in place in the event of a significant bleed. Foremost the patient should be instructed to place their head in the dependent position to prevent aspiration and then pressure should be applied to the affected side of the neck. Even if the patient becomes unconscious, the head of the patient should remain in the dependent position. Any bleed where the physician does not believe the bleed is superficial and can be treated with observation should go back to the operating room. The patient should then be intubated allowing the surgeon to carefully evaluate the source of bleeding and control it.

Neck Abscess

A neck abscess can result if, even with careful intraoperative evaluation, an orocervical communication occurs and is not repaired. The patient will present with swelling and erythema in the neck along with possible spontaneous rupture and drainage of the abscess. Treatment includes incision and drainage, obtaining cultures, and beginning broad-spectrum antibiotics while waiting for antibiotic susceptibilities from the culture. Wound care should include debridement and cleaning the wound with half-strength hydrogen peroxide followed by packing it with iodoform gauze. In order to allow the wound to heal by secondary intention, it should be packed twice daily, with slightly less gauze each time. If during evaluation of the cavity a pharyngocutaneous fistula is identified, an NGT should be placed so that the patient can be kept NPO for 10–14 days. Before oral intake can begin, the patient must show clinical improvement as well as undergo a swallow study demonstrating closure of the leak.

Dental Damage and Paresthesias of the Oral Cavity

Pressure is often placed on the teeth during surgery, and dental injuries or paresthesias can result. With the use of thermoplastic splints, dental damage occurs only rarely, but if a loose tooth is recognized it should be removed to prevent aspiration. Patients with large tongues, those with narrow mandibular arches, or those subjected to long operative times, are at a higher risk of developing paresthesias. It is important for the surgeon to keep this in mind and relax the retractor or scope when not operating. Treatment is usually conservative and resolves within a few days.

Rhinolalia and Velopharyngeal Insufficiency

In patients whose tumors have superior extension and undergo lateral pharyngectomy, or those who require palatectomy for extensive soft palate lesions, palatal insufficiency is not uncommon. When less than 50 % of the palate has been removed, conservative management is often sufficient, as the patient's symptoms will commonly improve over the next several months. On the other hand, if more than 50 % of the palate is resected without reconstruction at the time of the initial operation, then the patient can be given an obturator or return to the operating room for reconstruction. The risk of velopharyngeal insufficiency is higher in patients undergoing salvage surgery.

Aspiration and Pneumonia

Aspiration can occur in patients in the immediate operative period secondary to poor pulmonary toilet and swallow function. These patients can subsequently develop pneumonia and present with a rising leukocyte count, fever, as well as thick, foul-smelling tracheal secretions. Treatment involves aggressive pulmonary toilet, aspiration precautions, and starting proper antibiotic coverage.

Review of Data

Since its original introduction into the field of Otolaryngology in 2005, TORS and its application for oropharyngeal malignancies, primarily OPSCC, have provided a constant stream of information in the literature. Here we review how the use of TORS in oropharyngeal malignancies has continued to expand, again emphasizing the importance of establishing what patients are proper candidates. We will also address TORS' functional and oncologic outcomes, the more common complications in TORS, and lastly its use as salvage surgery.

In 2007, Weinstein and his colleagues published a prospective phase I clinical trial outlining the use of TORS for radical tonsillectomy in 27 patients [17]. This study buoyed the idea that TORS could be used for radical tonsillectomy in malignant disease. Even so, the authors had one unplanned tracheostomy, two patients with positive margins, and one case each of trismus, hypernasality, and postoperative mucosal bleeding. Since TORS offered the potential to not only decrease morbidity but also to provide better or equivalent long-term oncologic and functional outcomes when compared to open techniques, these acute morbidities were found to be acceptable.

With the expanding use of TORS in oropharyngeal pathology, as seen with Weinstein's use of TORS for radical tonsillectomy, surgeons became more comfortable with the technique and subsequently moved on to more complex resections. In 2009, Desai et al. published a prospective study on TORS lateral oropharyngectomy [35]. It was in that same year that Boudreaux et al. published a prospective, non-randomized clinical trial that in opposition to previous reports included T1–T4 tumors of the upper aerodigestive tract that were managed via the TORS approach [26]. Even with advanced tumors, Boudreaux achieved negative margins with outstanding functional results for the majority of cases. There were two patients in this series that were unable to undergo TORS due to technical issues with the robot, and two patients where inadequate exposure was obtained including a T2 vallecula and a T4 base of tongue. Deeply infiltrative tumor characteristics prevented two other patients from undergoing TORS resection. Although this study did expand the range of TORS surgery, it also emphasized certain limitations for oropharyngeal lesions including the value in proper preoperative patient selection.

Moore et al. have expanded on both what defines tumor candidacy as well as reported functional outcomes of TORS. He published a prospective series of 45 patients where TORS was performed for OPSCC with all patients undergoing complete resection [19]. With their prior experience using TLM, they reported that the T stage of the tumor was less crucial for adequate exposure than which adjacent structures were invaded by tumor. These findings helped to define the tumor candidacy for TORS as presented earlier in this chapter. Not only did this study show TORS to be a safe and efficacious method of surgically managing primary tumors, but it also argued against the need for staged surgical intervention by describing the feasibility of concomitant neck dissections. These were performed in 95.6 % of the patients (31 unilateral, 12 bilateral). A pharyngotomy was reported in 40 % of cases, all of which were repaired primarily. Only three patients (6.7 %) developed orocutaneous fistula and were treated conservatively without any further sequelae. In 2011, Moore et al. a retrospective review of 148 patients who underwent TORS for oropharyngeal malignancy along with a concomitant neck dissection [25]. In 42 patients (29 %), an orocervical communication was observed intraoperatively. All cases were managed surgically followed by conservative management in the postoperative period with only six patients developing a subcutaneous fluid collection that required incision and drainage. In no patient was postoperative adjuvant treatment delayed.

Another important complication to be aware of in the use of TORS for oropharyngeal malignancies is bleeding. This risk in minimally invasive surgical techniques is always important to assess as visibility and access is oftentimes limited when compared to the standard open technique. Pollei et al. presented a group of 906 patients whose OPSCC was treated transorally and reported postoropharyngectomy hemorrhage rates as well as associated risk factors. They reported an incidence of 5.4 % of postoperative bleeding, where 67.3 % required operative intervention. There was no significant difference in bleeding rate or severity when the transcervical external carotid system was ligated or not. In addition, no difference in bleeding rates was observed when comparing patients treated with laser versus the robot. It is important to note that patients with significantly higher T-stage tumors were treated with laser instead of robotic technique [34].

Although there is an abundance of data supporting the safety and efficacy of TORS for oropharyngeal malignancy, data of long-term oncologic outcomes for this technique are relatively recent. Weinstein et al. presented the first study with long-term data showing that even with advanced tumors, TORS offers disease control comparable to standard treatment protocols as well as similar survival. His study group was comprised of 47 patients who underwent TORS for advanced OPSCC (Stages III and IV) with an average follow-up of 26.6 months [10]. These outcomes only pertain to primarily treated oropharyngeal malignancies, which has been the focus of most authors when evaluating TORS.

Dean et al. did evaluate the use of TORS as a salvage option when he compared TORS for primary versus recurrent OPSCC with the use of open surgical approaches for recurrent disease [36]. A significant difference was seen between TORS and the open surgical groups with regard to length of hospital stay, postoperative diet, gastrostomy tube dependence, and tracheostomy tube dependence. They also reported that patients with primary OPSCC overall fared better functionally compared to those with recurrent OPSCC. Of note, no patient in either of the TORS treatment groups developed any immediate postoperative complications, but two postoperative wound infections and two hematomas were seen in the open resection group.

Future Directions

From the initial debut of TORS for oropharyngeal malignancies almost 20 years ago to today, we have made huge advances now allowing for access to difficult to reach tumors coupled with minimal morbidity and the possibility for reduced or no adjuvant therapy, but there is still more to be done. The future direction for TORS will most likely move towards advancements in instrumentation, real-time intraoperative imaging, and improved margin analysis.

Initial robotic arms and instrumentation were designed for use in the abdomen; thus the future for robotic instrumentation in the head and neck will move toward miniaturization of robotic arms as well as the creation of innovative robotic platforms tailored to the otolaryngologist's needs. There has even been a start in establishing the use of a highly flexible robotic for exploration of the oropharynx by Rivera-Serrano et al. [37]. This tele-operated robot was adapted from the CardioARM (Medrobotics, Inc, Raynaham, MA) and allows for 102-degrees-of-freedom while being steered on a nonlinear path that is self-supported. The benefit of this new technology is that it may eliminate the need for laryngeal suspension. The other possible benefit of a more flexible robotic arm is the potential to have patients positioned in the seated position during the procedure, as they are in the clinic for nasopharyngeal laryngoscopy. The seated position avoids the effects that gravity can have on anatomical structures and soft tissue while in the supine position. Looking to other specialties, the urology literature describes in vivo robots providing both video and illumination that have been trialed in both porcine and canine models performing intraperitoneal surgeries. Even with these moves toward perfecting instrumentation intraoperatively, surgeons still struggle to be able to identify important landmarks during surgery that have shifted from preoperative scans.

Preoperative imaging is an extremely useful tool to help the surgeon decide on the best surgical approach. However, many of the bony landmarks such as the mandible, which are seen on initial imaging, are mobile and become unreliable points of reference intraoperatively with the placement of retractors. There has been some research focusing on overcoming this limitation. King and his colleagues evaluated the use of intraoperative cone-beam CT with a mobile C-arm. Although it would be useful in situations with complex 3D anatomy seen in oropharyngeal surgeries, its primary focus is bony anatomy and less detail is seen of the soft tissues, which is also important during transoral surgery. Another approach to intraoperative real-time imaging in TORS of oropharyngeal malignancies is the adaptation of image guidance systems such as BrainLAB, which was explored by Desai, Sung, and Genden in 2008 [38]. Image guidance potentially provides the surgeon with orientation in regard to pertinent vasculature. Desai and his colleagues concluded that it is a reliable method to assess tumor extent, but did warn that soft tissues shift throughout the procedure due to repositioning compared to preoperative scans, as does the mandible. The idea of using an intraoperative 3D-navigation system can also be used in combination with PET/CT image fusion since it has the ability of showing the surgeon areas of hypermetabolic activity. This method was used in patients undergoing major head and neck resection and successfully identified four patients with residual positive margins.

Leaving behind positive margins leads to a very poor prognosis; thus much emphasis has been placed on developing a method of identifying microscopically positive margins, which is both efficient and improves patient outcomes. Photothermal imaging was used in an in vivo study by Jakobsohn et al. for the detection of head and neck neoplasms, where cancer cells were targeted by gold nanoparticle therapy with the goal of improving real-time margin analysis [39]. With a similar goal in mind, Keereweer and his associates studied the ability to target epidermal growth factor receptors or glucose receptors in a murine model using tumor-specific near-infrared fluorescent agents [40]. Both of these studies address the hope to eventually be able to directly visualize positive margins while in the operating room.

Conclusions

Transoral robotic surgery has developed into an important tool in the armamentarium of the oncologic surgeon who treats head and neck malignancies. The procedure is just that: a tool that can be utilized to expedite transoral removal of tumors in an effort to achieve complete margin negative resection and decrease the morbidity associated with more extensive "open" approaches. The surgeon should not be so firmly attached to this one technique as to abandon other transoral approaches, transhyoid pharyngotomy, or even mandibulotomy if that will provide superior access, safety, or efficacy. Some tumors will be best treated with TORS, some with other surgical approaches, and some with nonoperative means. With all of these options at the surgeon's disposal, the best care will be delivered to that individual patient in a way that optimizes their outcome.

References

1. Harreus U. Cummings otolaryngology: head & neck surgery. 5th ed. Philadelphia: Mosby, Inc.
2. Charturvedi AK, Engels EA, Pfeiffer RM, et al. Human papillomavirus and rising oropharyngeal cancer incidence in the United States. J Clin Oncol. 2011;29:4224–30.
3. Chen AY, Schrag N, Hao Y, Stewart A, Ward E. Changes in treatment of advanced oropharyngeal cancer, 1985–2001. Laryngoscope. 2007;117(1):16–21. doi:10.1097/01.mlg.0000240182.61922.31.
4. Van Abel KM, Moore EJ. The rise of transoral robotic surgery in the head and neck: emerging applications. Expert Rev Anticancer Ther. 2012;12(3):373–80.
5. Moore EJ, Henstrom DK, Olsen KD, Kasperbauer JL, McGree ME. Transoral resection of tonsillar squamous cell carcinoma. Laryngoscope. 2009;119(3):508–15. doi:10.1002/lary.20124.
6. Holsinger FC, McWhorter AJ, Menard M, Garcia D, Laccourreye O. Transoral lateral oropharyngectomy for squamous cell carcinoma of the tonsillar region: I. Technique, complications, and functional results. Arch Otolaryngol Head Neck Surg. 2005;131(7):583–91. doi:10.1001/archotol.131.7.583.
7. Steiner W, Ambrosch P. Endoscopic laser surgery of the upper aerodigestive tract with special emphasis on cancer surgery. Stuttgart, Germany: Thieme; 2000.
8. Steiner W, Fierek O, Ambrosch P, Hommerich CP, Kron M. Transoral laser microsurgery for squamous cell carcinoma of the base of tongue. Arch Otolaryngol Head Neck Surg. 2003;129:36–43.

9. Moore EJ, Olsen SM, Laborde RR, et al. Long-term functional and oncologic results of transoral robotic surgery for oropharyngeal squamous cell carcinoma. Mayo Clin Proc. 2012;87(3):219–25. doi:10.1016/j.mayocp.2011.10.007.
10. Weinstein GS, O'Malley BW, Cohen MA, Quon H. Transoral robotic surgery for advanced oropharyngeal carcinoma. Arch Otolaryngol Head Neck Surg. 2010;136(11):1079–85.doi:10.1001/archoto.2010.191.
11. Malley O, Jr BW, Weinstein GS, Snyder W, Hockstein NG. Transoral robotic surgery (TORS) for base of tongue neoplasms. Laryngoscope. 2006;116(8): 1465–72.
12. Hockstein NG, Nolan JP, Malley O, Jr BW, Woo YJ. Robot-assisted pharyngeal and laryngeal microsurgery: results of robotic cadaver dissections. Laryngoscope. 2005;115:1003–8. doi:10.1212/01.WNL.0000164714.90354.7D.
13. Hockstein NG, Malley O, Jr BW, Weinstein GS. Assessment of intraoperative safety in transoral robotic surgery. Laryngoscope. 2006;116(2):165–8. doi:10.1097/01.mlg.0000199899.00479.75.
14. Weinstein GS, O'Malley Jr BW, Magnuson JS, et al. Transoral robotic surgery: a multicenter study to assess feasibility, safety, and surgical margins. Laryngoscope. 2012;122(8):1701–7. doi:10.1002/lary.23294.
15. White HN, et al. Transoral robotic-assisted surgery for head and neck squamous cell carcinoma: one and 2-year survival analysis. Arch Otolaryngol Head Neck Surg. 2010;136(12):1248–52.
16. Moore EJE, Janus JJ, Kasperbauer JJ. Transoral robotic surgery of the oropharynx: clinical and anatomic considerations. Clin Anat. 2012;25(1):135–41. doi:10.1002/ca.22008.
17. Weinstein GS, et al. Transoral robotic surgery: radical tonsillectomy. Arch Otolaryngol Head Neck Surg. 2007;133(12):1220–6.
18. Chi JJ, Mandel JE, Weinstein GS, O'Malley BW. Anesthetic considerations for transoral robotic surgery. Anesthesiol Clin. 2010;28(3):411–22. doi:10.1016/j.anclin.2010.07.002.
19. Moore EJ, et al. Transoral robotic surgery for oropharyngeal squamous cell carcinoma: a prospective study of feasibility and functional outcomes. Laryngoscope. 2009;119(11):2156–64.
20. Park YM, Lee JG, Lee WS, Choi EC, Chung SM, Kim S-H. Feasibility of transoral lateral oropharyngectomy using a robotic surgical system for tonsillar cancer. Oral Oncol. 2009;45(8):e62–6. doi:10.1016/j.oraloncology.2009.02.012.
21. Hinni ML, Zarka MA, Hoxworth JM. Margin mapping in transoral surgery for head and neck cancer. Laryngoscope. 2013;123(5):1190–8. doi:10.1002/lary.23900.
22. Looser KG, Shah JP, Strong EW. The significance of "positive" margins in surgically resected epidermoid carcinomas. Head Neck Surg. 1978;1(2):107–111. Available at: http://eutils.ncbi.nlm.nih.gov/entrez/eutils/elink.fcgi?dbfrom=pubmed&id=755803&retmode=ref&cmd=prlinks.
23. Howard BE, Hinni ML, Nagel TH, Chang YH, Cheng MR, Hayden RE. Submandibular gland preservation during concurrent neck dissection and transoral surgery for oropharyngeal squamous cell carcinoma. Otolaryngol Head Neck Surg. 2014;150(4):587–93. doi:10.1177/0194599813519041.
24. Moore EJ, Ebrahimi A, Price DL, Olsen KD. Retropharyngeal lymph node dissection in oropharyngeal cancer treated with transoral robotic surgery. Laryngoscope. 2013;123(7):1676–81. doi:10.1002/lary.24009.
25. Moore EJ, Olsen KD, Martin E. Concurrent neck dissection and transoral robotic surgery. Laryngoscope. 2010;121(3):541–4.
26. Boudreaux BA, et al. Robot-assisted surgery for upper aerodigestive tract neoplasms. Arch Otolaryngol Head Neck Surg. 2009;135:397–401.
27. Salass JR, et al. Postoperative bleeding in transoral laser microsurgery for upper aerodigestive tract tumors. Otolaryngol Head Neck Surg. 2008;139(3): 453–9.
28. Woodley DT. Woodley: The Molecular and Cellular Biology of Wound…—Google Scholar. 1996.
29. Kramer S, Gelber RD, Snow JB, et al. Combined radiation therapy and surgery in the management of advanced head and neck cancer: final report of study 73-03 of the radiation therapy oncology group. Head Neck Surg. 1987;10:19–30.
30. Cooper J, et al. Postoperative concurrent radiotherapy and chemotherapy for high-risk squamous cell carcinoma of the head and neck. N Engl J Med. 2004;250: 1937–44.
31. Ang KK, et al. Human papilloma virus and survival of patients with oropharyngeal cancer. N Engl J Med. 2010;363(1):24–35.
32. Olsen SM, Moore EJ, Laborde RR, et al. Transoral surgery alone for human-papillomavirus-associated oropharyngeal squamous cell carcinoma. Ear Nose Throat J. 2013;92(2):76–83.
33. Weinstein GS, Quon H, Newman HJ, et al. Transoral robotic surgery alone for oropharyngeal cancer: an analysis of local control. Arch Otolaryngol Head Neck Surg. 2012;138(7):628–34. doi:10.1001/archoto.2012.1166.
34. Pollei TR, Hinni ML, Moore EJ, et al. Analysis of postoperative bleeding and risk factors in transoral surgery of the oropharynx. JAMA Otolaryngol Head Neck Surg. 2013;139(11):1212–8. doi:10.1001/jamaoto.2013.5097.
35. Desai SC, Sung C-K, Jang DW, Genden EM. Transoral robotic surgery using a carbon dioxide flexible laser for tumors of the upper aerodigestive tract. Laryngoscope. 2008;118(12):2187–9. doi:10.1097/MLG.0b013e31818379e4.
36. Dean NR, Rosenthal EL, Carroll WR, et al. Robotic assisted surgery for primary or recurrent oropharyngeal carcinoma. Arch Otolaryngol Head Neck Surg. 2010;136(4):380–4.

37. Serrano CR, Johnson P, Zubiate B. A transoral highly flexible robot. Laryngoscope. 2012;122(5):1067–71.
38. Desai SC, Sung C-K, Genden EM. Transoral robotic surgery using an image guidance system. Laryngoscope. 2008;118(11):2003–5. doi:10.1097/MLG.0b013e3181818784.
39. Jakobsohn K, Motiei M, Sinvani M, Popovtzer R. Towards real-time detection of tumor margins using photothermal imaging of immune-targeted gold nanoparticles. Int J Nanomedicine. 2012;7:4707–13. doi:10.2147/IJN.S34157.
40. Keereweer S, Kerrebijn JDF, Mol IM, et al. Optical imaging of oral squamous cell carcinoma and cervical lymph node metastasis. Head Neck. 2012;34(7):1002–8. doi:10.1002/hed.21861.

Transoral Robotic Surgery of the Larynx and Airway

Abie Mendelsohn, Georges Lawson, and Marc Remacle

Introduction

Robotic-assisted surgery is one of the fastest growing areas of Head and Neck surgery, specifically transoral robotic surgery (TORS) for pharyngeal and laryngeal procedures has shown early and rapid acceptance. While early clinical trials had focused mainly on oropharyngeal tumors [1], technologic advances have improved the reach and access of robotic instruments and visualization and advanced the application of TORS beyond the oropharynx and into the larynx. The following chapter will review the specifics of robotic-assisted surgery for the larynx and airway, describe clinical applications, and comment on future applications for robotic surgery of the larynx and airway.

A. Mendelsohn, M.D. (✉)
Department of Head and Neck Surgery, David Geffen School of Medicine at UCLA, 924 Westwood Blvd, Suite #515, Los Angeles, CA 90024, USA
e-mail: Amendelsohn@mednet.ucla.edu

G. Lawson, M.D. • M. Remacle, M.D., Ph.D.
Department of Otolaryngology, Head and Neck Surgery, Louvain University Hospital of Mont-Godinne, Therasse Avenue, No 1, 5530 Yvoir, Belgium
e-mail: Georges.Lawson@uclouvain.be; marc.remacle@uclouvain.be

The da Vinci Robotic Surgical System

The da Vinci robotic surgical system is a complex surgeon-driven instrument which will be discussed in detail elsewhere in this textbook. Though the newer da Vinci models (*S*, *Si*, *Xi*) provide four independent robotic arms, anatomic narrowing currently restricts TORS to the use of three arms. The central arm is equipped with a robotic endoscope containing two visual channels along with multiple light apertures (See Fig. 1). Currently, there are two endoscope diameters are available: 12 mm or 8.5 mm. With the limited access to the larynx, the 8.5 mm endoscope is strongly recommended to improve operative access. Endoscopes are also available with a straight (0°) view or with an angled (30°) view. The angled endoscope can be quite useful when accessing anterior-most portions of the larynx. The endoscope can be positioned with the angled view anteriorly (up looking) or posteriorly (down looking). However, as with endoscopic sinus surgery, use of angled endoscopes can alter the expected position of anatomic landmarks and should be used with caution.

The arms on each side of the central endoscope are equipped with robotic instruments. With well over 30 types of instrument designs, identifying the optimal surgical instrument can sometimes be laborious. Instruments are broadly categorized by their diameter and by their function. The first generation of robotic instruments maintained 8 mm

G.A. Grillone and S. Jalisi (eds.), *Robotic Surgery of the Head and Neck: A Comprehensive Guide*, DOI 10.1007/978-1-4939-1547-7_9, © Springer Science+Business Media New York 2015

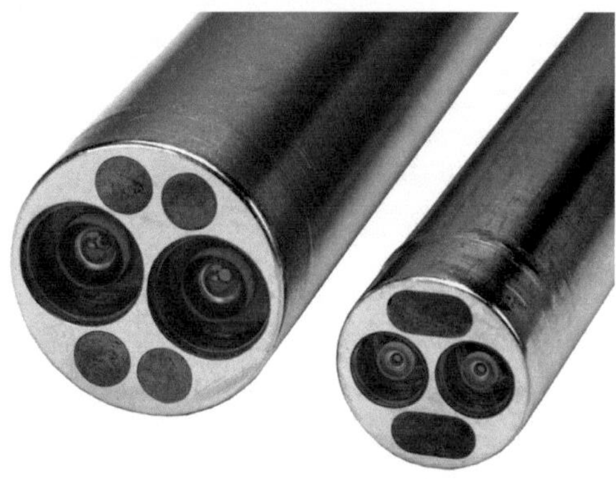

Fig. 1 Transoral robotic surgery endoscopes. Depicts the dual camera system of the robotic endoscopes which provides a three-dimensional high definition display. The endoscope on the *left* maintains a diameter of 12 mm and the *right* maintains 8.5 mm diameter

outer diameter, which included a right-angled jointed instrument. However, newer instruments now maintain a smaller 5 mm outer diameter. The 5 mm instruments are recommended within the tight spacing of the pharynx and larynx. The newer 5 mm instruments are also designed with a wristed joint to allow for improved reach and dexterity.

The instrument function can be categorized as either *cutting* or *retracting*. Given the specialized tissue of the larynx and airway, the cutting energy options should be reviewed. The most common cutting energy instrument is the Bovie monopolar cautery, which can be delivered by either a spatula or hooked tip. TORS is routinely performed with the use of the spatula tip. Bipolar cautery instruments were previously only available in 8 mm diameter, but a 5 mm bipolar cautery forceps has recently been made available for clinical use. Bipolar will likely become adapted within TORS procedures as clinical experience collects.

Harmonic scalpel (Ethicon Endo-Surgery, Inc., Cincinnati, Ohio, USA) robotic instrument is available in both 8 mm and 5 mm diameters; however, complexity in energy delivery has prevented the harmonic scalpel from obtaining the same degree of wristed angulation that is typical of the other robotic instruments. As such, its description has to date been limited to blood vessel control within cervical compartment surgeries. With improved degrees of motion, the harmonic scalpel will likely have a larger role in laryngeal TORS, specifically endoscopic ligation of the superior laryngeal artery.

Laser integrated instruments make up the last group of cutting instruments. *Intuitive Surgical* only offers the thulium laser fiber delivery as an integrated robotic instrument. While a positive experience with the thulium laser in the larynx and pharynx has been described [2, 3], popular use is still limited. This underutilization may be related to relative unfamiliarity with the thulium wavelength or perhaps from the capital requirement of purchasing a new thulium laser system in addition to the robotic system. Third party laser adapters have allowed for the conversion of standard retracting instruments into robotic-assisted CO_2 laser delivery systems. Specifically, *Lumenis Inc*. (Yokneam, Israel) producing the *FiberLase Robotic Drop-in Guide* and *OmniGuide Inc* (Cambridge, Massachusetts, USA) producing the *FlexGuide Ultra* provide CO_2 fiber delivery instruments. Overall, both systems provide a flexible fiber guide that is fitted for robotic graspers (recommended instrument is the 5 mm needle driver) (See Fig. 2). The fiber can be delivered and removed as needed throughout each procedure. On a practical level, both systems offer individual differences that can be considered when comparing the laser system.

The most distinct difference between the *Omniguide* and *FiberLase* by *Lumenis* is the laser energy dispersion. Energy dispersion is seen when the laser spot widens as the tip of the fiber is moved away from the target. The energy dispersion reduces the final laser power density or cutting efficiency. However, the energy dispersion also helps coagulate small diameter (~1 mm) blood vessels. *OmniGuide* laser energy typically has a wider field of energy dispersion than the *FiberLase*. This increased dispersion can be seen as an advantage for either system depending on surgeon preference. A more dispersed energy beam will coagulate more effectively while a more focused energy beam will offer a more precise incision line. Another difference between the two fiber laser systems is that the FiberLase provides a HeNe aiming beam, similar to standard articulated

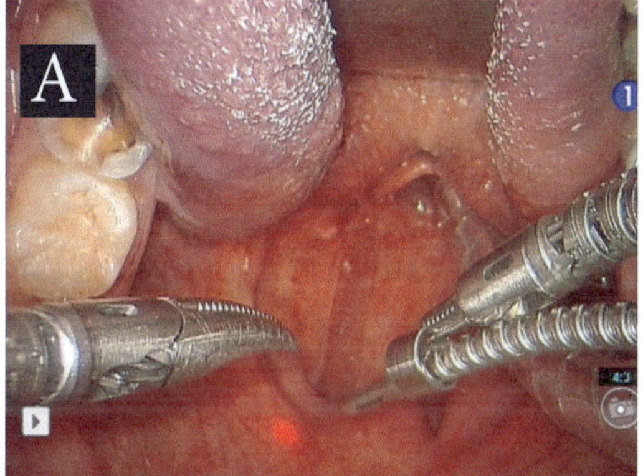

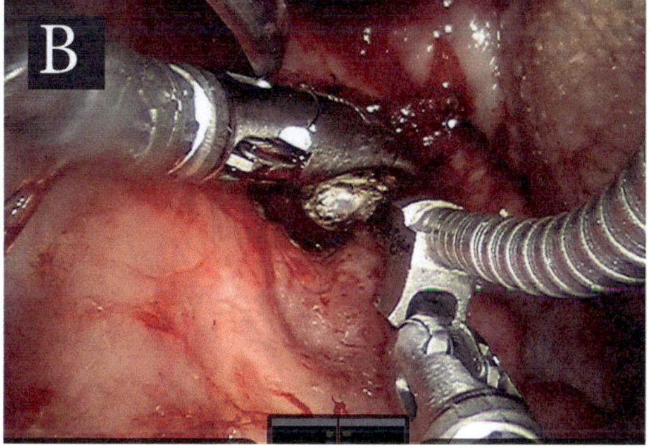

Fig. 2 CO_2 laser flexible fiber delivery systems. Third party CO_2 laser delivery systems are shown. *Lumenis* provided *Fiberlase* system (**a**) and *Omniguide* provided *FlexGuide* system (**b**) are adapted to robotic needle drivers. One of the main differences between the systems is the presence of the aiming HeNe beam of the *Fiberlase* (**a**) system

armed CO_2 delivery systems. Both robotic-assisted CO_2 laser systems have been reported with good early clinical experience [4, 5]. Table 1 reviews the general advantages and disadvantages of the available cutting instruments.

TORS and Microsuspension Laryngoscopy

A TORS approach for laryngeal and airway surgery is typically suggested as an alternative to standard microsuspension Direct Laryngoscopy (mDL) with either laser or cold knife surgery. The same contraindications that have been well described for mDL surgery are applicable for laryngeal TORS. Specifically, potential patients must:

- Maintain overall health to undergo the strains of general anesthesia
- Accept cervical spinal extension without vertebral precautions
- Demonstrate acceptable mandibular excursion
- When malignancy is present, the tumor must be amenable to endoscopic resection (e.g., an absence of vocal fold fixation)

Surgical risk profiles are similarly described between mDL and TORS, including but not limited to chipped teeth, tongue numbness, taste alterations, airway swelling, or bleeding. It is common for patients to undergo diagnostic mDL prior to proceeding to laryngeal TORS so that the patients may have an understanding of the requirements and risk profile.

However, there are also noticeable advantages that TORS offers over the mDL approach. The high-definition wide-angle endoscope of the robotic system offers a superior visualization of the operative field. As demonstrated (See Fig. 3), TORS can offer wide-field visualization of the entire operative field while still being able to magnify the area of interest. The difference in field of view can be minimal in the case of lesions confined to the glottis, yet larger lesions which extend beyond the anatomic boundaries of the glottis typically exceed the view of standard direct laryngoscopes. The robotic visualization is also enhanced by a three-dimensional (3D) dis play which is superior to that of binocular display of the operative microscopes. Adjusting the operative view is also improved with the robotic system. The surgeon-controlled endoscope (by way of the console foot pedal) can rapidly recenter the surgical view without effort or disruption to the surgical momentum which is in contrast to the surgical disruption required for microscope readjustments.

TORS also provides improvement in surgical dexterity. With degrees of freedom at the instrument wrist, angled surgical motion can achieve improved direction of retraction and cutting over that of the static directionality of long-handled mDL instruments. Additionally, the long-handled mDL instruments enhances physiologic hand tremor. However, the movement scaling of the robotic system provides a tremor-free surgical

Table 1 Summary of strengths and limitations of TORS cutting instrumentation

	Surgical precision	Thermal damage	Blood vessel coagulation
Flexible fiber CO_2 laser	++++	++	++
Thulium laser	++	+++	+++
Electrocautery	+	++++	++++
Cold knife	++++	–	–

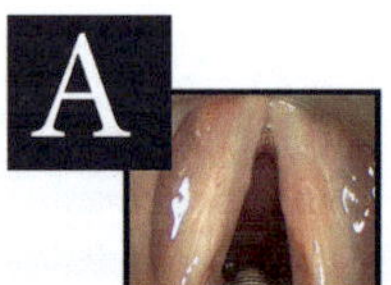

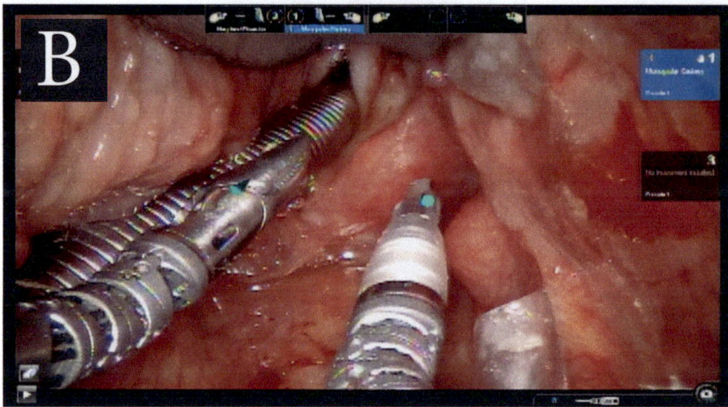

Fig. 3 Comparative views of Microdirect laryngoscopy and TORS. Direct laryngoscopes provide microscopic magnification of lesions of the glottis (**a**). Robotic endoscopes can provide similar magnified view of the glottis while still providing wide-field view of the supraglottis, hypopharynx, and oropharynx in the same frame (**b**). The *small blue cones* seen in **b** are produced by the teaching console of the dual console robotic system

action along with graded motion. Finally, the placement of the cutting instrument in the field of surgery (as in the spatula bovie arms) provides a two-handed surgical experience. In contrast, when an articulated-arm laser system is used, one hand is required for beam aiming leaving only one surgical instrument in the surgical field.

Laryngeal TORS approach also adds improvement with education and training of future surgeons. mDL procedures can prove to be challenging to observe with frequent microscope adjustments and limited field of view. In comparison, the wide field view of TORS will typically provide an improved observing experience for students and surgeons-in-training. The newer (*Si, Xi*) generations of the robotic system provide an additional layer of training with the dual console. Now, surgeons-in-training can observe the surgical procedures from the exact perspective of the operative surgeon. The observing personnel can also move the surgical controls along with the surgery as a "rehearsal." When the nonoperating console moves the surgical controls, visual markers are displayed across the digital displays as blue pointers (See Fig. 3b). When the surgeon-in-training achieves sufficient experience, operative control of the robotic instruments may be alternated between the two consoles, between the two surgeons, so that initial surgical experiences may be provided in a controlled manner (See Fig. 4). Finally, the computer-based simulator of the robotic system allows for standardized skills training and objective trainee metrics. In all, the transition from mDL to TORS approach when appropriate may allow for improved training of the next generation of laryngeal surgeons.

Clinical Applications

From the technical advantages, a number of robotic-assisted surgical approaches have been adapted to the larynx and airway. This chapter will now discuss more frequently described

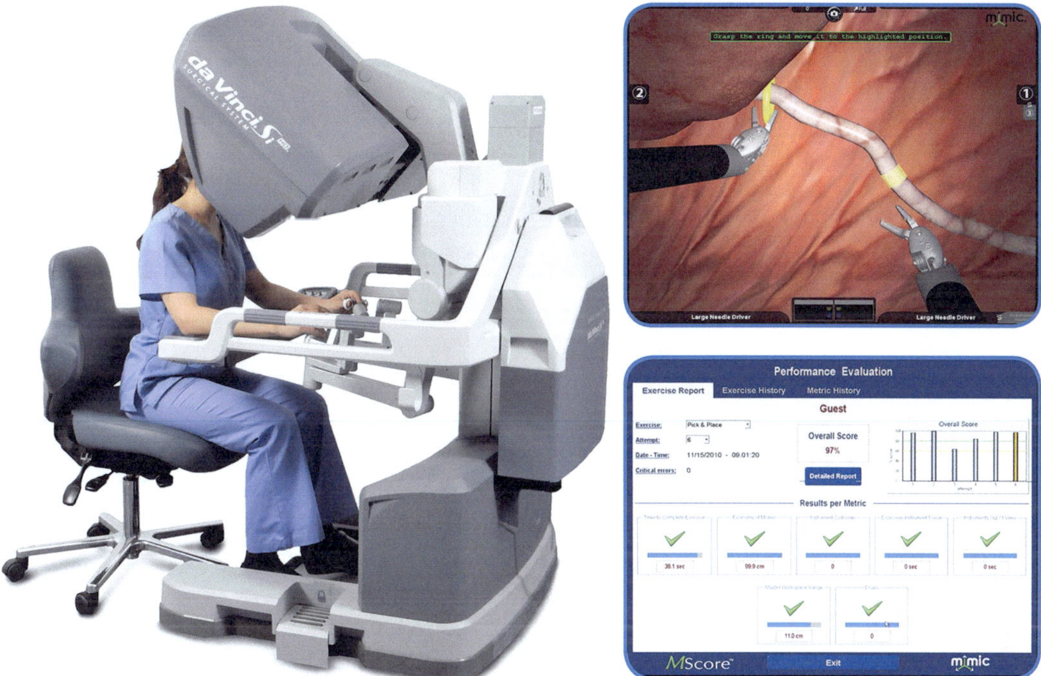

Fig. 4 Training surgical simulation. As the surgeon-in-training is seated at the operative console (*left*), example screen shot of surgical simulation is displayed (*upper right*). Objective training measures (*lower right*) are also recorded and are available for supervising surgeon review

applications. The surgical approaches described require extensive training. Endoscopic laryngeal and airway surgery experience will also clearly enhance the transition to endoscopic robotic surgcry. An "insidc-out" undcrstating of laryngcal neurovascular anatomy is critical in order to avoid major surgical complications [6]. These approaches also require specialized head and neck training for the robotic system concentrating on transoral exposure and transoral placement of instrumentation to access the larynx and airway [7]. Additionally, robotic surgery programs should allow surgeons the appropriate time to progress through the expected learning curve [8] and should plan cases more proximal in the head and neck, such as the palatine tonsillar fossa, reserving laryngeal robotic surgery for only the experienced robotic surgeon.

Supraglottic Laryngectomy

For many tumors of the supraglottis primary surgical resection may offer an excellent treatment option. While the most common malignancy of the supraglottis is squamous cell carcinoma, surgical resection can also be commonly recommended for other tumors of the supraglottis such as nerve sheath tumors [9], paragangliomas [10], and carcinoid tumors [11].

Operative Technique

The operative technique for TORS supraglottic laryngectomy parallels the techniques for endoscopic CO_2 laser supraglottic laryngectomy [12]. Variations in technique are required based on the anatomic location and extent of tumor progression. Recommendations for surgical excision have therefore been divided

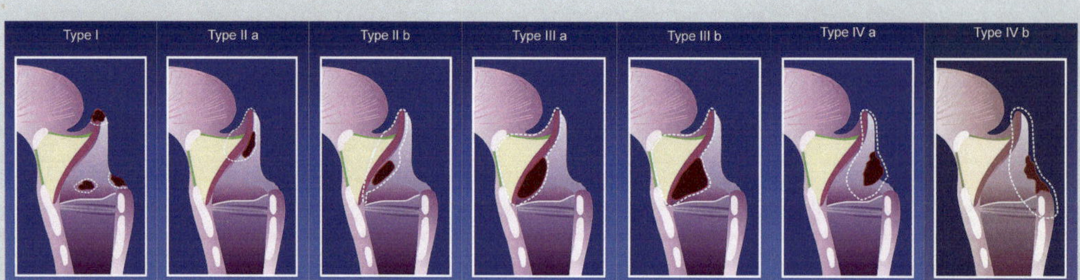

Fig. 5 European Laryngological Society (ELS) Supraglottic laryngectomy classifications. Depicts the European Laryngological Society (ELS) classification scheme for endoscopic supraglottic laryngectomy. The classification scheme, though designed for endoscopic CO_2 laser supraglottic resections, has successfully been adapted to TORS laryngectomy

according to the classification scheme of the European Laryngological Society (ELS) (See Fig. 5) [13].

Exposure is obtained utilizing the operative pharyngoscope of choice. The authors use the Laryngeal Advanced Retraction System (LARS) pharyngoscope. Resections limited to the suprahyoid epiglottis can be exposed with a tongue blade fitted into the vallecula (See Fig. 6a). The remaining resections including deeper portions of the supraglottis, such as the aryepiglottic fold or false vocal folds, should be first exposed with a laryngeal (long, narrow width) tongue blade fitted at the petiole (See Fig. 3b). With this configuration, the posterior-most boundaries may be incised first before blood can obscure the dependent portions of the operative field. If needed, the epiglottis can then be released from retraction with minor adjustments to the pharyngoscope for epiglottic or vallecular incisions.

A "Limited Excision" (type I) supraglottic laryngectomy entails excision of small superficial tumors on the free border of the epiglottis, the aryepiglottic fold, the arytenoids, or the ventricular fold or any other part of the supraglottis. In cases of small and superficial T1 tumors of the laryngeal surface of the epiglottis located above the hyoid bone, the resection includes half of the suprahyoid epiglottis. This procedure is a "Limited Medial" supraglottic laryngectomy without resection of the preepiglottic space (type IIa).

"Medial" supraglottic laryngectomy without resection of the preepiglottic space (type IIb) should be applied for T1 tumors of the laryngeal surface of the epiglottis extending below the hyoid bone. In these cases, a total epiglottectomy is performed. The incision line goes through the preepiglottic space without its complete excision. The pharyngoepiglottic, aryepiglottic, and ventricular folds are preserved.

The resection of T1 or T2 tumors extending to the petiole of the epiglottis must include the preepiglottic space. This procedure is the "Medial supraglottic laryngectomy with Resection of the Preepiglottic Space" (type IIIa) (See Fig. 6). The incision is guided along the valleculae until the hyoid bone is reached. The incision line moves caudally from the hyoid bone toward the thyrohyoid membrane until the upper border of the thyroid cartilage is exposed. From this point, the whole entity of the preepiglottic space is removed along the inner surface of the lamina of the thyroid cartilage together with the epiglottis, toward the anterior commissure of the vocal folds.

T1–T2 tumors of the infrahyoid epiglottis extending to the ventricular fold can be resected with the same technique (type IIIb). The ventricular folds can be completely dissected from the thyroid cartilage along the inner surface toward the ventricle of Morgagni.

In cases of tumors of the aryepitglottic fold (also known as marginal tumors) with possible

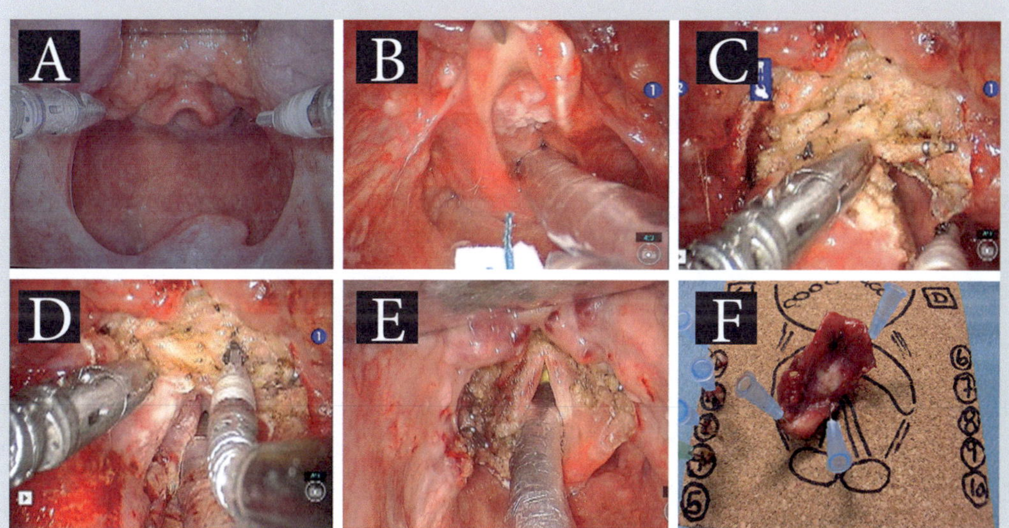

Fig. 6 TORS medial supraglottic laryngectomy with resection of preepiglottic space (type IIIa). The robotic-assisted images display the critical steps of type IIIa supraglottic laryngectomy. (**a**) demonstrates initial placement of operative pharyngoscope (LARS system used here) exposing the vallecula and larynx. (**b**) shows the T2 squamous cell carcinoma on the laryngeal surface of the epiglottis. (**c**) is following surgical clipping of the right superior laryngeal vessels. Following which, (**d**) transects the vessels and resects the preepiglottic space fat, extending inferiorly to the level of the laryngeal ventricles. (**e**) demonstrates the post-resection larynx with minimal glottal edema. (**f**) shows en-bloc resection specimen oriented for accurate pathologic analysis; intraoperative margin assessment is performed by the additional specimens (seen with the number labels on the left side of figure)

extension to the ventricular folds, the resection includes the free edge of the epiglottis, the three folds' region, and the ventricular fold. This procedure is the "Lateral" supraglottic laryngectomy (type IVa).

The "Lateral supraglottic laryngectomy with Arytenoid Resection" (type IVb) was proposed in case of extension to the mobile arytenoids; the arytenoid is included in the resection. The resection may include the inner or medial and anterior part of the pyriform sinus.

As much as possible en bloc resections should be performed. The specimen is examined, but frozen sections are typically taken from the laryngeal margins after tumor resection. Tracheostomy is not a recommended portion of this surgery. Cervical nodal basins also require intervention, either through selective neck dissections or through sentinel lymph node biopsy [14]. The details of these procedures are beyond the scope of this text but should be part of the surgical plan. The authors routinely perform the neck surgeries during the same anesthetic administration as the robotic-assisted resection.

Postoperative care includes intravenous steroid, or steroid nebulization, for 8–10 days, preventive antibiotics for 3–4 days, and proton pump inhibitors until the healing is completed. Oral intake with a pureed diet is resumed the day after surgery under speech therapist guidance.

The authors' previously published experience with TORS supraglottic laryngectomy currently described 18 patients who underwent robotic-assisted surgical resection (See Fig. 7) [15]. There were no (0 %) tracheostomies performed at any point during treatment. Overall, patients required an average of 4.5 days for safe swallow for solids and 5.5 days for safe swallow

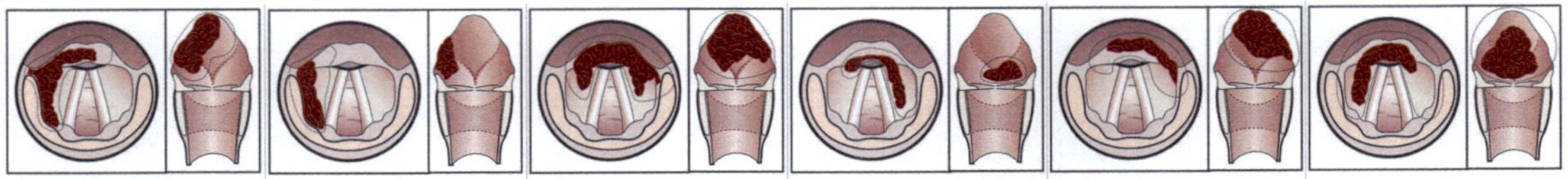

ClinicoRadiographic Stage	$T_2N_{2c}M_0$	$T_1N_0M_0$	$T_2N_0M_0$	$T_2N_0M_0$	$T_1N_1M_0$	$T_2N_{2c}M_0$
ELS Supraglottic Classification	IVa	IVa	IVa	IVa	III+ IVa	IIIb
Time to Solid/Liquid Diet (Days)	3/5	3/5	5/5	2/2	2/3	5/11
Clinical Follow up (Months)	51	20	43	42	42	40
Pathologic Stage Modification					$T_1N_{2b}M_0$	$T_3N_{2c}M_0$

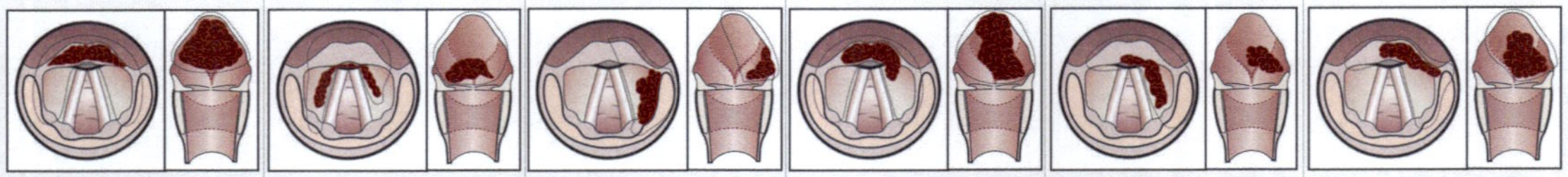

ClinicoRadiographic Stage	$T_2N_{2b}M_0$	$T_3N_{2b}M_0$	$T_2N_1M_0$	$T_3N_{2c}M_0$	$T_3N_{2b}M_0$	$T_2N_0M_0$
ELS Supraglottic Classification	IIIb	III + IVa	IVa	IIIb	IIIb	IIIb
Time to Solid/Liquid Diet (Days)	3/3	24*/31*	19*/28*	29*/45*	26*/34*	20*/36*
Clinical Follow up (Months)	29	28	23	23	21	19
Pathologic Stage Modification			$T_2N_{2b}M_0$			

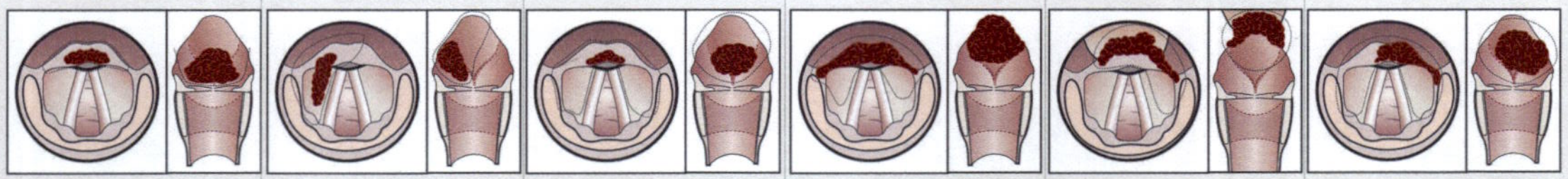

ClinicoRadiographic Stage	$T_1N_0M_0$	$T_1N_0M_0$	$T_1N_{2b}M_0$	$T_2N_0M_0$	$T_2N_0M_0$	$T_2N_{2b}M_0$
ELS Supraglottic Classification	IIIb	IVa	IIIb	IIIb	IIIb	IIIb
Time to Solid/Liquid Diet (Days)	3/4	3/5	4/6	3/5	7/32	10/29
Clinical Follow up (Months)	19	43	20	16	13	13
Pathologic Stage Modification					$T_4N_{2b}M_0$	$T_2N_0M_0$

*Temporary postoperative vocal fold hypomobility

Fig. 7 Clinical experience with TORS supraglottic laryngectomy. For each of the 18 patients reported, tumor extent is illustrated along with dotted line borders of surgical resection. For each case, presenting clinicoradiographic stage is listed along with the ELS classification. Functional outcome of diet is listed separately for solid and liquid diet advancement

for thin liquids. Female gender, advanced pathologic T-stage (III/IV), simultaneous neck dissection, and temporary postoperative vocal fold hypomobility were associated with significant delays in return of swallow function. There were no gastrostomies tubes placed at any point during treatment. Over a 2-year follow up period, there were no local recurrences leading to a local control rate of 100 %. Three (16.7 %) patients developed regional recurrences. Four (22.2 %) developed distant metastases. Only overall cancer stage IV was found to be significantly associated with the development of distant metastasis. Two patients died during the follow-up period (cardiopulmonary failure) leading to a 2-year overall survival of 88.9 %. The authors' positive experience with TORS supraglottic laryngectomy has been confirmed with additional studies demonstrating good functional and oncologic outcomes [16–18].

Total Laryngectomy

The authors introduced total laryngectomy as a new TORS technique designed to decrease treatment-related morbidities and to increase postoperative quality of life [19]. Shortly following, several case reports were published with additional experience with this technique [20, 21]. The common motivation from these reports was to provide a minimally invasive approach which could potentially improve healing and to speed recovery time following total laryngectomy.

Operative Technique

The procedure begins with a standard tracheostomy skin incision, approximately 4 cm in length, midway between the cricoid cartilage and the sternal notch. After the superior subplatysmal skin flap is raised, the strap muscles are divided along the midline raphe to expose the trachea and cricoid cartilages. A thyroid isthmusectomy is performed, and the lateral lobes are dissected off of the lateral tracheal walls. A complete transection of the trachea is placed at the third tracheal space with rising posterior tracheal mucosal cuts. Inferior stomal stitches are placed to secure the caudal trachea. The 4-cm skin incision allows ample visualization to dissect around the remaining rostral trachea and cricoid cartilage, which includes sectioning bilateral recurrent laryngeal nerves. At this point, heavy braided sutures are placed around the lateral walls of the rostral trachea and are threaded atraumatically through glottis for intraoral retraction. The stoma site is then covered with sterile drapes to minimize contamination from the transoral portion.

Initial placement of the LARS pharyngoscope uses the intraoral retractor blade retracting the epiglottis at the petiole. After optimal visualization is obtained, the initial incision is positioned along the superior-most aspect of the arytenoid mucosa. With the dissector forceps holding the postcricoid mucosa posteriorly, the Bovie separates this mucosal layer from the underlying cricoid cartilage. Subsequently, the epiglottis is then released from retraction, and the vallecula incision is made along lingual surface of the epiglottis in the direction toward the superior border of thyroid cartilage. Extending the vallecular incision laterally and posteriorly, the superior laryngeal vessels are encountered as they course through the thyrohyoid membrane. Multiple clips are placed on the vessels and divided. Dissection is continued caudally until the thyroid cartilage is encountered. Keeping the hyoid bone retracted underneath the intraoral retractor blade, the thyrohyoid membrane is transected. The instruments are directed along the external thyroid cartilage perichondrium. As progress continues inferiorly, tension will be required on the previously placed inferior tracheal retraction sutures. These sutures will give a rostral pull to the inferior portion of the laryngeal skeleton, as well as allowing for lateral deflection of the specimen to improve visualization. Dissection continues caudally until the larynx is freed from its attachments. The larynx is then delivered orally.

The pharyngotomy is closed endoscopically by approximating the pharyngeal mucosa to the base of tongue with 3-0 braided absorbable sutures placed with the use of the 5-mm robotic needle holder and dissecting forceps. In our experience, given the extensive mucosal preservation, the pharyngotomy can be closed in a horizontal orientation. Following a watertight closure, fibrin glue is placed over the incision transorally. At this time, optional steps of salivary bypass tube placement or primary tracheal–esophageal prosthesis placement may be performed in a typical manner depending on surgeon preference. Intraoral retraction is released.

With the skin flap in superior retraction, the pharyngotomy may be bolstered with placed sutures along the cervical aspect of tongue base musculature. The strap muscles are reapproximated over the pharyngotomy site. A small suction drain is placed superior to the stoma site. The superior skin flap is released, and the superior stomaplasty is performed using braided absorbable suture. At the conclusion of the procedure, the endotracheal tube is replaced with a standard laryngectomy tube.

More than a demonstration of technologic capacity, the application of TORS for total laryngectomy was proposed to address two specific surgical concerns of standard open approach for total laryngectomy. The first is the standard open pharyngotomy. The incision lines of open laryngectomy, even with optimal pyriform sinus mucosal preservation, results in pharyngotomy defects of considerable size. Some authors have proposed closing the large pharyngotomy defects in a "T" pattern as opposed to the more conventional linear closure [22]. Conventional practice continues with linear pharyngotomy closures; however, the risk of psuedodiverticula formation and post-laryngectomy dysphagia remains [23]. The endoscopic TORS approach allows for substantial reduction in pharyngotomy size with maximal mucosa-sparing incisions. In fact, the pharyngotomy is closed in a completely horizontal linear orientation. The initial experience of the authors has not identified psuedodiverticula or persistent dysphagia; however, additional cases and longer follow-up are required to make conclusions comparing swallowing outcomes between surgical approaches.

The second motivating factor to transition laryngectomy to TORS is to improve the formation of pharyngocutaneous fistulae. Fistula formation is the most common major complication following total laryngectomy [24]. Most commonly seen in post-radiated larynges, fistula formation is thought to be secondary to decreased blood supply, tissue necrosis, and subsequent pharyngeal suture line breakdown. Along with prolonged hospitalizations with IV antibiotics, fistula contents can ultimately track laterally in the neck to the carotid sheath and artery. The infected salivary contents weaken the arterial wall risking psuedoaneurysm formation and carotid rupture [25]. The TORS approach targets this potential complication in two ways. First, the limited pharyngotomy closure reduces the area of sutured mucosa at risk for breakdown. Second, without lateral surgical dissection of an open approach, fascial barriers remain intact between the neopharynx and the carotid sheath following the peri-laryngeal dissection of TORS. The elimination of natural drainage paths between the pharyngeal suture line and carotid artery targets the lethal laryngectomy complication of carotid rupture. Though TORS laryngectomy patients in the several clinical reports have experienced fistula formation, this patient population is comprised of extremely poor laryngeal tissue quality with diffuse fibrosis from high dose chemoradiotherapy. Fistula contents following the midline dissection path maintain a medial drainage path, away from the lateral neck contents supporting the surgical proposal.

The first clinical reports of TORS total laryngectomy has demonstrated feasibility and safety. For oncologic indications, TORS total laryngectomy has also demonstrated clear pathologic margins. While the initial outcomes are promising following TORS, long-term follow-up and additional case series are needed to understand the benefits of this minimally invasive approach.

Glottic Surgery

Though it is the opinion of the authors that in its current state robotic surgery does not match the advantages of CO_2 laser microsurgery, there have been several reports of TORS glottic surgery [26, 27]. With glottic surgery confined to the laryngeal introitus, the ability to quickly adjust the robotic endoscope plays a smaller role as compared to more involved surgery of the supraglottic larynx. Additionally while the angled robotic endoscope could be used to visualize a larynx not readily exposed with direct line of site, the depth of an anatomically restricted glottis typically prevents robotic instrument reach to the level of the glottis. TORS for both benign and malignant lesions of the vocal folds have been suggested; however, published benign vocal fold lesion experience to date has been limited to the laboratory (animal or cadaver) [28–30]. Robotic vocal fold cordectomy for glottic carcinoma have demonstrated successful achievement of negative margins; however, the experience is also complicated with infrequent feeding tube and tracheostomy tube placement [27] which is typically not seen with mDL CO_2 laser cordectomy.

TORS can be combined with flexible fiber CO_2 delivery to improve the critical thermal damage which Bovie cautery transmits within the specialized tissue of the glottis [31]. However, until further experience with TORS CO_2 laser glottic surgery can be shared, it is unclear how this combined robotic and laser approach offers a noticeable improvement from standard microscopic laser glottic surgery.

Laryngeal Cleft

Laryngeal clefts are rare congenital anomalies. Type I involves a defect between the arytenoids and can extend to the level of the true vocal folds; type II clefts extend below the level of the true vocal folds and into the cricoid; type III clefts involve the entire cricoid cartilage into the cervical trachea; type IV extends into the posterior wall of the thoracic trachea [32, 33]. Clinical presentation may vary and includes coughing, choking, stridor, feeding difficulty, respiratory distress, and recurrent aspiration pneumonias [33, 34].

Endoscopic repair has been recommended for type I or II clefts, while open repair has been reserved for more advanced type III or IV clefts [35]. Successful robotic-assisted surgical closure for types I and II have been reported [36]. while several additional unreported laryngeal cleft repair cases have been shared with the authors [*Personal Communications*].

Operative Technique

Exposure of the larynx is obtained with a appropriate oral retractor depending on the patient age and size (See Fig. 8). Based on the authors' experience, Crowe-Davis tonsil retractor is typically sufficient in the pediatric population. 8.5 mm, 30° angled endoscope should be utilized. The authors recommend using flexible fiber robotic-assisted CO_2 laser delivery (described earlier) system at a setting of 4–6 W to ablate the internal mucosal surfaces of the cleft. A flexible fiber CO_2 system allows for precise mucosal ablation down to the apex of the cleft. Following the ablation, any charred tissue should be removed utilizing oxymetazoline-soaked pledgets.

The mucosal layers are then approximated using 4-0 braded absorbable suture in

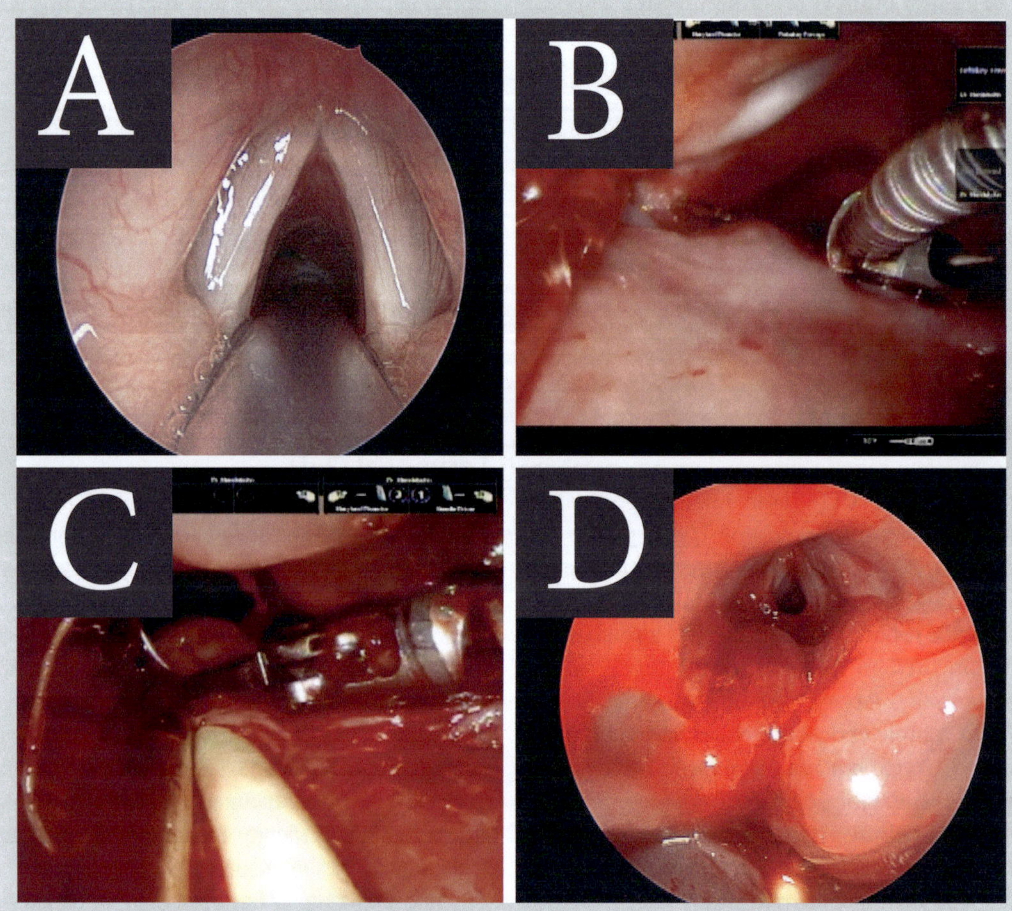

Fig. 8 TORS repair of pediatric laryngeal cleft. (**a**) displays the preoperative diagnostic bronchoscopy/laryngoscopy with a suction catheter within the laryngeal cleft splaying the arytenoid bodies apart. (**b**) displays the robotic-assisted view of the flexible fiber CO_2 laser delivery system used to ablate the medial mucosal surfaces of the cleft. (**c**) demonstrates the improved dexterity of the robotic system allowing for instrument wristing and placement of sutures deep within the laryngeal cleft. (**d**) displays the postoperative laryngoscopy demonstrating nasogastric feeding tube within the esophageal inlet without evidence of persistent cleft

a simple interrupted fashion. If there is limitation of rotation of the needle, a smaller 5-0 stitch may be used. Using the robotic instruments, the first suture is placed at the apex of the cleft by passing the needle posterior to anterior, and then anterior to posterior. This allowed the knot to be tied on the posterior surface to decrease the formation of granulation tissue in the airway [33]. A second suture is then placed more proximally to close the defect. Immediate postsurgical microlaryngobronchoscopy should be performed to ensure complete closure. After surgery, the patients should be kept NPO until oral intake can be examined by modified barium swallow study.

The advantages of robotic-assisted surgery over traditional endoscopic surgery include 3D visualization, surgeon tremor filtration, but mainly improved surgical dexterity. Endoscopic suture placement is extremely challenging and with the wristed motion of the robotic instruments, this procedure is improved significantly. The lack of tremor and increased freedom of instrument movement allowed for precise handling of the tissue and controlled surgical closure of the cleft that extended into the cervical trachea.

A major challenge of laryngeal cleft repair is maintaining the patient under anesthesia with spontaneous ventilation. An endotracheal tube can interfere with visualization and instrumentation of the defect. In some cases the patients may already be tracheostomy tube dependent, which may obviate the need to maintain spontaneous ventilation or to intermittently utilize an endotracheal tube.

A second challenge in pediatric robot-assisted surgery is introducing the robotic arms into the smaller pharynx, as robotic instrumentation specialized for pediatric-sized patients is not readily available. Exposure with a Crowe-Davis retractor allowed for adequate space for the robotic arms and instrumentation in our experience. While endoscopic pediatric laryngeal surgery is challenging the inclusion of robotic assistance has offered improvements, but continued advancement of the robotic technology will only continue to allow for additional surgical airway applications. Ultimately, robotic-assisted approach with combined flexible fiber CO_2 laser delivery holds promise as a minimally invasive approach for selected laryngeal cleft repairs.

Future of Laryngeal and Airway TORS

Although this chapter discussed many advantages and applications of TORS to surgery of larynx and the airway, robotic-assisted procedures are still hampered by the underlying necessity of access. Many patients anatomically will not be able to accept the robotic instrumentation and as such the benefits of TORS still cannot be applied universally. Smaller and more flexible instruments provided by *Intuitive Surgical* for the *da Vinci* system would help improve this shortcoming. However, at this time it does not appear that new TORS equipment will be offered within the next few years. Therefore, other surgical robotic systems may be required to achieve access to the larynx.

Research and development from the University of Pittsburg have developed a novel system which offers a flexible endoscope which can be set in a rigid position when arriving at the area of interest, such as the glottis [37, 38]. The endoscope, having conformed to the patient's individual anatomic variability, can then guide the microsurgical instruments through the newly set course through the pharynx. The robotic controls for this system more closely resemble that of endoscopic sinus surgery with the operative surgeon positioned at the patient's head as compared with the classic surgeon's console of the *da Vinci* system. This new *Medrobotics Flex System* is undergoing clinical testing and FDA approval process. This system may directly address the inadequacies of the larger robotic system applied to the limited area of the larynx.

In a similar strategy, another robotic-assisted microsurgical instrument system has been described which is fixated to a rigid laryngoscope [39]. Though this system has not been shown to be effective in the clinical setting, the approach of the curved-frame robotic system mimics that of Transoral Videolaryngscopic Surgery (TOVS), which combines laryngeal endoscopy and laparoscopic instrumentation to achieve magnified visualization of the glottis and bimanual operative instrumentation [40].

Conclusions

Surgeries of the supraglottis, larynx, and airway have been affected by the rapid expansion of robotic-assisted surgery in the head and neck. Specifically, transoral robotic supraglottic laryngectomy has demonstrated good functional and oncologic outcomes. Transoral robotic total laryngectomy and laryngeal cleft repair are early in their clinical description and both show good promise as minimally invasive approaches. As technology improves, or new systems become available, more procedures for the larynx and beyond into the airway will continue to be established with robotic assistance.

References

1. Weinstein GS, O'Malley Jr BW, Snyder W, Sherman E, Quon H. Transoral robotic surgery: radical tonsillectomy. Arch Otolaryngol Head Neck Surg. 2007;133(12):1220–6.
2. Benazzo M, Canzi P, Occhini A. Transoral robotic surgery with laser for head and neck cancers: a feasibility study. ORL J Otorhinolaryngol Relat Spec. 2012;74(3):124–8.
3. Van Abel KM, Moore EJ, Carlson ML, Davidson JA, Garcia JJ, Olsen SM, Olsen KD. Transoral robotic surgery using the thulium:YAG laser: a prospective study. Arch Otolaryngol Head Neck Surg. 2012;138(2): 158–66.
4. Desai SC, Sung CK, Jang DW, Genden EM. Transoral robotic surgery using a carbon dioxide flexible laser for tumors of the upper aerodigestive tract. Laryngoscope. 2008;118(12):2187–9.
5. Remacle M, Matar N, Lawson G, Bachy V, Delos M, Nollevaux MC. Combining a new CO_2 laser wave guide with transoral robotic surgery: a feasibility study on four patients with malignant tumors. Eur Arch Otorhinolaryngol. 2012;269(7):1833–7.
6. Goyal N, Yoo F, Setabutr D, Goldenberg D. Surgical anatomy of the supraglottic larynx using the da Vinci robot. Head Neck. 2014;36:1126–31. doi:10.1002/hed.23418.
7. De Virgilio A, Park YM, Kim WS, Baek SJ, Kim SH. How to optimize laryngeal and hypopharyngeal exposure in transoral robotic surgery. Auris Nasus Larynx. 2013;40(3):312–9.
8. Lawson G, Matar N, Remacle M, Jamart J, Bachy V. Transoral robotic surgery for the management of head and neck tumors: learning curve. Eur Arch Otorhinolaryngol. 2011;268(12):1795–801.
9. Kayhan FT, Kaya KH, Yilmazbayhan ED. Transoral robotic approach for schwannoma of the larynx. J Craniofac Surg. 2011;22(3):1000–2.
10. Tülin Kayhan F, Hakan Kaya K, Altıntas A, Fırat P, Sayin I. First successful transoral robotic resection of a laryngeal paraganglioma. J Otolaryngol Head Neck Surg. 2012;41(6):E54–7.
11. Muderris T, Bercin S, Sevil E, Acar B, Kiris M. Transoral robotic surgery for atypical carcinoid tumor of the larynx. J Craniofac Surg. 2013;24(6): 1996–9.
12. Remacle M, Lawson G, Hantzakos A, Jamart J. Endoscopic partial supraglottic laryngectomies: techniques and results. Otolaryngol Head Neck Surg. 2009;141(3):374–81.
13. Remacle M, Hantzakos A, Eckel H, Evrard AS, Bradley PJ, Chevalier D, Djukic V, de Vincentiis M, Friedrich G, Olofsson J, Peretti G, Quer M, Werner J. Endoscopic supraglottic laryngectomy: a proposal for a classification by the working committee on nomenclature, European Laryngological Society. Eur Arch Otorhinolaryngol. 2009;266(7):993–8.
14. Lawson G, Matar N, Nollevaux MC, Jamart J, Krug B, Delos M, Remacle M, Borght TV. Reliability of sentinel node technique in the treatment of N0 supraglottic laryngeal cancer. Laryngoscope. 2010;120(11): 2213–7.
15. Mendelsohn AH, Remacle M, Van Der Vorst S, Bachy V, Lawson G. Outcomes following transoral robotic surgery: supraglottic laryngectomy. Laryngoscope. 2013;123(1):208–14.
16. Park YM, Kim WS, Byeon HK, Lee SY, Kim SH. Surgical techniques and treatment outcomes of transoral robotic supraglottic partial laryngectomy. Laryngoscope. 2013;123(3):670–7.
17. Ozer E, Alvarez B, Kakarala K, Durmus K, Teknos TN, Carrau RL. Clinical outcomes of transoral robotic supraglottic laryngectomy. Head Neck. 2013;35(8): 1158–61.
18. Olsen SM, Moore EJ, Koch CA, Price DL, Kasperbauer JL, Olsen KD. Transoral robotic surgery for supraglottic squamous cell carcinoma. Am J Otolaryngol. 2012;33(4):379–84.
19. Lawson G, Mendelsohn AH, Van Der Vorst S, Bachy V, Remacle M. Transoral robotic surgery total laryngectomy. Laryngoscope. 2013;123(1):193–6.
20. Smith RV, Schiff BA, Sarta C, Hans S, Brasnu D. Transoral robotic total laryngectomy. Laryngoscope. 2013;123(3):678–82.
21. Dowthwaite S, Nichols AC, Yoo J, Smith RV, Dhaliwal S, Basmaji J, Franklin JH, Fung K. Transoral robotic total laryngectomy: report of 3 cases. Head Neck. 2013;35(11):E338–42.
22. Davis RK, Vincent ME, Shapshay SM, Strong MS. The anatomy and complications of "T" versus vertical closure of the hypopharynx after laryngectomy. Laryngoscope. 1982;92:16.
23. Deschler DG, Blevins NH, Ellison DE. Postlaryngectomy dysphagia caused by an anterior neopharyngeal diverticulum. Otolaryngol Head Neck Surg. 1996;115(1):167–9.
24. Ganly I, Patel S, Matsuo J, Singh B, Kraus D, Boyle J, Wong R, Lee N, Pfister DG, Shaha A, Shah J. Postoperative complications of salvage total laryngectomy. Cancer. 2005;103(10):2073–81.
25. Weber RS, Berkey BA, Forastiere A, Cooper J, Maor M, Goepfert H, Morrison W, Glisson B, Trotti A, Ridge JA, Chao KS, Peters G, Lee DJ, Leaf A, Ensley J. Outcome of salvage total laryngectomy following organ preservation therapy: the radiation therapy oncology group trial 91-11. Arch Otolaryngol Head Neck Surg. 2003;129(1): 44–9.
26. Lallemant B, Chambon G, Garrel R, Kacha S, Rupp D, Galy-Bernadoy C, Chapuis H, Lallemant JG, Pham HT. Transoral robotic surgery for the treatment of T1-T2 carcinoma of the larynx: preliminary study. Laryngoscope. 2013;123(10):2485–90.
27. Kayhan FT, Kaya KH, Sayin I. Transoral robotic cordectomy for early glottic carcinoma. Ann Otol Rhinol Laryngol. 2012;121(8):497–502.

28. Lalich IJ, Olsen SM, Ekbom DC. Robotic microlaryngeal surgery: feasibility using a newly designed retractor and instrumentation. Laryngoscope. 2014;124:1624–30. doi:10.1002/lary.24443.
29. O'Malley Jr BW, Weinstein GS, Hockstein NG. Transoral robotic surgery (TORS): glottic microsurgery in a canine model. J Voice. 2006;20(2):263–8.
30. Hockstein NG, Nolan JP, O'Malley Jr BW, Woo YJ. Robot-assisted pharyngeal and laryngeal microsurgery: results of robotic cadaver dissections. Laryngoscope. 2005;115(6):1003–8.
31. Blanco RG, Ha PK, Califano JA, Saunders JM. Transoral robotic surgery of the vocal cord. J Laparoendosc Adv Surg Tech A. 2011;21(2):157–9.
32. Benjamin B, Inglis A. Minor congenital laryngeal clefts: diagnosis and classification. Ann Otol Rhinol Laryngol. 1989;98(6):417–20.
33. Watters K, Ferrari L, Rahbar R. Minimally invasive approach to laryngeal cleft. Laryngoscope. 2013;123(1): 264–8.
34. Thiel G, Clement WA, Kubba H. The management of laryngeal clefts. Int J Pediatr Otorhinolaryngol. 2011;75(12):1525–8.
35. Rahbar R, Chen JL, Rosen RL, et al. Endoscopic repair of laryngeal cleft type I and type II: when and why? Laryngoscope. 2009;119(9):1797–802.
36. Rahbar R, Ferrari LR, Borer JG, Peters CA. Robotic surgery in the pediatric airway: application and safety. Arch Otolaryngol Head Neck Surg. 2007;133(1): 46–50.
37. Rivera-Serrano CM, Johnson P, Zubiate B, Kuenzler R, Choset H, Zenati M, Tully S, Duvvuri U. A transoral highly flexible robot: novel technology and application. Laryngoscope. 2012;122(5):1067–71.
38. Johnson PJ, Rivera Serrano CM, Castro M, Kuenzler R, Choset H, Tully S, Duvvuri U. Demonstration of transoral surgery in cadaveric specimens with the medrobotics flex system. Laryngoscope. 2013;123(5): 1168–72.
39. Kwon YS, Tae K, Yi BJ. Suspension laryngoscopy using a curved-frame trans-oral robotic system. Int J Comput Assist Radiol Surg. 2013;9:535–40.
40. Tomifuji M, Araki K, Yamashita T, Shiotani A. Transoral videolaryngoscopic surgery for oropharyngeal, hypopharyngeal, and supraglottic cancer. Eur Arch Otorhinolaryngol. 2014;271:589–97.

Robotic-Assisted Microvascular Surgery of the Head and Neck

Laureano A. Giraldez-Rodriguez, Brett Miles, and Eric M. Genden

Traditional treatment of the majority of oropharyngeal squamous cell carcinoma has relied on multimodality therapy, including chemoradiation or open surgical approaches with postoperative radiotherapy. Both treatment strategies may result in significant functional morbidity: The combination of chemoradiotherapy is associated with significantacute and long term toxicity that may leave up to 20 % of patientgastrostomy tube dependent and up to 11 % of patients reliant on a tracheostomy. The use of a lip splitting incision combined with a transmandibular approach and pharyngotomy to the oropharynx is also a morbid procedure associated with an extensive postoperative recovery [1–7]. In some studies, the morbidity of midline mandibulotomy with a lip splitting incision has been as high as 20–48 % [8, 9], while other investigations have not found the functional impact as devastating as previously expected, especially when reconstructive techniques are used appropriately and when compared with the functional outcomes of concurrent chemoradiation [10, 11]. Prior the era of free tissue transfer large defects in the oropharynx required large and bulky regional pedicled flaps (i.e., pectoralis major muscle flap (PMMF)). This required in decreased mobility of the base of tongue and the pharyngeal wall which in turn resukted in increased dysphagia and occassionally gastrostomy tube dependence [12]. Improved reconstructive techniques utilizing free tissue transfer have dramatically improved these outcomes; however, the functional results remain suboptimal due to issues related to surgical access and traditional transmandibular or transcervical approaches [1, 13, 14]. Concurrent chemoradiation was introduced as an organ preserving strategy for treatment of oropharynx carcinoma because of improved functional outcomes with comparable survival outcomes to open surgery followed by adjuvant radiation or chemoradiation [15]. Nonetheless, organ preservation still carries a high risk of dysphagia and functional disturbances related to the therapy [2, 3, 16].

L.A. Giraldez-Rodriguez, M.D.
Department Otolaryngology Head and Neck Surgery, Icahn School of Medicine at Mount Sinai, One Gustave L. Levy Place, Box 1189, New York, NY 10029, USA

B. Miles, D.D.S., M.D.
Department Otolaryngology Head and Neck Surgery, Icahn School of Medicine at Mount Sinai, One Gustave L. Levy Place, Box 1189, New York, NY 10029, USA

Department Oral and Maxillofacial Surgery, Icahn School of Medicine at Mount Sinai, One Gustave L. Levy Place, Box 1189, New York, NY 10029, USA
e-mail: brett.miles@mountsinai.org

E.M. Genden, M.D. (✉)
Department Otolaryngology Head and Neck Surgery, Icahn School of Medicine at Mount Sinai, One Gustave L. Levy Place, Box 1189, New York, NY 10029, USA

The Head Neck, and Thyroid Center, The Mount Sinai Medical Center, New York, NY 10029, USA
e-mail: ericgenden@mountsinai.org

G.A. Grillone and S. Jalisi (eds.), *Robotic Surgery of the Head and Neck: A Comprehensive Guide*,
DOI 10.1007/978-1-4939-1547-7_10, © Springer Science+Business Media New York 2015

The primary goal of contemporary treatment of oropharyngeal malignancy is to achieve equivaent with non- surgical modaliteis, but locoregional control and overall survival with improved functional outcomes, notably in terms of speech and swallowing. Transoral robotic surgery (TORS) has been introduced as an alternative to open surgery and organ preservation. Compared to the previously mentioned treatment modalities, review of the TORS literature demonstrates superb functional outcomes and the potential for decreased adjuvant therapy [17–22]. TORS offers several advantages for the management of oropharyngeal carcinoma. The view of the oropharynx afforded by the three-dimensional camera coupled with the ability to use two-handed instrumentation via the endo-wrist manipulator has contributed to the recent popularity of TORS [19, 22]. In addition, improved functional outcomes have been reported when TORS is compared to standard concurrent chemoradiation strategies in the management of oropharyngeal malignancy [17, 19, 22–24]. The coincident epidemic of human papilloma virus (HPV)-associated oropharyngeal carcinoma, lends itself to surgical management [19, 20, 22]. While the FDA has approved TORS for the management of early stage oropharyngeal carcinomas, there has been an evolution to apply this technology to more advanced stages of disease. This has resulted in more extensive defects in the oropharynx that often involve multiple anatomic regions, including the soft palate, tonsil, base of tongue, and pharynx. Our experience suggests that there are four approaches to the management of oropharyngeal defects after TORS. Healing by secondary intention, primary closure, local regional reconstruction, or reconstruction via free tissue transfer.

Postablative defects associated with smaller tumors are generally managed with secondary intention and left to remucosalize. This approach is used in the majority of isolated defects of the tonsillar fossa, tongue base, and pharynx. The primary advantage of remucosalization is that the resulting surface is native sensate mucosa, which improves swallowing sensation, decreases aspiration risk, and improves the overall functional dynamic of the pharynx. In contrast, defects associated with advanced disease can be moderate to large defects and may require formal reconstruction. Local advancement flaps as well as regional and free tissue transfer may be necessary to achieve the following goals: closure of pharyngocervical communication, coverage of carotid artery closure of extensive palatal defects, and transfer of vascularized free tissue to an irradiated bed in order to improve local wound healing.

Although most early staged oropharyngeal carcinomas can be surgically resected and left to heal by secondary intention, defects resulting from advanced staged tumors and salvage surgery represent unique circumstances that may benefit from reconstruction. The complex neuromuscular anatomy of the oropharynx is critical to speech and swallowing. Following TORS, the alteration of the anatomy often disturbs both the oral and pharyngeal phases of swallowing. During the oral phase of swallowing, the tongue drives the food bolus back into the oropharynx. Concomitantly, the velopharyngeal sphincter provides the closure necessary to propel food downward towards the lower oropharynx. The oropharyngeal phase of swallowing relies on both the muscular drive of the tongue and complex coordinated peristalsis of the upper pharynx that relies on pressure gradients produced by adequate velopharyngeal closure and complex muscular coordination [25]. Any disruption in either the bulk or muscular contraction of the tongue will lead to dysphagia and/or dysarthria. Similarly, any disturbance in velopharyngeal competence or pharyngeal contraction will result in dysphagia. Prior to the popularization of TORS, reconstruction of the oropharynx was necessary to achieve separation of the visceral compartment from the neck and restore function. The literature is replete with studies celebrating the impact of free tissue transfer on function, and an associated body of work has been dedicated to evaluating the impact of sensory re-innervation on function. A review of this literature suggests that free and pedicle flap reconstruction provides superior functional results when compared with primary closure, skin grafts, and adjacent tissue transfer for extensive defects [1, 13, 26, 27]. However, it is also clear that the asensate and adynamic properties of free tissue may hinder function. Free tissue transfer is often necessary to partition the oropharynx from the neck but paradoxically; the interposition of this tissue may hinder function. Choosing the appropriate defect and the appropriate modality of reconstruction is key to optimal outcomes.

The four ultimate principles to consider when evaluating extensive TORS defects for free tissue transfer reconstruction are closure of pharyngocervical communication, coverage of carotid artery exposure, closure of extensive palatal defects, and transfer of vascularized free tissue to an irradiated bed in order to improve local wound healing.

Classification of Oropharyngeal Robotic Defects

In order to guide reconstruction, our institution developed a Classification for Oropharyngeal Robotic Defects (CORD) to serve as a reconstructive algorithm [28] in an effort to optimize TORS reconstruction. This classification system is based on the site of the defect, number of subsites involved, exposure of the internal carotid artery, communication with the oropharynx, and if resection of more than 50 % of the palate was performed. Defects are categorized from Class I to IV in order of increasing defect complexity with higher classifications requiring more advanced reconstructive techniques. As with any reconstructive effort, reconstructive goals should include structural and functional considerations when reconstructing oropharyngeal defects following transoral robotic surgery. Structural considerations include preventing cervicopharyngeal fistula by creating an adequate barrier separating the neck and pharynx and ensuring adequate coverage of the vascular structures of the neck. Functional considerations include restoration of swallowing function, preservation of speech and articulation, and maintaining velopharyngeal competence (Tables 1 and 2). The CORD system accounts for both functional and structural considerations by dividing defects into four classes.

Table 1 Classification of oropharyngeal robotic defects

Class I—one subsite of the oropharynx, no adverse features
Class II—involves more than one subsite, no adverse features
Class III—only one subsite, adverse features
Class IV—involve more than one subsite, adverse features
Subsites of the oropharynx: base of tongue, tonsil, soft palate
Adverse features: carotid artery exposure, communtication with the neck, >50 % soft palate resection
Table 1 Illustration I CORD Classification System for TORS defects

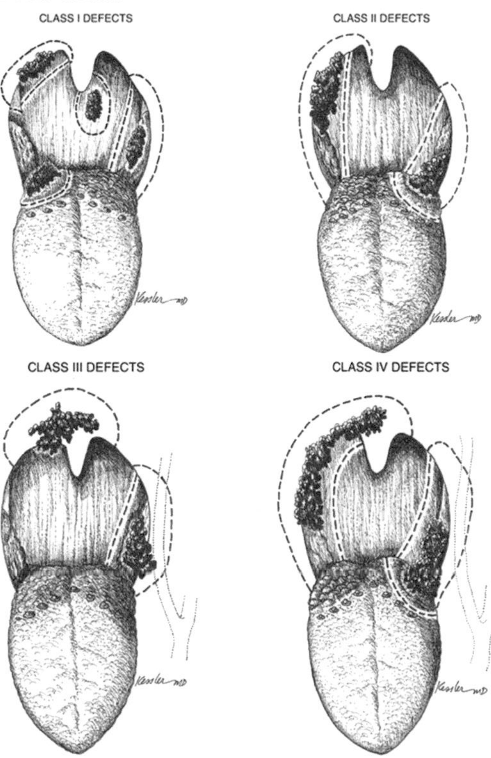

Class I defects include any single subsite of the oropharynx without any complicating features such as carotid artery exposure, pharyngocervical communication, or extensive palatal defect. The majority of these defects are typically left to remucosalize secondarily and often do so with minimal functional morbidity (Fig. 1). For tongue base defects, exposed deep intrinsic tongue muscles serve as the vascularized bed for remucosalization. Posterior pharyngeal defects

Table 2 Structural and functional considerations of TORS reconstruction

Structural Considerations
Create an anatomic barrier between the neck and the pharynx
Carotid artery coverage
Functional Considerations
Restore swallowing function
Preserve speech and articulation
Prevent aspiration
Maintaining velopharyngeal competence

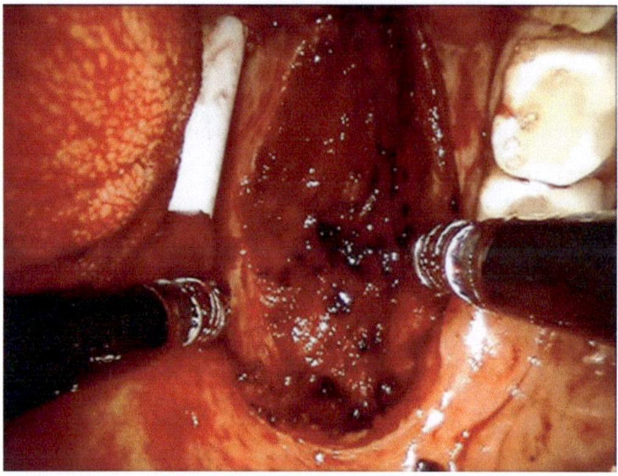

Fig. 1 Class I defect involving only one subsite of the oropharynx (tonsil) with no complicating defects

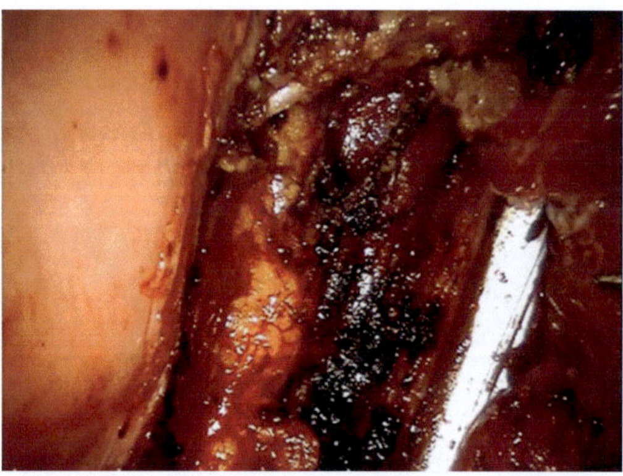

Fig. 2 Parapharyngeal fat outpouching from the lateral pharyngeal wall after TORS resection (*blue arrow*)

wherein the prevertebral fascia is exposed, mucosa will reline the area within several weeks. After pharyngectomy, fat from the parapharyngeal space provides vessel coverage and a surface for epithelialization (Fig. 2). Small defects of the palate, however, may require a series of sutures to close the free edge of the remaining palate to the posterior pharyngeal wall, thus closing the enlarged nasopharyngeal aperture. The goal of this technique is to minimize velopharyngeal insufficiency to improve speech and swallowing.

Seikaly et al. described reconstruction of the palate using a size-based classification system with defects classified into one of three categories [14]. For defects of less than one-fourth of the palate, they suggest primary closure of the palate to the posterior pharyngeal wall. In their series of 22 patients with small defects closed primarily, only one patient complained of nasopharyngeal regurgitation at 1 year after operation. In the same cohort, one patient remained gastric tube dependant and three required nutritional supplementation.

Class II defects are similar to class I defects in that they have no complicating features; however, they are more advanced in that more than one subsite is involved. Rarely do class II defects require a regional or free flap for reconstruction. Defects involving the tongue base extending into the tonsil are often left to heal secondarily. For defects of the tonsillar–palatal complex, a local musculomucosal flap may be used to seal the nasopharyngeal port. This flap is typically based on the mucosa and the superior constrictor muscle of the posterior pharyngeal wall. A monopolar cautery or contact laser is typically mounted in one of the robotic arms and used to raise this flap in the submuscular plane carefully to avoid potential injury to the internal carotid artery. This flap can then be rotated toward the posterior edge of the palate and sutured in order to reduce the size of the nasopharyngeal port. This technique has been previously described by Gehanno [29] and has also been referred to as a superior constrictor advancement rotation flap. The advantage of this local flap is that it is theoretically a neurotized flap and can preserve the dynamic function of the constrictor muscles during swallowing.

Class III defects were classified as those that involved one subsite of the oropharynx, but had adverse features such as internal carotid artery exposure in the pharynx, communication with the neck, or >50 % soft palate resection (Fig. 3).

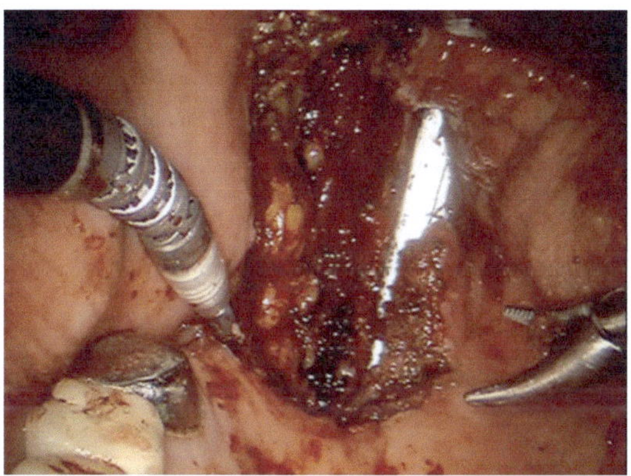

Fig. 3 Class 3 defect involving a portion of the soft palate, the tonsil, base of tongue. This patient also had communtication with the neck after the TORS resection

Class IV defects involved multiple subsites of the oropharynx and one or more of the adverse features mentioned in Class III (Table 1). We advocate regional or free flap reconstruction for class III and class IV defects or smaller defects in patients who have received prior radiotherapy. In a recent review of 92 patients TORS patients at Mount Sinai Medical Center the majority of the patients fell in the Class II category ($n=45$, 49 %), while Class I, III and IV defects were 34 % ($n=31$), 3 % ($n=3$), and 14 %($n=13$), respectively [30].

Rationale and Goals of Transoral Robotic Surgery Assisted Microvascular Reconstruction

Pharyngocervical Communication

When TORS is performed with a concomitant neck dissection, a pharyngocutaneous fistula may develop inadvertently or as part of the planned resection. A recent study by Moore and colleagues showed that 29 % of patients had a pharyngocervical communication intraoperatively, while only 4 % of these developed a permanent communication [31]. While some have advocated for a staged neck dissection to reduce the risk of fistula formation, tumors invading through the pharyngeal constrictor muscles may require a resection resulting in a surgically created fistula. Several techniques have been advocated for management of a fistula in the acute setting; however, in large defects or in patients who have received previous external beam radiotherapy, regional or free tissue transfer may represent the only reliable method of reconstruction. Flap reconstruction may be accomplished with the use of local flaps such as the infrahyoid or sternocleidomastoid muscle flap (Fig. 4a, b) or the submental island flap (Fig. 5) [32, 33]. Irrespective of the technique used to reconstruct the defect it is important to separate the upper aero digestive tract from the neck, to prevent postoperative fistula and vascular complications associated with the great vessels of the neck.

Carotid Artery Exposure

Rupture of the carotid artery is a well-known complication following surgery when the great vessels are exposed to salivary contaminants and or in the setting of prior external beam radiotherapy. It can occur in 3–14 % [34, 35] of patients after oropharyngeal surgery. In most cases of tonsil cancer resection, the parapharyngeal fat is left in place protect the carotid artery and provide a vascularized surface or remucosalization. In advanced cancers of the pharynx, the fat pad may require resection resulting in exposure of the carotid artery. In such cases, it is important to provide coverage and protection of the great vessels. A recent survey of TORS surgeons across the United States revealed the rate of postoperative hemorrhage ranges between 2.5 and 4.5 % in a total of 2015 reported procedures. They also reported 6 deaths within 30 days after TORS, all from hemorrhage related to the surgery [36]. While the majority of these events are likely related to branches of the external carotid the importance of vessel coverage cannot be underestimated.

Extensive Palatal Defects

Defects of the soft palate that involve more than 50 % of the soft palate represent a unique func-

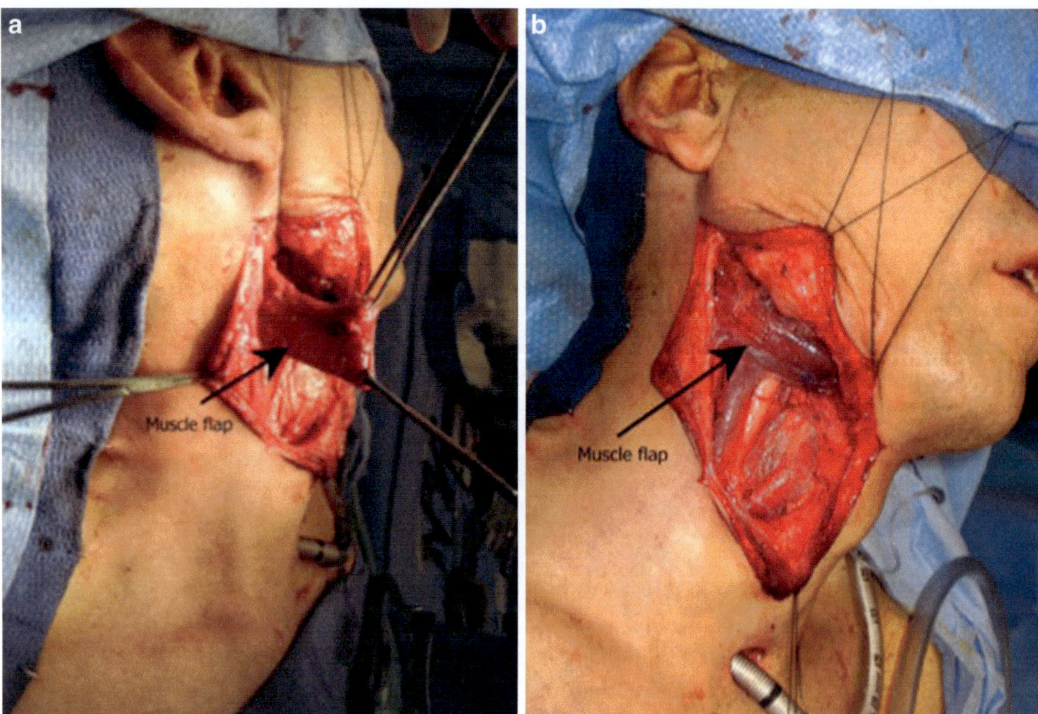

Fig. 4 (**a**) Sternocleidomastoid muscle flap raised in the neck for inset into the oropharynx. (**b**) Sternocleidomastoid muscle flap positioned in the neck to reinforce the robotic defect

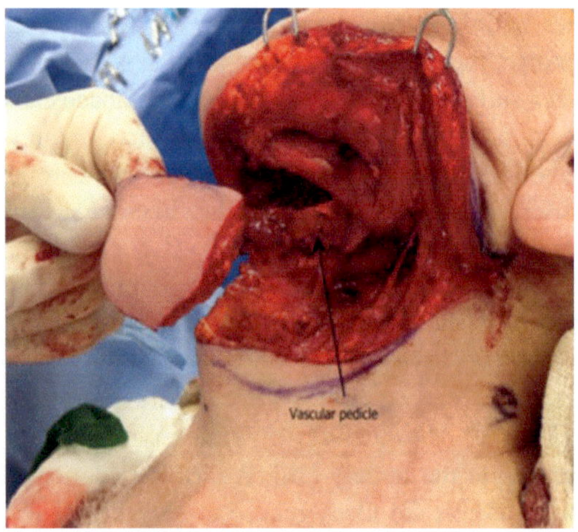

Fig. 5 Pedicled submental island flap for oropharynx reconstruction after a TORS resection

tional problem [26]. It has been shown that such defects of the soft palate result in high rates of velopharyngeal insufficiency, dysphagia, and a compromise in quality of life [37]. These defects often require a velopharyngoplasty in addition to soft tissue reconstruction. The velopharynoplasty can typically be achieved using a posterior-based musculomucosal flap that is approximated with the cut edge of the soft palate. The soft tissue reconstruction is best achieved with a regional or free tissue transfer to provide the appropriate soft tissue coverage. This is approach has proven effective in reestablishing speech and swallowing [14].

Radiotherapy

The impact of external beam radiotherapy on wound healing has been well documented. In patients who have undergone prior external beam radiotherapy, transoral robotic salvage surgery can be fraught with complications if the surgical defect is not managed appropriately [38]. Because the tissue has been compromised and the wound healing is suboptimal, free tissue transfer provides an opportunity to interpose well-vascularized tissue into the defect. This approach is been shown safe and effective for the management of these complex wounds [39]. In contrast to the extensive defects described previously, we advocate the use of free tissue transfer for modest defects of the pharynx because of the high risk of fistula, great vessel exposure, and catastrophic complications. In our experience, failure to reconstruct these patients with free tissue transfer leads to adverse scarring, are high risk of fistula formation, and significant compromise and decreased functional performance.

Surgical Technique

TORS-assisted microvascular reconstruction requires planning and a coordinated effort. Preoperative assessment is important in anticipating the defect. The use of gadolinium-enhanced MRI as well as contrast-enhanced CT scan may be necessary to assess the extent of tumor involvement of the oropharynx. In patients undergoing salvage surgery after radiotherapy, we start by selecting the optimal donor site in the event that a comples reconstruction is required. In most cases, the radial forearm donor site provides a source of thin and pliable tissue that can be manipulated to achieve the native contouring of the oropharynx. In select cases the anterolateral thigh or lateral arm donor sites may be appropriate. Most importantly, preoperative coordination the instrumentation and room set up is critical. Ideally a large OR should be utilized to provide space for robotic and microscopic instrumentation, and we have noted that when bringing the microscope into the room after resection of the primary tumor, neck dissection, and identification of the donor vessels while the flap harvest is already underway provides better logistical use of the OR space and prevents congestion. For large tumors, we perform the superior mucosal incisions around the tumor with the robot and in combination with a transcervical pharyngotomy with the inferior mucosal incisions while palpating the tumor in order to achieve safe inferior mucosal and deep margins. If a combined transcervical approach is warranted, we then remove the patient from suspension and proceed with neck dissection, mobilization of the hypoglossal nerve, and transcervical pharyngotomy with completion of the inferior resection.

After flap harvest and obtaining negative mucosal margins, the inset is performed. Defects that are confined to the soft palate and the tonsil can be closed transorally with traditional transoral or robotic techniques the majority of the time. However, as the defect extends inferiorly into the base of tongue, the glossotonsillar sulcus, and the pharyngeal wall at the level of the pyriforms sinus, the robotic instrumentation becomes essential for visualization and water-tight closure of the defect. It should be noted that once the tumor has been excised, we place two to four sutures at the inferior apex of the defect in order to use them as a guide for the most inferior edge of the mucosa were the flap needs to be sutured for a water tight closure. Commonly, these sutures are placed transcervically to achieve a reliable distal mucosal closure. If the defect is very inferior, we recommend placing the initial two or three sutures transcervically and then pushing the flap into the defect. This will allow for positioning of the vascular pedicle as it is tunneled into the neck as well. The robot is then brought into place and the patient is suspended. If we decide that the defect can be closed with the robot completely then using a 30° camera, the caudal aspect of the flap can be sutured to the adjacent native tissue of the hyopharynx (Fig. 6). Then, complete inset of the flap is performed before microvascular anastomosis. Robotically placed sutures should be trimmed to avoid tangling with instrumentation, which complicates robotic knot throwing. In tight spaces, urologic needles may be used which have a smaller radius and aid dramatically in robotic suturing.

It is our experience that in TORS-assisted microvascular free flap reconstruction, the robot provides the access, visualization, and dexterity necessary to achieve complex microvascular reconstruction without the need for mandibulotomy. In more than half of the cases, a portion of the closure was achieved transcervically. This

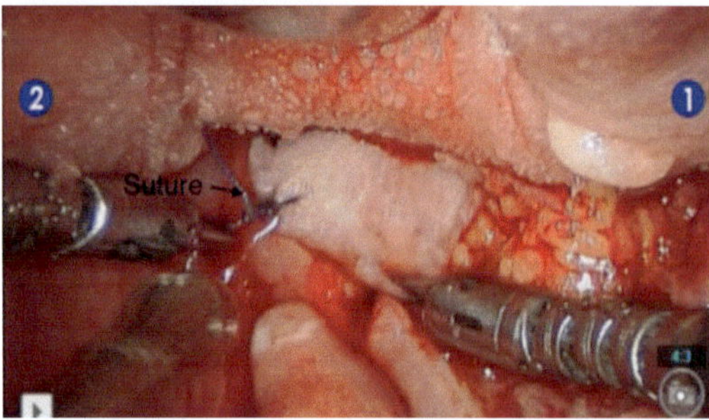

Fig. 6 Inset of radial forearm flap with robotic needle holders

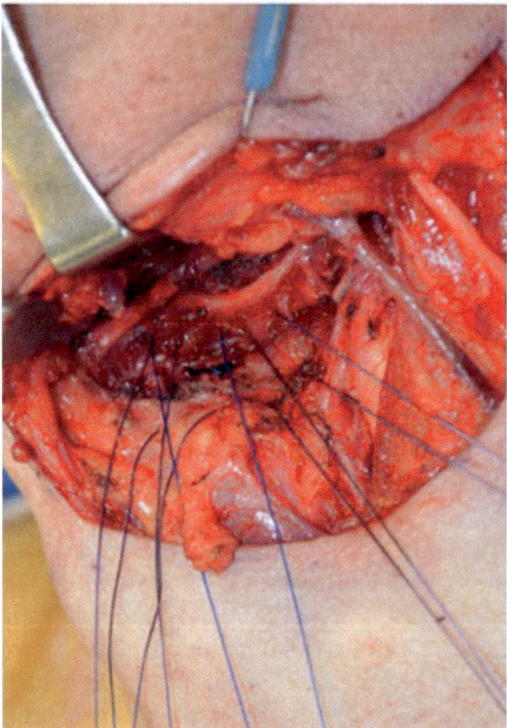

Fig. 7 Sutures placed along the inferior periphery of the pharyngotomy defect aids in the closure

is often done to assure a reliable caudal closure. This is often accomplished by placing a series of sutures peripherally around the defect (Fig. 7). The flap can then be placed into position and reliably sutured into the defect. Once the flap is inset, the microvascular anastomosis is performed.

Outcomes and Function

Much of the data related to TORS-assisted free flap reconstruction are in the process of analysis, and initial data seem to indicate that the technique provides an excellent tool to manage complex and extensive defects of the oropharynx. However, data demonstrate that with the exception of the extensive soft palate defect, the functional performance following free tissue transfer is rarely equivalent to local musculomucosal flap reconstruction. Patients healing by secondary intention or reconstructed with local musculomucosal flaps performed significantly better than patients requiring a free flap reconstruction [2, 40]. However, older studies suggest the same when comparing speech and swallowing outcomes of oropharyngeal reconstruction with primary closure or secondary intention healing versus flap reconstruction [41]. Although the size of the defect and tumor stage have been well documented to impact functional outcome in open surgery, in the TORS group, age (>50 year) and preoperative functional performance status had a significant impact on early (<30 days) and long-term (>30 days) function as assessed by the need for a gastrostomy [42]. As such, patients with potential indications for TORS-assisted free flap reconstruction should be counseled regarding the risk of gastrostomy dependence.

Our early unpublished experience data suggests that the risk of flap failure, fistula formation, or wound infection in the TORS-assisted free flap reconstruction group is not statistically different from age-matched, stage-matched, and performance-matched patients treated with open surgery. The length of hospital stay is less in the former group and although not quantified, patients value an opportunity to forgo a mandibulotomy and lip-splitting incision (Fig. 8).

Conclusion and Future Directions

TORS provides an outstanding opportunity to treat disease of the oropharynx, particularly in an era dominated by HPV-associated disease. Unlike

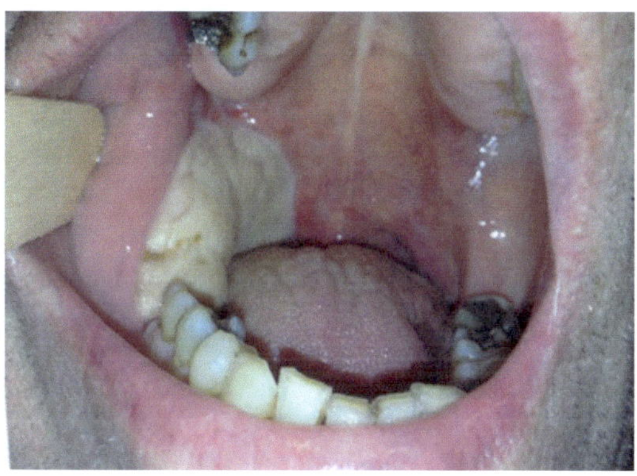

Fig. 8 Healed radial forearm free flap 6 months after TORS and microvascular reconstruction

tobacco-related carcinoma the surrounding tissue rarely demonstrates field effect dysplasia, and HPV-associated oropharyngeal carcinoma is commonly a focal entity. For this reason, HPV-associated disease is more amenable to surgical resection. Local-regional recurrence rates are significantly lower than documented in tobacco-related disease. Transoral surgical resection can be achieved through transoral laser microsurgery (TLM), TORS, or direct transoral approaches. While there are merits of each approach, TORS provides the unique ability to manipulate and suture tissue using a "two-handed approach." The design of the robotic instrumentation provides the operator the advantage of the ability to manipulate the tissue with one instrument while driving the suture with the second instrument. Because of this unique advantage, TORS is the only transoral technique that allows for complex reconstruction of the deep oropharynx, supraglottic larynx, and base of tongue. TORS-assisted free flap reconstruction provides a reliable method to achieve a safe reconstruction without the functional and aesthetic disturbance associated with traditional transmandibular approaches. As discussed, the rate of short-term and long-term gastrostomy dependence rises when free tissue reconstruction is required, and patients should be aware of this risk.

In its current form, the DaVinci robotic system has many limitations for head and neck reconstruction. Until the instrumentation is designed for transoral application, the acute angles of approach necessary to access the deep recess of the hypopharynx limit what can be achieved. For this reason, we often place the caudal sutures using a combination of transcervical and transoral approaches. In spite of these limitations, TORS-assisted reconstruction hold great promise by obviating the need for a mandibulotomy. Future goals will be directed toward improved instrumentation and modifications in technique that provide improved access to the hypopharnx.

References

1. Rieger JM, Zalmanowitz JG, Li SY, Sytsanko A, Harris J, Williams D, Seikaly H. Functional outcomes after surgical reconstruction of the base of tongue using the radial forearm free flap in patients with oropharyngeal carcinoma. Head Neck. 2007;29:1024–32.
2. Logemann JA, Pauloski BR, Rademaker AW, McConnel FM, Heiser MA, Cardinale S, Shedd D, Stein D, Beery Q, Johnson J, et al. Speech and swallow function after tonsil/base of tongue resection with primary closure. J Speech Hear Res. 1993;36:918–26.
3. Jantharapattana K. Oncologic and functional outcomes in advanced laryngeal and hypopharyngeal cancer treated with concurrent chemoradiation versus primary surgery followed by adjuvant treatment. J Med Assoc Thai. 2013;96:1164–8.
4. Suntornpong N, Sukkasem M, Uwattanasombat C, Samasanti N, Thephamongkol K. The effectiveness of clinical practice guideline for nasopharyngeal and oropharyngeal cancer to reduce acute treatment toxicity from concurrent chemoradiation. J Med Assoc Thai. 2011;94:585–91.
5. Barkati M, Fortin B, Soulieres D, Clavel S, Despres P, Charpentier D, Tabet JC, Guertin L, Olivier MJ, Coulombe G, Donath D, Nguyen-Tan PF. Concurrent chemoradiation with carboplatin-5-fluorouracil versus cisplatin in locally advanced oropharyngeal cancers: is more always better? Int J Radiat Oncol Biol Phys. 2010;76:410–6.
6. Boscolo-Rizzo P, Stellin M, Fuson R, Marchiori C, Gava A, Da Mosto MC. Long-term quality of life after treatment for locally advanced oropharyngeal carcinoma: surgery and postoperative radiotherapy versus concurrent chemoradiation. Oral Oncol. 2009;45:953–7.
7. Machtay M, Rosenthal DI, Hershock D, Jones H, Williamson S, Greenberg MJ, Weinstein GS, Aviles VM, Chalian AA, Weber RS. Penn cancer center clinical trials G: organ preservation therapy using induction plus concurrent chemoradiation for advanced resectable oropharyngeal carcinoma: a University

of Pennsylvania phase II trial. J Clin Oncol. 2002;20:3964–71.
8. Dubner S, Spiro RH. Median mandibulotomy: a critical assessment. Head Neck. 1991;13:389–93.
9. Shah JP, Kumaraswamy SV, Kulkarni V. Comparative evaluation of fixation methods after mandibulotomy for oropharyngeal tumors. Am J Surg. 1993;166: 431–4.
10. Dziegielewski PT, O'Connell DA, Rieger J, Harris JR, Seikaly H. The lip-splitting mandibulotomy: aesthetic and functional outcomes. Oral Oncol. 2010;46:612–7.
11. Dziegielewski PT, Mlynarek AM, Dimitry J, Harris JR, Seikaly H. The mandibulotomy: friend or foe? Safety outcomes and literature review. Laryngoscope. 2009;119:2369–75.
12. Tsue TT, Desyatnikova SS, Deleyiannis FW, Futran ND, Stack Jr BC, Weymuller Jr EA, Glenn MG. Comparison of cost and function in reconstruction of the posterior oral cavity and oropharynx. Free vs pedicled soft tissue transfer. Arch Otolaryngol Head Neck Surg. 1997;123:731–7.
13. Bozec A, Poissonnet G, Chamorey E, Laout C, Vallicioni J, Demard F, Peyrade F, Follana P, Bensadoun RJ, Benezery K, Thariat J, Marcy PY, Sudaka A, Dassonville O. Radical ablative surgery and radial forearm free flap (RFFF) reconstruction for patients with oral or oropharyngeal cancer: postoperative outcomes and oncologic and functional results. Acta Otolaryngol. 2009;129:681–7.
14. Seikaly H, Rieger J, Zalmanowitz J, Tang JL, Alkahtani K, Ansari K, O'Connell D, Moysa G, Harris J. Functional soft palate reconstruction: a comprehensive surgical approach. Head Neck. 2008;30:1615–23.
15. Gillespie MB, Brodsky MB, Day TA, Lee FS, Martin-Harris B. Swallowing-related quality of life after head and neck cancer treatment. Laryngoscope. 2004;114: 1362–7.
16. Bhayani MK, Hutcheson KA, Barringer DA, Lisec A, Alvarez CP, Roberts DB, Lai SY, Lewin JS. Gastrostomy tube placement in patients with oropharyngeal carcinoma treated with radiotherapy or chemoradiotherapy: factors affecting placement and dependence. Head Neck. 2013;35:1634–40.
17. Hutcheson KA, Holsinger FC, Kupferman ME, Lewin JS. Functional outcomes after TORS for oropharyngeal cancer: a systematic review. Eur Arch Otorhinolaryngol. 2014.
18. Sinclair CF, McColloch NL, Carroll WR, Rosenthal EL, Desmond RA, Magnuson JS. Patient-perceived and objective functional outcomes following transoral robotic surgery for early oropharyngeal carcinoma. Arch Otolaryngol Head Neck Surg. 2011;137:1112–6.
19. Moore EJ, Olsen KD, Kasperbauer JL. Transoral robotic surgery for oropharyngeal squamous cell carcinoma: a prospective study of feasibility and functional outcomes. Laryngoscope. 2009;119: 2156–64.
20. Hurtuk A, Agrawal A, Old M, Teknos TN, Ozer E. Outcomes of transoral robotic surgery: a preliminary clinical experience. Otolaryngol Head Neck Surg. 2011;145:248–53.
21. Genden EM, Park R, Smith C, Kotz T. The role of reconstruction for transoral robotic pharyngectomy and concomitant neck dissection. Arch Otolaryngol Head Neck Surg. 2011;137:151–6.
22. Weinstein GS, O'Malley Jr BW, Cohen MA, Quon H. Transoral robotic surgery for advanced oropharyngeal carcinoma. Arch Otolaryngol Head Neck Surg. 2010;136:1079–85.
23. Iseli TA, Kulbersh BD, Iseli CE, Carroll WR, Rosenthal EL, Magnuson JS. Functional outcomes after transoral robotic surgery for head and neck cancer. Otolaryngol Head Neck Surg. 2009;141:166–71.
24. Weinstein GS, O'Malley Jr BW, Desai SC, Quon H. Transoral robotic surgery: does the ends justify the means? Curr Opin Otolaryngol Head Neck Surg. 2009;17:126–31.
25. Giraldez-Rodriguez LA, Johns 3rd M. Glottal insufficiency with aspiration risk in dysphagia. Otolaryngol Clin North Am. 2013;46:1113–21.
26. Seikaly H, Rieger J, Wolfaardt J, Moysa G, Harris J, Jha N. Functional outcomes after primary oropharyngeal cancer resection and reconstruction with the radial forearm free flap. Laryngoscope. 2003;113: 897–904.
27. Arce K, Bell RB, Potter JK, Buehler MJ, Potter BE, Dierks EJ. Vascularized free tissue transfer for reconstruction of ablative defects in oral and oropharyngeal cancer patients undergoing salvage surgery following concomitant chemoradiation. Int J Oral Maxillofac Surg. 2012;41:733–8.
28. de Almeida JR, Genden EM. Robotic assisted reconstruction of the oropharynx. Curr Opin Otolaryngol Head Neck Surg. 2012;20:237–45.
29. Gehanno P, Guedon C, Veber F, Perreau P, Alalouf P, Moisy N. Velopharyngeal rehabilitation after transmaxillary buccopharyngectomy extending to the soft palate. Ann Otolaryngol Chir Cervicofac. 1985;102: 135–7.
30. de Almeida JR, Park RC, Villanueva NL, Miles BA, Teng MS, Genden EM. A reconstructive algorithm and classification system for transoral oropharyngeal defects. Head Neck. 2013.
31. Moore EJ, Olsen KD, Martin EJ. Concurrent neck dissection and transoral robotic surgery. Laryngoscope. 2011;121:541–4.
32. Selber JC, Robb G, Serletti JM, Weinstein G, Weber R, Holsinger FC. Transoral robotic free flap reconstruction of oropharyngeal defects: a preclinical investigation. Plast Reconstr Surg. 2010;125: 896–900.
33. Perrenot C, Berengere P, Mastronicola R, Gangloff P, Dolivet G. Infrahyoid myocutaneous flap for reconstruction after robotic transoral surgery for oropharyngeal tumors. Plast Reconstr Surg. 2014;133:236–7.

34. Marks JE, Freeman RB, Lee F, Ogura JH. Pharyngeal wall cancer: an analysis of treatment results complications and patterns of failure. Int J Radiat Oncol Biol Phys. 1978;4:587–93.
35. Righini CA, Nadour K, Faure C, Rtail R, Morel N, Beneyton V, Reyt E. Salvage surgery after radiotherapy for oropharyngeal cancer. Treatment complications and oncological results. Eur Ann Otorhinolaryngol Head Neck Dis. 2012;129:11–6.
36. Chia SH, Gross ND, Richmon JD. Surgeon experience and complications with transoral robotic surgery (TORS). Otolaryngol Head Neck Surg. 2013;149:885–92.
37. Rieger J, Dickson N, Lemire R, Bloom K, Wolfaardt J, Wolfaardt U, Seikaly H. Social perception of speech in individuals with oropharyngeal reconstruction. J Psychosoc Oncol. 2006;24:33–51.
38. Teknos TN, Myers LL, Bradford CR, Chepeha DB. Free tissue reconstruction of the hypopharynx after organ preservation therapy: analysis of wound complications. Laryngoscope. 2001;111:1192–6.
39. Fung K, Teknos TN, Vandenberg CD, Lyden TH, Bradford CR, Hogikyan ND, Kim J, Prince ME, Wolf GT, Chepeha DB. Prevention of wound complications following salvage laryngectomy using free vascularized tissue. Head Neck. 2007;29:425–30.
40. Pauloski BR, Logemann JA, Rademaker AW, McConnel FM, Stein D, Beery Q, Johnson J, Heiser MA, Cardinale S, Shedd D, et al. Speech and swallowing function after oral and oropharyngeal resections: one-year follow-up. Head Neck. 1994;16:313–22.
41. McConnel FM, Pauloski BR, Logemann JA, Rademaker AW, Colangelo L, Shedd D, Carroll W, Lewin J, Johnson J. Functional results of primary closure vs flaps in oropharyngeal reconstruction: a prospective study of speech and swallowing. Arch Otolaryngol Head Neck Surg. 1998;124:625–30.
42. Dziegielewski PT, Teknos TN, Durmus K, Old M, Agrawal A, Kakarala K, Marcinow A, Ozer E. Transoral robotic surgery for oropharyngeal cancer: long-term quality of life and functional outcomes. JAMA Otolaryngol Head Neck Surg. 2013;139:1099–108.

Transoral Robotic Surgery for Parapharyngeal Space Tumors

Tom Thomas and Donald J. Annino Jr.

Introduction

The parapharyngeal space (PPS) with its complex anatomy is a rare location for head and neck neoplasms. This location accounts for only 0.5 % of all head and neck tumors [1, 2]. The majority of these tumors are benign and have their origin in the salivary glands or in neurogenic tissue [1, 3]. It is mainly an adult disease, but it has been reported in the pediatric population [4]. Several studies have found there was a slight male predominance of PPS tumors [3]. The anatomic location and lack of or subtlety of symptoms early in the disease process can make the diagnosis challenging. Over the last several decades, various imaging modalities have proven to be invaluable in the diagnosis of many of the PPS tumors. In addition, they provide critical anatomical information for treatment planning. Surgery remains the primary modality of treatment for parapharyngeal space tumors. However, surgery in this location can lead to surgical or tumor related morbidity that can have moderate to devastating consequences. Transoral robotic surgery is one of the newest surgical approaches to minimize morbidity and allow complete tumor resection in the parapharyngeal space.

T. Thomas, M.D., M.P.H. (✉)
Center for Head and Neck Oncology,
Dana Farber Cancer Institute, 450 Brookline Avenue, Boston, MA, 02215, USA
e-mail: tthomas9@partners.org

D.J. Annino Jr., M.D., D.M.D.
Brigham and Women's Hospital,
Division of Otolaryngology, 45 Francis Street, ASB-2, Boston, MA 02115, USA

Anatomy

The PPS is complex due to its location and the structures that occupy the space. A thorough understanding of the complex anatomy of the parapharyngeal space is of utmost importance. It allows the clinician to assemble a logical differential diagnosis, appropriate laboratory and imaging studies, and select the most appropriate treatment option for the patient.

Although it is called the parapharyngeal "space," it is a potential space since it is not enclosed on all sides by fascia. It is most commonly described as an "upside down" or "inverted" pyramid. The base of the pyramid, the superior margin, is at the skull base and involves part of the temporal bone, but not the middle cranial fossa [5, 6]. The apex of the upside down pyramid that forms the inferior extent is made up of the posterior belly of the digastric muscle and greater cornu of the hyoid bone. The lateral boundary consists of medial pterygoid muscle fascia, the deep lobe of the parotid, and mandibular ramus. Its medial border is continuous with the lateral aspect of the retropharyngeal space and is located lateral to each side of the pharynx. It is made up of fascia over the superior constrictor muscle, tensor, and levator

G.A. Grillone and S. Jalisi (eds.), *Robotic Surgery of the Head and Neck: A Comprehensive Guide*, DOI 10.1007/978-1-4939-1547-7_11, © Springer Science+Business Media New York 2015

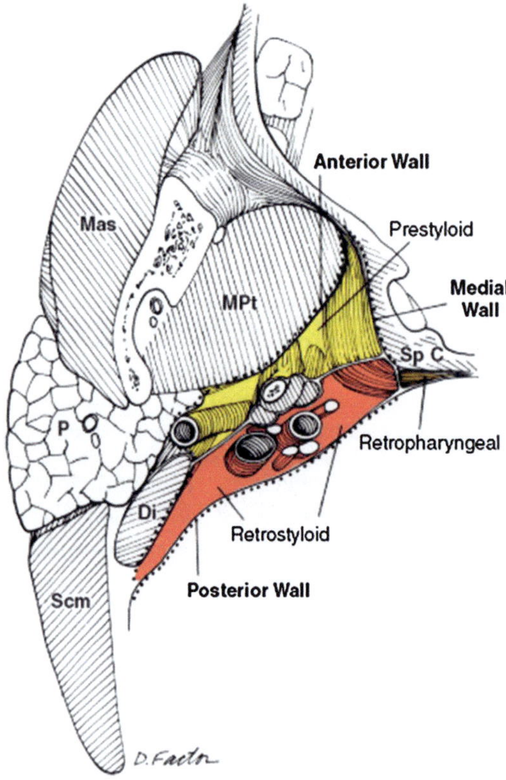

Fig. 1 Anatomic borders of the parapharyngeal space (*area outlined by dots*). *Di* Digastric muscle, *Mas* Masseter muscle, *Mpt* Medial pterygoid muscle, *P* Parotid gland, *Scm* Sternocleidomastoid muscle, *Spc*, Superior constrictor muscle (Courtesy of the Mayo Foundation, Rochester, Minn. Copy Right obtained from Mosby Elsevier)

veli palatine muscles. The posterior aspect of the pyramid is formed by paraspinal muscles and the fascia over the spinal column.

The parapharyngeal space is divided into an anterolateral space, also known as the pre-styloid compartment and the posterolateral space called the post or retro-styloid compartment by the fascia that extends from the styloid process to the tensor veli palatini muscle on each side (Fig. 1) [7]. The pre-styloid compartment contains the deep lobe of the parotid gland, auriculotemporal nerve, and internal maxillary and ascending pharyngeal artery besides adipose tissue and lymph nodes. The post-styloid compartment contains more important structures such as the Internal Carotid Artery (ICA), Internal Jugular vein (IJV), Cranial Nerves IX, X, XI, XII, cervical sympathetic chain, glomus bodies and rarely parotid tissue.

Epidemiology

Parapharyngeal space tumors account for 0.5 % of all head and neck neoplasms. The majority (>80 %) of these PPS tumors are benign and a minority (<20 %) are malignant [1, 3]. See Table 1 for a more inclusive list. A recent systematic review of the literature on parapharyngeal space tumors by Riffat et al. reiterated this occurrence. The study found the most common primary PPS tumor originates in the salivary gland (45 %) and is found in the pre-styloid area [1, 3]. Pleomorphic adenomas were the most common benign salivary gland tumors (64 %) in the PPS [1, 3]. The second most common PPS tumors were found to be the neurogenic tumors (41 %) located mainly in the post-styloid area [1, 3]. The most common benign neurogenic tumor of the PPS was paragangliomas (52 %) followed by schwannomas (27 %) and neurofibromas (9 %). Prior studies reported schwannomas to be the most common neurogenic tumor [8]. The most common paragangliomas of the PPS were Vagus nerve in origin followed by carotid body tumors and glomus jugulare tumors [1].

Less than 20 % of the PPS tumors were malignant [1, 3]. Out of all the salivary gland tumors in the PPS, 23 % were malignant. Adenoid cystic carcinomas (7 %) and mucoepidermoid carcinomas (4 %) were the most common malignant salivary gland neoplasms. Out of all the neurogenic tumors, 5 % were malignant. Metastatic disease is a rare occurrence in the PPS. Only 3 % of the tumors in the PPS were metastatic lesions [1]. However, this could be the result of incomplete data collection and reporting. Thyroid carcinoma is the most common metastatic lesion (20 %) of all the PPS cancers [1].

Clinical Presentation and Workup

It is more common for a clinician to encounter an asymptomatic patient presenting to the clinic with an incidentally found mass during a physical examination or on imaging that was performed as part of another workup. Approximately 50 % of patients are asymptomatic at presentation [9].

Table 1 Parapharyngeal tumors

Origin	Benign	Malignant
Salivary	Pleomorphic adenoma Warthins tumor Oncocytoma Lymphoepithelial cyst	Carcinoma ex-pleomorphic adenoma Adenoid cystic carcinoma Mucoepidermoid carcinoma Adenocarcinoma Acinic cell carcinoma
Neurogenic	Carotid body tumor Vagal paraganglioma Neurofibroma Neurilemoma	Neurofibrosarcoma
Lymphovascular	Hemangioma Hemangioepithelioma Venous malformation Lymphatic malformation	Lymphoma Hemangiopericytoma Plasmacytoma
Metastatic		Thyroid Carcinoma Squamous Cell Carcinoma
Other	Lipoma Rhabdomyoma Leiomyoma Branchial cleft cyst Teratoma Meningioma Carotid artery aneurysm	Liposarcoma Rhabdomyosarcoma Chondrosarcoma Fibrosarcoma

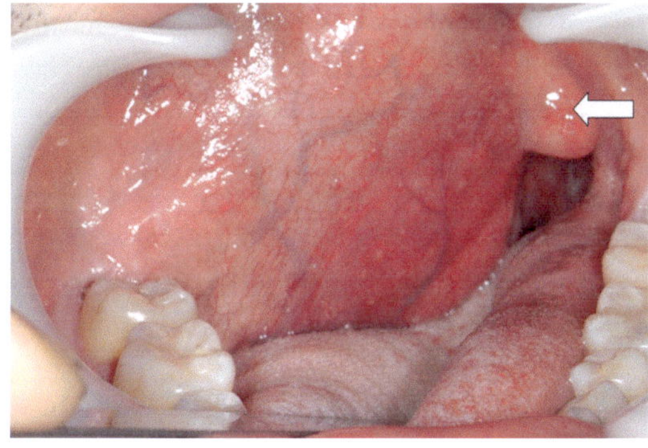

Fig. 2 Right oropharyngeal mass at presentation. *Arrow* points to displaced uvula

The most common sign (50 %) is intraoral swelling (Fig. 2), followed by a cervical mass (44 %) [1]. The PPS tumor is usually at least 2.5 cm before it is palpable as a cervical mass. When a post-styloid mass enlarges, it can compress the surrounding tissue, especially cranial nerves IX, X, XI, and XII. Cranial nerve neuropathy was reported as the third most common sign (18 %) behind neck mass and intraoral swelling [1]. The Vagus nerve was most commonly affected and was seen in 7 % of cases [1]. Medial enlargement of the mass combined with cranial nerve deficit produced dysphagia (11 %) and dysphonia (9 %) [1]. Although clinically interesting, Horner syndrome, known by the triad of ptosis, miosis, and anhydrosis of the ipsilareral face, was seen in only 2 % of cases [1]. Hearing loss and middle ear effusion are seen when superior enlargement of the mass causes Eustachian tube compression.

Imaging

Cross sectional, anatomic imaging studies are of paramount importance in diagnosing and developing treatment plans for patients with PPS tumors. The complex anatomic location prevents complete assessment of any PPS mass with physical examination and endoscopy alone. Computed tomography (CT) scan with contrast and magnetic resonance imaging (MRI) with gadolinium are the most widely used imaging modalities for PPS tumors. CT and MRI scans are complimentary in the evaluation since CT scans can provide better bony details such as skull base erosion and MRI scans provide better soft tissue detail without the need for ionizing radiation (Fig. 3) [3, 10]. Given that the majority

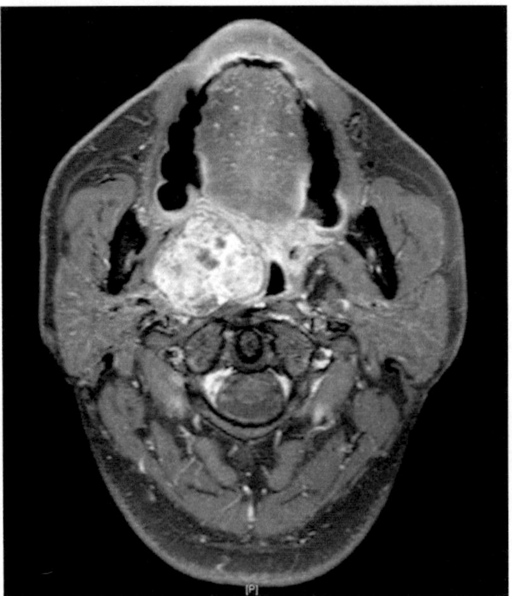

Fig. 3 Magnetic resonance image: right PPS pleomorphic adenoma

of the PPS tumors are of salivary or neurogenic origin, MRI with gadolinium is the preferred imaging tool. Besides providing the size, shape, extent of disease, and adjacent structures, it also provides the location (pre- and post-styloid) based on the displacement of the parapharyngeal fat, internal carotid artery and internal jugular vein (Table 2) [10]. However, PPS fat can be less discerning with increasing tumor size. CT and MRI scans can indicate malignancy in the presence of irregular tumor margins and invasion into the surrounding tissue plane. Schwannomas and paragangliomas have specific imaging and enhancing characteristics such as "salt and pepper" appearance on MRI for paragangliomas. In addition, CT and MR angiography can be valuable in assessing vascularity of the tumor and/or vascular invasion by the tumor.

Table 2 Image findings in pre and post-styloid contents

PPS Location	Image findings
Pre-styloid	1. Mass in the anterior PPS, displacing the PPS fat medially and posteriorly 2. Displacement of the posterior belly of the digastric and styloid muscle group posteriorly 3. Location medial to and separable from the medial pterygoid muscle 4. Mass is anterior to the ICA and IJV
Post-styloid	1. Mass in the posterior or medial PPS 2. Extension posterior to the styloid process rather than anteriorly via the stylomandibular tunnel 3. Lateral and anterior displacement of the posterior belly of the digastric and styloid muscle group 4. Anterior displacement of the ICA and IJV

Diagnosis

Having a tissue diagnosis is invaluable in making treatment decisions. It will also help with obtaining consent from the patient for surgery, discussing morbidity, cure rate, and recurrence. Fine needle aspiration (FNA) Biopsy of the PPS mass has mixed published results. It is, however, the least morbid or invasive way to obtain a diagnosis when feasible. In our institution, when an Ultrasound guided FNA is not possible due to the tumor location, CT guided FNA has been successful in obtaining a diagnosis. Open biopsy, whether it is transoral or transcervical, has been universally discouraged [11, 12]

Treatment

The primary treatment modality for PPS tumors is surgery [1, 3]. Over the decades, several surgical approaches to PPS tumors have been developed. In the most recent systematic review of the past 20 years of literature on PPS tumors, the transcervical approach was the most commonly used (48 %) followed by cervical-parotid approach (27 %), cervical approach with mandibulotomy (9 %), and the transoral approach (2 %) [1]. The best and safest approach is chosen after careful deliberation of tumor size, pathology, location within the PPS along with the best surgical access.

The PPS tumors located in the inferior aspect can be approached via the cervical approach. It provides the best direct access with good visualization of the cranial nerves and the great vessels. PPS tumors located in the middle and upper aspect

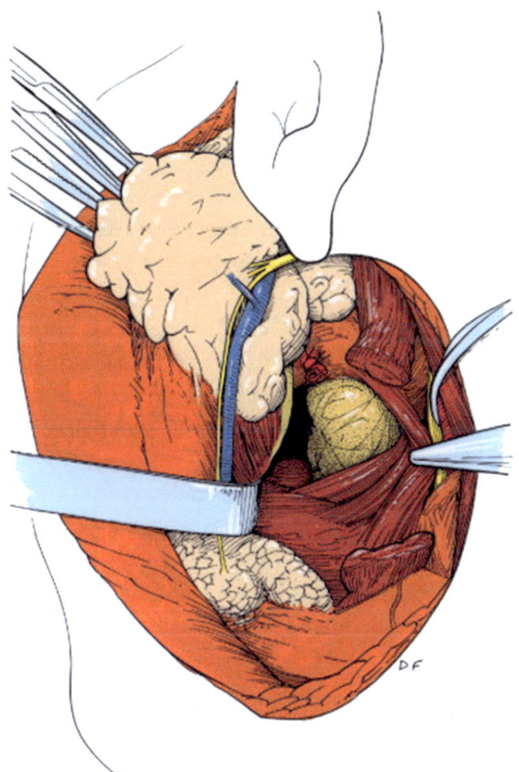

Fig. 4 Cervical-parotid approach

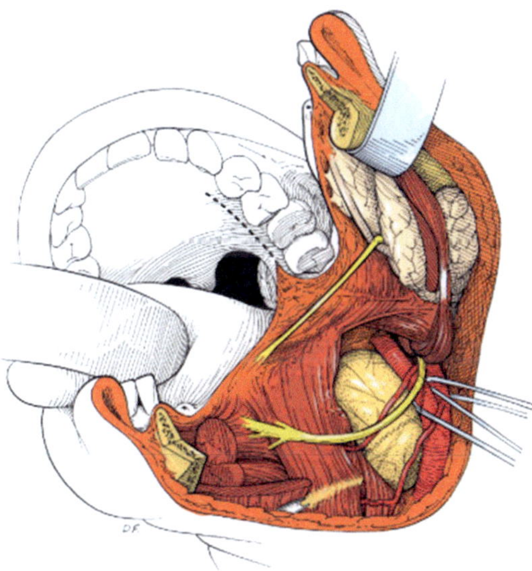

Fig. 5 Cervical-parotid approach with midline mandibulotomy

with facial nerve involvement can be accessed via the cervical-parotid approach (Fig. 4) [7]. This approach allows access to the deep lobe of the parotid and the great vessels [3, 6, 11]. Large tumors located in the upper PPS can be accessed via the cervical approach with a median or a paramedian mandibulotomy (Fig. 5) [3, 6, 7, 11].

In order to overcome some of the disadvantages of the open surgery, Duvvuri et al recently described a novel transcervical, minimally invasive, video assisted, image guided technique [13]. It facilitated resection of the PPS mass using bony landmarks for guidance in four patients with good outcomes and showed its feasibility [13]. However, long-term follow-up in a larger cohort is needed.

In general, the larger the tumor, the larger the surgical incision and the higher the potential for tumor or surgery related complications. Given the complex location of the PPS tumors, their removal can result in short- or long-term morbidity anywhere from 10 to 40 % [1, 7]. Some of the published complications are tumor rupture, positive margins, damage to cranial nerves causing dysphonia, dysphagia, aspiration, airway compromise requiring emergency tracheostomy, facial paralysis, Frey syndrome, first bite syndrome, and Horner syndrome [1, 3, 7, 14]. Mandibulotomy can cause malocclusion, malunion, nerve injury, wound infection and salivary fistula [1, 7]. Vascular injury can lead to hemorrhage, cerbrovascular accident, or even death [1, 7].

Another approach that can avoid an external cervical incision and can access the parapharyngeal space directly is the transoral approach. It is only used in 2 % of surgical cases with small benign, intraoral PPS tumors [1, 15]. This is due to limited visualization of the great vessels and a limited operative space resulting in higher tumor rupture, incomplete tumor removal, and difficulty in controlling any possible hemorrhage [16].

Since the development of Transoral robotic surgery at the University of Pennsylvania to resect oropharyngeal, hypopharyngeal, supraglottic, and glottic tumors, there is renewed interest in the transoral approach to PPS tumors [15, 17–20]. The da Vinci Surgical Robotic System (Intuitive Surgical, Sunnyvale, CA) has the ability to provide the surgeon with a 3-dimensional view of the surgical site with high definition and magnification [21]. It provides direct or angled views of the surgical field using a 0° or 30° scopes [21]. The da Vinci robot's capacity for motion scaling and tremor filtration is advantageous in performing careful dissection around the "pseudo capsule" of a pleomorphic adenoma. Reported disadvantage of the TORS approach is lack of tactile feedback [21]. A recent systematic review of the literature of 40 TORS cases of the PPS showed that it is safe and feasible [22]. In addition, TORS cases are comparable or better than the cervical approach in operating time, blood loss, time to oral diet, and length of stay [18, 22]. However, they found total unintended capsule violation of pleomorphic adenomas to be much higher than open approaches [22]. This could, however, be secondary to a small sample size. Only long-term follow-up will provide data on the recurrence rate from tumor spillage.

Preoperative Considerations

A detailed history and documentation of any overt or subtle symptoms involving breathing, voice, and swallowing are of utmost importance. A thorough physical examination of the head and neck region including cranial nerves and sympathetic chain related symptoms should be noted. The physical examination is not complete without an upper endoscopy, carefully inspecting for any obvious or subtle mucosal or submucosal mass causing contour deformity of the upper aerodigestive tract. Endoscopy also helps with evaluation of airway status and aspiration risk.

Both contrast enhanced CT and MRI scans are important to assess the mass, surrounding neurovascular and bony structures. MR can be useful in patients with dental amalgam. Also the PPS is a fat filled space where the direction of displacement of the fat by the tumor can be key in identifying the location of tumor origin. Further imaging such as an MR or CT angiogram or PET scan can be obtained if the mass involves vasculature or there is a concern for metastatic disease.

A careful review of the various imaging results should be undertaken, paying close attention to the tumor and its relationship to the ICA and IJV. If these structures are displaced medially by the tumor, the transoral robotic approach should not be considered [23]. If the patient has any signs of bone invasion or metastatic disease to the neck that require the management of the neck disease or need for any free flap reconstruction, he/she should be excluded from the transoral approach [23]. TORS should be avoided in any paragangliomas of the neck given their intimate involvement with the surrounding neurovascular structures.

It is important to have a detailed conversation with the patient regarding the potential expected and unexpected complications of the procedure and its short- and long-term sequelae. Informed consent should include the rationale for the transoral approach and the possibility of an external approach in case there are any intraoperative findings that make the transoral approach not feasible. If the risk of the surgery outweighs benefit of the surgery then nonsurgical options should be pursued, especially in patients with slow growing or benign tumors with prohibitive comorbidities. In addition, evaluating the patient in a multidisciplinary (radiation and medical oncology) setting will help with preoperative workup, adjuvant treatment decisions, and long-term cancer surveillance. Bradley et al. concluded in their 2011 article "Update on the management of parapharyngeal tumors" that intraoral surgery should be performed in only highly select small benign tumors and only by expert head and neck surgeons who have the expertise to convert to a cervical approach when necessary [11].

Intraoperative TORS Setup [17, 23, 24]

The patient undergoes general endotracheal anesthesia utilizing a wire reinforced #6.0 endotracheal tube. Orotracheal intubation rather than naso-tracheal intubation is used usually to avoid nasal trauma and epistaxis.

The endotracheal tube is swept to the opposite side and secured in place to the lower nasolabial fold or lateral submental crease using a 2.0 silk suture.

The OR table is rotated 180° away from the anesthesia equipment to ensure working space.

The patient's eyes are protected with Opti-Gard to prevent inadvertent damage to the cornea and globe.

A head wrap, shoulder roll and Foley catheter are placed at this time. The patient is prepped and draped in a sterile manner, but the neck can be covered with a sterile towel to avoid any accidental contamination. This also prepares one to be ready in case of an intraoral hemorrhage that requires an emergent open cervical approach.

The patient's oral cavity is retracted open with a Crowe-Davis mouth gag or modified F–K retractor and it is suspended onto a Mayo stand or Storz scope holding arm.

A second stitch can be placed intraorally at the retromolar trigone, anterior tonsillar pillar, or lateral tongue to displace the ET tube out of the surgical area.

Then the mass is visualized, palpated, and marked as needed.

The daVinci robotic system is brought into the surgical field.

The 0° telescope is used for most of the case. However, a 30° scope is useful once the superior and inferior dissection requires an angled view ("view around the corners"). The scope is advanced into the oral cavity as close as possible to the mass without touching it. Then the 5-mm monopolar spatula tip electrocautery is placed to the ipsilateral aspect of the tumor and the 5-mm Maryland dissector is placed on the contralateral arm. This can be switched as the surgery progresses for better access and tissue handling (Fig. 6).

The bedside surgical assistant is important to help with suction and retraction. Hemostasis can be achieved using endoscopic surgical clips or suction cautery.

The incision is determined by the size and location of the tumor. A generous incision is made to obtain access and exposure (Fig. 7a). Gentle dissection is then performed circumferentially with the spatula tip electrocautery while paying attention to the tumor capsule (Fig. 7b, c). Blunt dissection can be achieved by replacing the electrocautery arm with a second 5-mm Maryland dissector holding Kittner dissector sponge ("peanut"). Given the lack of tactile feedback with the robotic arm, at times it is necessary for the surgeon to gently finger dissect an area where unusual adherence to the surrounding tissue is noted. Any visualized vasculature is ligated using endoscopic surgical clips. A 30° scope is useful for the superior and inferior aspect of the tumor visualization before transecting the specimen from these areas. Then the tumor is removed transorally.

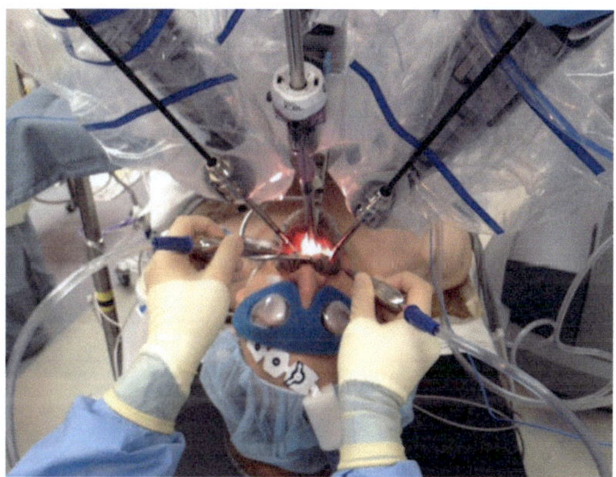

Fig. 6 Transoral robotic surgery: Intraoperative view

A careful evaluation of the tumor capsule under loop magnification will help to decide if complete tumor resection was achieved. Then the oral cavity is irrigated with sterile saline. If tumor spillage is noted, irrigation with sterile water is used. Hemostasis can be achieved using electrocautery (Fig. 7d). If incomplete excision is suspected or confirmed, transoral or transcervical approach should be used to extirpate the tumor completely.

Then using 3.0 Vicryl interrupted stitches, the incision is closed. This can be done manually or using the robotic arm.

A drain is not routinely placed in the surgical defect due to extubation, transferring process, or patient movement that can dislodge the drain. Attempting reinsertion of the drain in an awake patient, even with good visualization, can cause inadvertent trauma and bleeding.

At this point the patient's bed is turned back 180° and the care is transferred to the

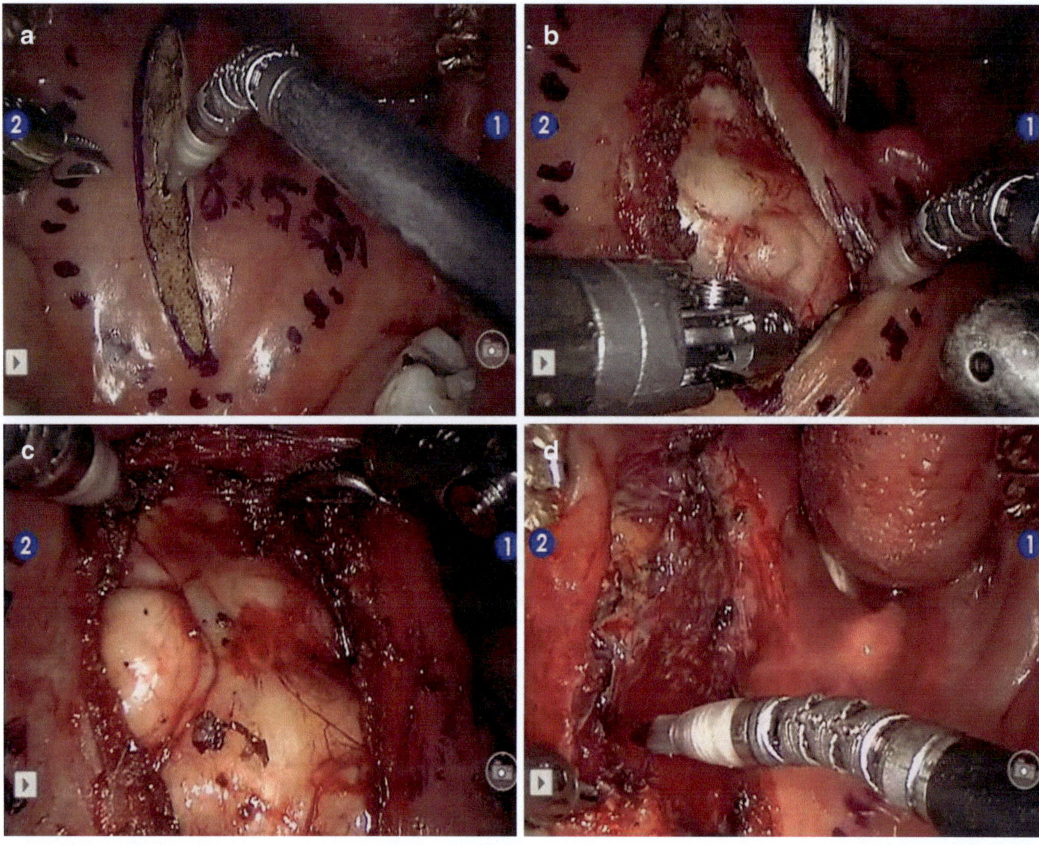

Fig. 7 (**a**) Transoral robotic surgery: intraoperative view, mucosal incision (Courtesy of Dr. Kim, Copyright obtained from Mary Ann Liebert, Inc). (**b**, **c**) Transoral robotic surgery: intraoperative view (Courtesy of Dr. Kim, Copyright obtained from Mary Ann Liebert, Inc). (**d**) Transoral robotic surgery: intraoperative view. Surgical defect (Courtesy of Dr. Kim, Copyright obtained from Mary Ann Liebert, Inc)

anesthesia team for extubation. If there is a concern for significant airway edema and possible airway compromise, delayed extubation in the Surgical Intensive Care Unit (SICU) is preferred.

Postoperative Care

Depending on the size and extent of the resection, over night observation of the airway in the SICU and IV steroids are recommended.

Enteral nutrition is started on postoperative day one and advanced as tolerated.

The patient is educated prior to discharge about any potential serious complications such as oropharyngeal hemorrhage or airway distress and to seek immediate medical help by calling 911.

Summary

The parapharyngeal space is one of the most complex anatomic locations in the head and neck. The tumors of the PPS are uncommon given that they account for only 1/200 of the head and neck cancers. The majority are benign and of salivary gland origin but malignancy can have significant morbidity. A detailed history, physical examination, fine needle aspiration, and imaging can help with diagnosis and treatment planning. Surgery is the mainstay treatment for PPS tumors. There are several surgical approaches that have been published. They are all variations of the transoral or the transcervical approach. All of these techniques are a sincere effort by surgeons to achieve complete tumor extirpation with minimal short- and or long-term morbidity to patients. Transoral robotic resection of a parapharyngeal space tumor is one such approach that avoids an external incision. It is safe and feasible with minimal morbidity. It offers an unparallel 3-dimensional-magnified visualization and articulated arms with thin instruments that provide degrees of freedom for manipulating tissue in a confined space that was not possible in the past. However, it lacks the tactile feedback that is critical in this complex anatomic location. In addition, the literature is sparse with cases and case series without long-term follow-up data. As of now, the Transoral Robotic approach can make the traditional transoral approach safer by overcoming several of its past limitations. However, even with all of its advantages, this approach is not for every patient.

References

1. Riffat F, Dwivedi RC, Palme C, Fish B, Jani P. A systematic review of 1143 parapharyngeal space tumors reported over 20 years. Oral Oncol. 2014;50(5):421–30. doi:10.1016/j.oraloncology.2014.02.007. Epub 2014 Feb 28.
2. Batsakis JG, Sneige N. Pathology consultation: parapharyngeal and retropharyngeal space diseases. Ann Otol Rhinol Laryngol. 1989;98:320–1.
3. Zhi K, Ren W, Zhou H, et al. Management of parapharyngeal tumors. J Oral Maxillofac Surg. 2009;67:1239–44.
4. Starek I, Mihal V, Novak Z. Paediatric tumours of the parapharyngeal space. Int J Pediatr Otorhinolaryngol. 2004;68:601–6.
5. Maheshwar AA, Kim E-Y, Pensak ML, Keller JT. Roof of the parapharyngeal space: defining its boundaries and clinical implications. Ann Otol Rhinol Laryngol. 2004;113:283–8.
6. Olsen KD. Tumours and surgery of the parapharyngeal space. Laryngoscope. 1994;104:1–28.
7. Moore EJ, Olsen KD. Complications of surgery of the parapharyngeal space (Chapter 21). In: Eisele DW, Smith RV, editors. Complications in head and neck surgery. 2nd ed. St. Louis: Mosby Elsevier; 2009. p. 241–50.
8. Luna-Ortiz K, Navarrete-Alemán JE, Granados-García M, Herrera-Gómez A. Primary parapharyngeal space tumors in a Mexican cancer center. Otolaryngol Head Neck Surg. 2005;132(4):587–91.
9. Carrau RL, Mayer EN, Johnson JT. Management of tumors arising in PPS. Laryngoscope. 1990;100:583.
10. Mafee MF, Venkatesan MD, Ameli N, et al. Tumours of the parotid and parapharyngeal space: role of computed tomography and magnetic imaging. Oper Tech Otolaryngol Head Neck Surg. 1996;7:348–57.
11. Bradley PJ, Bradley PT, Olsen KD. Update on the management of parapharyngeal tumours. Curr Opin Otolaryngol Head Neck Surg. 2011;19(2):92–8.
12. Eisele DW, Richmon JD. Contemporary evaluation and management of parapharyngeal space neoplasms. J Laryngol Otol. 2013;127(6):550–5.
13. Beswick DM, Vaezi A, Caicedo-Granados E, Duvvuri U. Minimally invasive surgery for parapharyngeal space tumors. Laryngoscope. 2012;122:1072–8.
14. Caldarelli C, Bucolo S, Spisni R, Destito D. Primary parapharyngeal tumours: a review of 21 cases. Oral Maxillofac Surg. 2014;18:283–92.
15. Hockstein NG, Nolan JP, O'Malley Jr BW, et al. Robot-assisted pharyngeal and laryngeal microsurgery: results of robotic cadaver dissections. Laryngoscope. 2005; 115:1003–8.
16. Papadogeorgakis N, Petsinis V, Goutzanis L, et al. Parapharyngeal space tumors: surgical approaches in a series of patients. Int J Oral Maxillofac Surg. 2010;39:243–50.
17. Mendelsohn AH. Transoral robotic assisted resection of the parapharyngeal space. Head Neck. 2014 May 2. doi:10.1002/hed.23724. [Epub ahead of print].
18. O'Malley Jr BW, Quon H, Leonhardt FD, Chalian AA, Weinstein GS. Transoral robotic surgery for parapharyngeal space tumors. ORL J Otorhinolaryngol Relat Spec. 2010;72:332–6.
19. Goodwin Jr WJ, Chandler JR. Transoral excision of lateral parapharyngeal space tumors presenting intraorally. Laryngoscope. 1988;98:266–9.
20. Arshad H, Durmus K, Ozer E. Transoral robotic resection of selected parapharyngeal space tumors. Eur Arch Otorhinolaryngol. 2013;270(5):1737–40.
21. Hans S, Delas B, Gorphe P, Ménard M, Brasnu D. Transoral robotic surgery in head and neck cancer. Eur Ann Otorhinolaryngol Head Neck Dis. 2012;129(1): 32–7.
22. Chan JY, Tsang RK, Eisele DW, Richmon JD. Transoral robotic surgery of the parapharyngeal space: a case series and systematic review. Head Neck. 2013 Nov 29. doi: 10.1002/hed.23557. [Epub ahead of print].
23. Weinstein GS, O'Malley BW, Leonhardt FD, Quon H. Robotic resection of parapharyngeal space tumors (Chapter 11). In: Weinstein GS, O'Malley BW (eds) Transoral robotic surgery (TORS). Plural Publishing, San Diego, CA; 2005; 135–146.
24. Park YM, De Virgilio A, Kim WS, Chung HP, Kim S-H. Parapharyngeal space surgery via a transoral approach using a robotic surgical system: transoral robotic surgery. J Laparoendoscopic Adv Surg Tech. 2013;23(3):231–6.
25. Mendelson AH, Bhuta S, Calcaterra TC, et al. Parapharyngeal space pleomorphic adenoma: a 30-year review. Laryngoscope. 2009;119:2170–4.

Robotic Thyroid Surgery

William S. Duke and David J. Terris

Introduction

Thyroid surgery remained largely unchanged for nearly 100 years after Kocher refined the traditional thyroidectomy technique utilizing his eponymous incision. During the late 1990s, significant advances in endoscopic technology and favorable experiences with minimally invasive parathyroid surgery prompted exploration into ways to reduce the cosmetic impact of the Kocher incision. While some authors pursued minimally invasive anterior cervical approaches to the thyroid gland, other groups developed remote access procedures, which completely remove the incision from the visible portion of the anterior neck. The initial remote access approaches utilized endoscopic techniques and equipment, which limited their popularity and applicability in Western practices. The surgical robot was subsequently introduced into remote access thyroid surgery to overcome these limitations, significantly increasing the international feasibility and appeal of these techniques.

W.S. Duke, M.D. • D.J. Terris, M.D., F.A.C.S. (✉)
Department of Otolaryngology,
Georgia Regents University,
1120 Fifteenth Street, BP-4109,
Augusta, GA 30912-4060, USA
e-mail: wduke@gru.edu; dterris@gru.edu

Advantages of Remote Access Robotic Thyroidectomy

Despite the advances that minimally invasive anterior cervical approaches have made in recent years in reducing the cosmetic burden of thyroid surgery, these procedures still leave a visible scar on the neck. While many patients find this small scar an acceptable side effect of removing their disease, there are other patients who, for either personal or professional reasons, place a premium on avoiding any public stigma of surgery. For these individuals, remote access procedures offer the distinct advantage of completely removing the thyroidectomy scar from the visible portion of the neck.

The earliest remote access techniques typically involved endoscopic approaches from the anterior chest or axilla to access the thyroid compartment [1–6]. These procedures required CO_2 insufflation to maintain the operative pocket and were restricted by two-dimensional visualization and long rigid instruments inherent in endoscopic procedures [7], factors which hampered their widespread adoption outside of specific Asian markets. To overcome these limitations, the surgical robot was introduced into remote access thyroid surgery in 2005 [8], with the first reported outcomes studies emerging in 2009 [7, 9].

Remote access robotic thyroid surgery offers several advantages over the endoscopic approaches, including a three-dimensional view of the surgical field, improved maneuverability

G.A. Grillone and S. Jalisi (eds.), *Robotic Surgery of the Head and Neck: A Comprehensive Guide*,
DOI 10.1007/978-1-4939-1547-7_12, © Springer Science+Business Media New York 2015

of articulating instruments, and proportional motion scaling for fine dissection [10]. Development of reliable, intuitive fixed retraction systems also allowed for gasless approaches to the thyroid compartment, obviating the need for CO_2 insufflation of the neck [9]. These advances, coupled with the cosmetic advantages of remote access approaches, helped popularize remote access robotic thyroid surgery on a global scale.

Remote Access Robotic Thyroidectomy Approaches

There are currently two main types of remote access robotic thyroid surgery available in Western practices (Fig. 1). The robotic axillary thyroidectomy (RAT) emerged in South Korea in 2009 [7]. This gasless approach utilizes an incision hidden in the axilla and was developed to directly overcome the limitations inherent in endoscopic-assisted remote access thyroid surgery. While RAT has been both successful and popular in some Asian markets, several serious limitations became apparent as it was implemented into Western patient populations, leading many groups to abandon this technique [11–13]. To overcome these limitations, a gasless robotic facelift thyroidectomy (RFT) that utilizes a postauricular incision was developed in 2010 [14, 15].

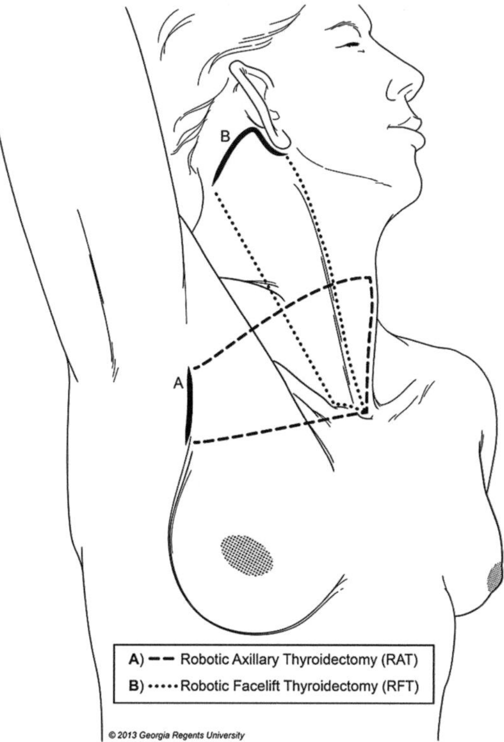

Fig. 1 Comparison of the robotic axillary thyroidectomy (RAT) and robotic facelift thyroidectomy (RFT) remote access approaches. From Dukews, Terris DJ. Alternative approaches to the thyroid gland. Endocrinal Metab Clin North Am. 2014; 43(2): 459–474. Used with permission

Robotic Axillary Thyroidectomy

RAT Advantages and Disadvantages

As with all remote access techniques, the robotic axillary approach leaves no trace of thyroid surgery on the anterior neck. The incision is well hidden in the axilla, and unlike the other endoscopic remote access procedures it does not result in any anterior chest or breast scarring. These cosmetic attributes have made RAT a popular method of treating surgical thyroid disease in certain Asian markets, where hypertrophic scarring is prominent and the neck is considered a highly sensuous area [16–18]. RAT is associated with increased patient cosmetic satisfaction when compared to open procedures [19, 20]. Some authors have also reported decreased pain after RAT [19], while others have noted that reduced postoperative neck pain was accompanied by increased chest wall pain [20].

There are several disadvantages of the technique. The length of the dissection pocket makes stimulating the recurrent laryngeal nerve difficult with the commercial stimulators currently available. The vector of approach involves dissection across the axilla and anterior chest, regions that may be unfamiliar to most head and neck surgeons. Additionally, as the procedure was imported from Asia to Western practices, it has been noted to be more difficult to obtain adequate operative exposure in patients who are tall or obese [21, 22], and obesity contributes to increased operative time [23]. The procedure is most commonly performed utilizing surgical drains and inpatient observation, requirements that represent a step backwards from many of the advances achieved by the minimally invasive anterior cervical thyroidectomy approaches currently available. Finally, a number of serious complications have been reported using this technique in Western practices [21, 23, 24]. These factors, along with cost and several other considerations, have caused many surgeons in North America to question or altogether abandon this procedure [11–13, 25, 26].

RAT Patient Selection

No uniform selection criteria exist for the RAT [21, 24]. The procedure was first reported in patients with both benign and malignant thyroid conditions, with RAT reserved for patients with nodules ≤5 cm and malignant lesions ≤2 cm [7, 9]. Patients were excluded from consideration if they had prior neck surgery, "severe" Graves' disease, malignancy with extrathyroidal extension, multiple lateral neck nodal metastases, nodal extracapsular spread, or lesions in the dorsal aspect of the thyroid [9]. Patients with substernal or retropharyngeal extension have also been excluded [23].

While the procedure is primarily utilized for unilateral thyroid surgery, bilateral procedures [7, 9, 21, 22] and both central and lateral neck dissections have been reported with this approach [7, 9, 27]. Candidates for lateral neck dissection have metastatic disease limited to 1 or 2 nodes in a single nodal basin and no evidence of extracapsular spread [27].

RAT Operative Details

The remote access robotic axillary thyroidectomy procedure has been reported in detail [7, 9, 21]. The procedure has undergone some modifications and surgeon-specific refinements since its initial description, and a generalized description of the technique is outlined here. After appropriate positioning, the patient's arm is extended at the shoulder and a 5–6 cm vertical incision is marked in the anterior axilla. The arm is replaced into its natural position to ensure that the planned incision line will be hidden within the axilla. The arm is then extended again and secured to an armrest. Some authors advocate flexing the elbow to minimize the risk of positional nerve injury [21]. If desired, a 1 cm incision is marked on the patient's chest 2 cm above the nipple line and 2 cm lateral to midline, though many surgeons now omit this extra working port and introduce all the instruments through the axillary incision, as described below.

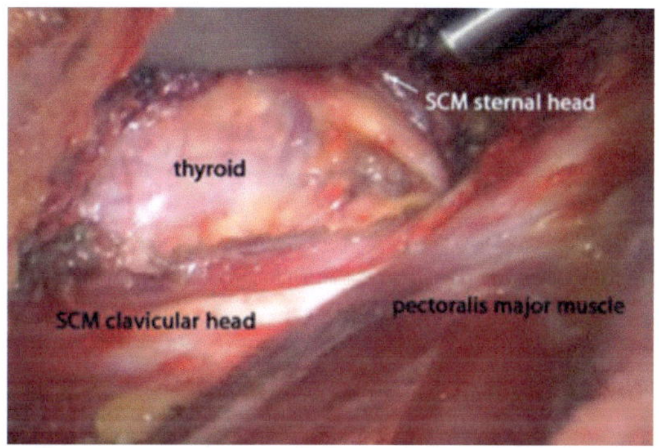

Fig. 2 View of the thyroid between the sternal and clavicular heads of the sternocleidomastoid muscle in the remote access robotic axillary thyroidectomy. From: Lewis CM, Chung WY, Holsinger FC. Feasibility and surgical approach of transaxillary robotic thyroidectomy without CO_2 insufflation. Head Neck. 2010;32:121–126. Used with permission

The axillary incision is made and continued down to the fascia overlying the pectoralis major muscle. A plane is developed between the subcutaneous tissue and the pectoralis major as dissection is continued medially to the midline and superiorly above the clavicle. The sternocleidomastoid muscle (SCM) is identified and the soft tissue overlying it is elevated from the clavicle and sternal notch superiorly. The space between the sternal and clavicular heads of the SCM is opened and the sternal head is retracted ventrally to expose the strap muscles, taking care to avoid injuring the internal jugular vein or its tributaries. The strap muscles are then elevated off the thyroid gland from the sternal notch to the superior pole and across the midline. The omohyoid may be divided if necessary to improve exposure. A fixed retractor system is employed to maintain the operative pocket (Fig. 2).

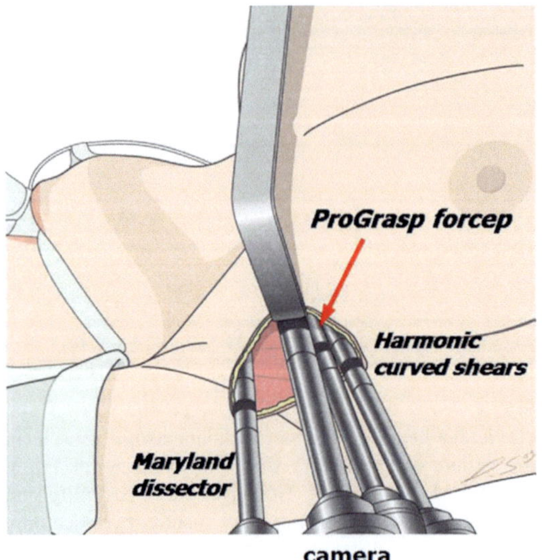

Fig. 3 Positioning of camera and instrument arms for single incision remote access robotic axillary thyroidectomy. From: Ryu HR, Kang SW, Lee SH, et al. Feasibility and safety of a new robotic thyroidectomy through a gasless, transaxillary single-incision approach. J Am Coll Surg. 2010;211(3):e13–e19. Used with permission

The robot console is then docked on the contralateral side of the operating table. A 30° downward facing camera is utilized. Harmonic shears (Ethicon Endosurgery Inc., Cincinnati, OH) are placed in the dominant arm, and ProGrasp forceps (Intuitive Surgical, Sunnyvale, CA) and a Maryland grasper are placed in the nondominant arms. The camera is inserted through the axillary incision so that the tip is oriented superiorly, while the instruments are inferiorly oriented (Fig. 3).

The superior pole is addressed first. The gland is retracted inferiorly, and the superior vascular pedicle is divided with the Harmonic device. The soft tissue attachments and vessels along the inferior aspect of the gland are divided and the gland is rotated medially. The recurrent laryngeal nerve (RLN) and parathyroid glands are identified and preserved. Once these structures have been secured, the isthmus and any remaining soft tissue attachments are divided and the lobe is removed. If a total thyroidectomy is indicated, the superior pedicle of the contralateral lobe is divided, and a subcapsular dissection between the thyroid and the trachea is performed to identify the contralateral RLN and liberate the gland. A surgical drain is placed and the wound is closed in layered fashion. Patients are generally admitted for inpatient observation after the procedure.

RAT Outcomes

RAT has been performed successfully in thousands of patients, mostly in Asia. The mean operative times for RAT vary from 115 to 168 min [7, 9, 28, 29]. Regardless of the approach used or the extent of surgery, remote access robotic thyroid surgery is consistently longer than conventional open thyroid surgery; a review of robotic axillary and bilateral axillo-breast procedures revealed a mean overall increase of 42 min for these approaches when compared to open surgery [20]. However, the overall hospital length of stay is shorter with remote access robotic thyroidectomy than with conventional open surgery [20].

Both central and lateral neck dissections have been described with the RAT approach using combined axillary and anterior chest incisions [9,27,30], with a mean of 6.1 lymph nodes removed from the central neck and 27.7 nodes removed from the lateral neck [27].

The completeness of surgical resection can be reflected in postoperative thyroglobulin (Tg) and ^{131}I uptake levels. Kang et al. [9] reported achieving postoperative Tg levels less than 1 ng/mL in 92 % of patients evaluated, with a mean Tg level of 4.9 ng/mL in the remaining 8 % of patients. A recent systematic review comparing 1,053 RAT patients with 794 open thyroidectomy patients showed no difference in the postoperative Tg levels between these two groups [20]. Kang et al. [30] reported no abnormal ^{131}I uptake levels in 209 patients undergoing total thyroidectomy by RAT followed by postoperative radioactive iodine therapy, though patients undergoing RAT have been reported to have higher postoperative Tg levels than patients having conventional surgery prior to radioactive iodine ablation [29].

RAT subjects patients to all the standard risks of thyroid surgery, and introduces several new ones. Complications such as hemorrhage, brachial plexus neuropathy, chyle leak, Horner's syndrome, conversion to an open procedure, and tracheoesophageal injury have been reported [9, 21, 23, 28]. Temporary RLN injury has been reported in 0.7–8 % of cases [28, 29], with a permanent RLN injury rate of 0.4 % [28]. Hematoma occurs in up to 2.6 % of cases [29]. Temporary hypocalcemia is seen in up to 41 % of cases [20, 29]. A recent systematic review showed that this risk of transient hypocalcemia was higher in remote access robotic procedures than in conventional thyroidectomy, but there were otherwise no differences in complication rates between the two types of approaches [20].

Robotic Facelift Thyroidectomy

RFT Advantages and Disadvantages

The remote access robotic facelift thyroidectomy offers several distinct advantages over the axillary approach. First, the relevant anatomy and route of dissection are familiar to head and neck surgeons [31]. Second, there is no risk of positional brachial plexus injury, as has been reported with the robotic axillary approach [21, 32]. Finally, the extent of dissection in the RFT approach is less than that of the axillary approach [14]. The shorter distance of dissection facilitates easily stimulation of the RLN, if required, while the reduced volume of dissection permits outpatient recovery without the need for postoperative drains [15].

Despite these advantages, the technique does have some limitations. First, the vector of approach and the robotic instruments currently available do not permit bilateral thyroid surgery through a single unilateral incision. Therefore, the procedure is indicated only in patients for whom unilateral surgery is expected. A completion procedure may be performed through a separate contralateral facelift incision if the final pathology mandates a total thyroidectomy. Second, transient dysfunction of the great auricular nerve is ubiquitous and patients should be counseled to expect temporary numbness of the ear. Third, while it may be technically feasible, no reports of neck dissection using the RFT approach have been published. Therefore this procedure is not recommended for patients who require a neck dissection [15]. Finally, the procedure generally takes longer than does a comparable operation performed via a minimally invasive anterior cervical approach [15, 33].

Table 1 Indications and contraindications for robotic facelift thyroidectomy

Indications	Contraindications
– Motivated patient willing to accept increased operative time, increased dissection, and transient ear numbness in exchange for no visible scar – ASA class I or II – No prior neck surgery – Unilateral disease	– Dominant nodule >4 cm – Morbid obesity – Associated lymphadenopathy – Substernal or extrathyroidal extension

RFT Patient Selection

Specific patient and disease criteria for RFT have been formalized to maximize the likelihood of operative success and minimize the risk of complications (Table 1) [34]. Patients should be generally healthy and able to tolerate general anesthesia for several hours. Patients should not be morbidly obese, but the presence of a slightly thicker layer of subcutaneous tissue helps protect the integrity of the soft tissue flap. They should have no prior history of neck surgery or radiation. Finally, the ideal patient is highly motivated to avoid a visible cervical scar, understands the limitations and risks of the procedure, and accepts the unlikely but possible chance that conversion to an anterior approach may be required.

The condition being assessed should also meet certain criteria to be considered appropriate for RFT [34]. Generally, the disease should be amenable to unilateral surgery, such as an enlarging or symptomatic benign nodule or a follicular lesion of undetermined significance. The largest nodule should not exceed 4 cm in its greatest dimension, and there should be no thyroiditis or prior history of thyroid compartment surgery. There should be no substernal component, and no

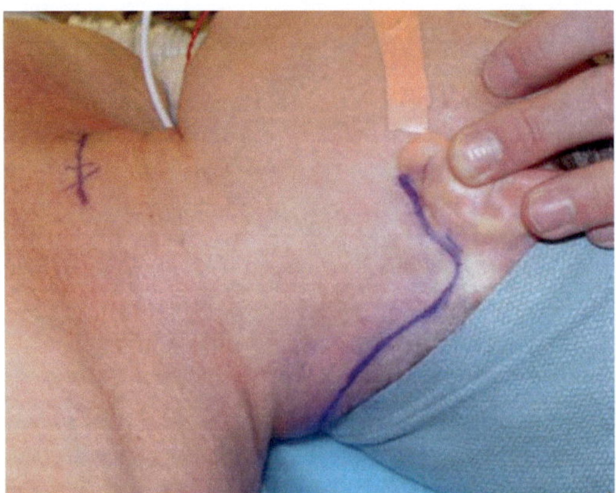

Fig. 4 Incision for remote access robotic facelift thyroidectomy. From: Terris D, Singer MC, Seybt MW. Robotic facelift thyroidectomy: patient selection and technical considerations. Surg Laparosc Percutan Tech. 2011;21(4): 237–242. Used with permission

evidence of a high-grade malignancy such as extrathyroidal extension of the lesion or concerning lymphadenopathy.

RFT Operative Details

The remote access robotic facelift thyroidectomy procedure has been described in detail [15, 34]. With the patient sitting upright in the preoperative holding area, a transverse anterior cervical incision is drawn in a natural neck crease in the unlikely event that conversion to an open procedure is necessary. The patient is then positioned just off-center of the operating table toward the side to be operated on. The top of the patient's head should be almost level with the top of the operating table.

General anesthesia is maintained with a propofol drip, which allows rapid titration of the anesthetic depth. A short-acting muscle relaxant, if necessary, is used to facilitate intubation. The patient is intubated with an EMG endotracheal tube (ETT) to permit intraoperative laryngeal nerve monitoring. A GlideScope (Verathon Inc, Bothell, WA) is useful during intubation so that all members of the operative team can confirm proper positioning of the EMG electrodes. A straight extension is placed on the anesthesia circuit to limit tension on the tubing. A 3-way stop-cock valve connects the CO_2 return tubing to the anesthesia circuit to prevent kinking of this tube. The bed is rotated 180° so that the patient's head is away from the anesthesia provider. The patient's arms are tucked at their sides and secured with wide silk tape. A formal safety strap that attaches to the table is not used above the patient's waist because the strap interferes with placement of the retractors. The patient's head is turned 20°–30° away from the surgical side, with the face supported with soft towels. The anesthesia circuit is taped to the operating table to prevent any excessive tension which might cause the endotracheal tube to twist or migrate.

One centimeter of the occipital hairline is shaved and the facelift incision is marked. The incision begins in the postauricular crease near the inferior extent of the earlobe, and is carried superiorly and then posteriorly into the shaved region of the occipital hairline in a gentle curve that will be obscured by the auricle (Fig. 4). This placement ensures the incision will be completely concealed once the hair regrows. The incision continues posteriorly and inferiorly as far as necessary to ensure adequate exposure.

The planned incision line is then infiltrated with 0.25 % bupivacaine with 1:200,000 epinephrine and the patient is prepped and draped in sterile fashion. The skin is incised with a knife and a guarded electrosurgical handpiece is used to develop a subplatysmal flap until the SCM is identified. Dissection then continues anteriorly and inferiorly along the SCM as a series of landmarks are encountered. The great auricular nerve (GAN) is the first structure identified. Further dissection superficial to the GAN exposes the external jugular vein and the anterior border of the SCM. The external jugular vein is preserved, though it may be divided if necessary to improve exposure. Dissection continues down the anteromedial border of the SCM to the clavicle. Placing the operating table in reverse Trendelenberg and rotating it away from the surgeon facilitates visualization during the deeper portion of the dissection.

A muscular triangle bounded by the anterior border of the SCM, the superior border of the omohyoid, and the posterior border of the sternohyoid

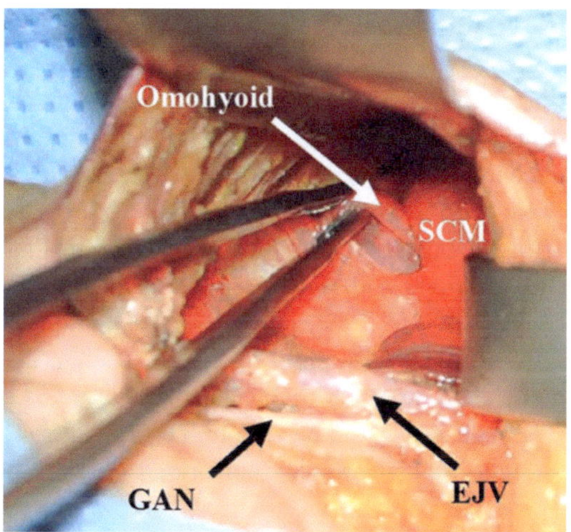

Fig. 5 Remote access robotic facelift thyroidectomy operative pocket showing the great auricular nerve (GAN), external jugular vein (EJV), omohyoid, and sternocleidomastoid (SCM). From: Terris DJ, Singer MC, Seybt MW. Robot facelift thyroidectomy: II. Clinical feasibility and safety. Laryngoscope. 2011;121:1636–1641. Used with permission

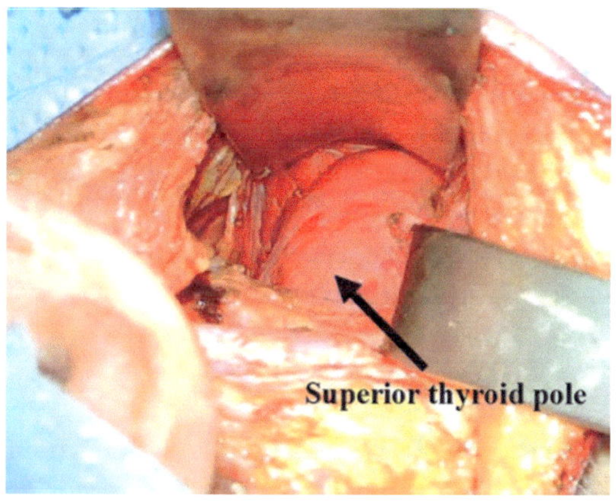

Fig. 6 View of superior pole of thyroid in the remote access robotic facelift thyroidectomy. From: Terris DJ, Singer MC, Seybt MW. Robot facelift thyroidectomy: II. Clinical feasibility and safety. Laryngoscope. 2011; 121:1636–1641. Used with permission

is defined (Fig. 5). The omohyoid, sternohyoid, and sternothyroid muscles are retracted ventrally to expose the superior pole of the thyroid gland (Fig. 6). The strap muscles are then elevated off of the rest of the thyroid lobe and the superior vascular pedicle is isolated. The lobe is mobilized as much as possible during this dissection. The

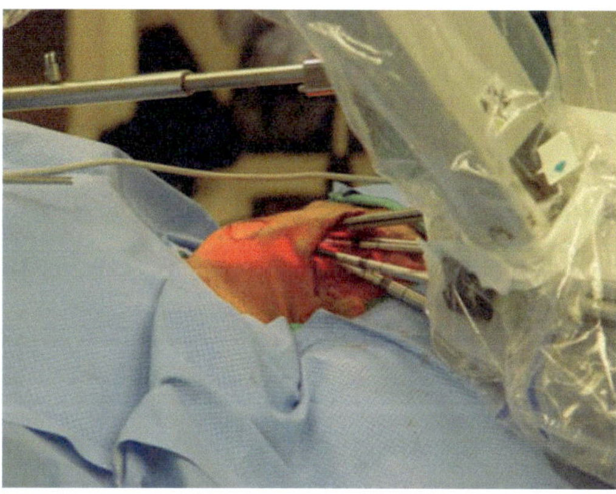

Fig. 7 Retractor and robotic arms positioned for a remote access robotic facelift thyroidectomy. From: Terris D, Singer MC, Seybt MW. Robotic facelift thyroidectomy: patient selection and technical considerations. Surg Laparosc Percutan Tech. 2011;21(4):237–242. Used with permission

modified Chung retractor (Marina Medical, Sunrise, FL) is positioned to retract the strap muscles ventrally. The retractor system is anchored to the operating table frame on the side opposite the lobe being resected. A Singer hook (Medtronic, Jacksonville FL) attached to a Greenberg retractor (Codman & Shurtleff, Inc, Raynham, MA) secured to the ipsilateral side of the table is used to retract the SCM laterally and dorsally, thereby securing the surgical pocket. The robotic cart is then deployed.

The robotic console is positioned near the operating table opposite of the side being dissected, with the pedestal angled 30° away from the table. Fine positioning adjustments are more easily accomplished by moving the table rather than by moving the robot console. The camera arm with a 30° down facing endoscope is positioned first, and the camera is advanced along the long axis of the modified Chung retractor. The camera arm is nearly fully extended so the elbow joints of the camera arm will not impede the movement of the other arms. A Harmonic device is placed in the dominant arm and a Maryland grasper is used in the nondominant arm (Fig. 7).

The robotic portion of the procedure begins by dividing the superior vascular pedicle with the Harmonic device. The superior thyroid pole is retracted inferiorly and ventrally to expose the

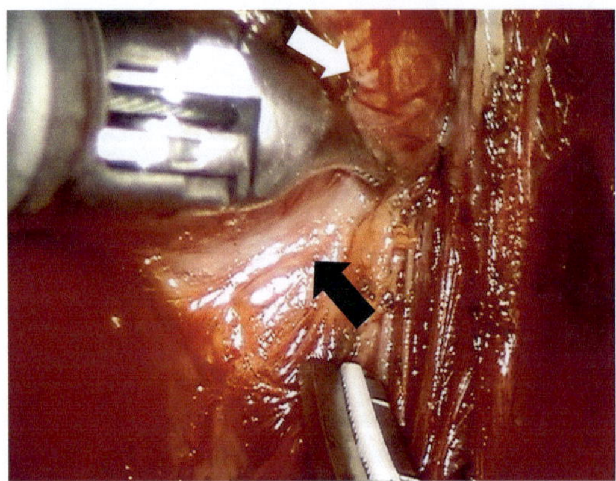

Fig. 8 View of recurrent laryngeal nerve (*black arrow*) and thyroid gland (*white arrow*) in the remote access robotic facelift thyroidectomy

inferior constrictor muscle. This muscle is traced inferiorly to its lower border, taking care to avoid injuring the superior laryngeal nerve. The superior parathyroid gland is identified on the posterior aspect of the thyroid and reflected away from the thyroid. The RLN is then identified laterally as it courses under the inferior constrictor (Fig. 8). The nerve is dissected inferiorly, exposing the ligament of Berry. With the nerve under direct visualization, the ligament is transected with the Harmonic device and the thyroid isthmus is divided. The middle thyroid vein is then divided. The inferior parathyroid gland is bluntly dissected inferiorly away from the thyroid, and the inferior vasculature is transected with the Harmonic device. Any remaining attachments between the thyroid lobe and the surrounding soft tissue or trachea are divided and the specimen is removed.

The robotic cart is removed. The surgical field is irrigated and Surgicel (Ethicon, Inc., Somerville, NJ) is placed into the thyroid bed. The incision is approximated using buried interrupted deep dermal 4-0 Vicryl sutures (Ethicon, Inc., Somerville, NJ). The skin edges are sealed with Dermaflex tissue adhesive (Chemence Medical Products, Inc., Alpharetta, GA) and ¼ inch Steri-Strips (3 M Corporation, St. Paul, MN) placed horizontally along the incision. No drains are utilized. Deep extubation is preferable to minimize coughing or straining on emergence from anesthesia.

RFT Outcomes

The RFT approach was first described in 2011, when Terris et al. [15] published a series of 14 patients undergoing 18 RFT procedures with a mean operative time of 155 min. One patient had a single-stage total thyroidectomy through bilateral incisions and three patients had a second completion RFT procedure to address malignancies identified at the initial surgery. Though the first patient treated with this technique received a drain and was admitted for observation, all subsequent procedures were performed on an outpatient basis without a drain. There were two seromas and one case of transient vocal fold weakness in this series. These conditions each resolved spontaneously without intervention. All patients experienced temporary hypesthesia of the great auricular nerve that resolved within several weeks after surgery. There were no instances of permanent vocal cord weakness or hypoparathyroidism. There were no conversions to a traditional open approach.

A follow-up study [34] expanded the patient selection criteria, including suggested limitations on the maximum nodule size appropriate for RFT as well as medical contraindications (discussed previously). This study also included an additional three patients undergoing unilateral RFT, none of whom experienced any complications. To date, a total of 22 RFT procedures in 18 patients have been reported in peer-reviewed publications [15, 34, 35].

More than 50 RFT procedures have now been accomplished in our center. These procedures were completed on an outpatient basis without drainage in all but the first patient. There have been no episodes of hypocalcemia and no conversions to an anterior approach. This experience has been repeated in at least four centers, with more than 100 procedures accomplished with the same safety profile as described in the original reports.

Two comparisons of the RFT and RAT techniques have been performed [14, 31]. In one study, morphometric analysis in cadaver models revealed that the RFT approach required a 38 % smaller area of dissection than the RAT [14].

In a study directly comparing the two techniques in patients, the mean operative time for the first ten RFT procedures was 156.9 min compared to 196 min for the five axillary approach procedures [31]. Though these differences were not of statistical significance in this small series, the operative time in the RFT group compared favorably with early reports of the remote access robotic axillary approach [9, 36] and steadily shortened throughout the study period, whereas the RAT times remained stable. All RAT patients were managed with drains as inpatients, while all but the first RFT patient were discharged on the day of surgery without drains. All patients treated with the axillary approach experienced chest wall numbness, while hypesthesia of the great auricular nerve distribution was ubiquitous in the RFT population. No major or permanent complications have been reported with the RFT approach. A large-scale multi-institutional review of the RFT experience in the United States is currently underway.

Current Considerations in Remote Access Robotic Thyroid Surgery

There is no doubt that some individual patients and patient groups place an extremely high value on the possibility of thyroid surgery without a visible neck scar. However, while remote access robotic thyroid surgery has been proven to be a safe, popular, and oncologically equivalent alternative to the traditional thyroidectomy in certain Asian markets, particularly South Korea, the concept has not fared as well in other countries. Despite early enthusiasm for this technology, a number of limitations and concerns surfaced as more surgeons and patients in Western practices gained experience with remote access robotic thyroidectomy techniques, in particular the RAT, which has proven to be dangerous for most American patients and most American practices [12, 13, 24] .

As discussed earlier, a number of new and sometimes catastrophic complications were encountered as this technique was implemented in the United States. The reasons for this are not completely clear, but may be related to differences in the body habitus or thyroid disease characteristics of Western patients or in the degree of surgical experience necessary to master these techniques. Many Western authors have suggested that RAT is more difficult in larger patients [18, 21, 23, 32]. According to the most recent World Health Organization data, over 60 % of the population in the United States is overweight or obese, versus South Korea, where over 60 % of the population has a normal BMI [37]. In a large study of South Korean RAT patients, the mean nodule diameter was 0.8 cm, while in many Western series the mean nodule size is consistently over 2.4 cm [23, 24, 26]. Careful patient selection may help overcome some of these differences. While specific nodule size limits have been proposed for RFT [34], no specific BMI or body habitus parameters have been established for safe remote access robotic thyroid surgery in Western patients.

There is a recognized learning curve in remote access robotic thyroid surgery. Kang et al. noted that their time spent operating at the robotic console stabilized after approximately 40–45 procedures [9]. Given that the vast majority of thyroid procedures are performed by low- to intermediate-volume surgeons [38] and given the low number of Western patients who are likely candidates for the procedure, it is doubtful that the majority of thyroid surgeons would achieve a consistently high caseload of remote access robotic thyroidectomies to overcome this learning curve and sustain their skillset to remain proficient in these procedures. A set of guidelines suggesting the minimum requirements for embarking on a safe robotic thyroidectomy program have been published [39].

Recent changes and uncertainty in the healthcare marketplace mandate evaluation of the financial and resource utilization implications when introducing new surgical technology. The surgical robot requires a large initial capital investment, as well as the cost of service contracts and disposable supplies. RAT has been shown to be significantly (1.5 times) more expensive than conventional thyroid surgery [11, 12], and this cost difference did not resolve until the RAT operative time was reduced to 68 min [11], an outcome that has not been achieved in any published series. While no direct comparison has been performed evaluating the cost of the RFT procedure, in a small series comparing RAT to RFT there was no significant difference in operative time between the two approaches [31], so it is reasonable to assume this procedure has a similar cost profile as the RAT approach, with the exception of the associated postoperative inpatient hospitalization costs.

Another important financial consideration in remote access robotic thyroid surgery is the issue of reimbursement. In South Korea, an endoscopic thyroidectomy is reimbursed at double the rate of conventional thyroid surgery, while robotic thyroidectomy receives four times the remuneration [18, 26]. In the United States reimbursement is based on the extent of the thyroid surgery performed, not the manner in which it is performed. This may lead some surgeons to question if it is financially reasonable to offer these procedures in their practice.

A final obstacle facing remote access robotic thyroid surgery in the United States relates to the current status of industry approval and Food and Drug Administration (FDA) approval of these techniques. In October, 2011, the manufacturer of the only commercially available surgical robot issued a statement that it would no longer support any activities associated with robotic thyroid surgery, pending further FDA approval [12, 13]. The status of this approval and renewed industry support for these procedures is currently unknown.

Despite these considerations, there is still considerable consumer demand for these procedures from patients who, either for personal or professional reasons, wish to make every effort to avoid an anterior neck scar. For these individuals the transient side effects, increased operative times, and potential risks of remote access robotic thyroid surgery are eclipsed by the possibility of living the rest of their lives without the visible stigma of neck surgery.

Conclusion

Remote access approaches represent the newest frontier in thyroid surgery. These procedures offer patients the possibility of treating their disease without the visible incision associated with more traditional thyroidectomy approaches. Though the remote access robotic axillary thyroidectomy approach has proven both successful and popular in certain Asian countries, the initial enthusiasm in Western markets for this technique has been tempered by factors such as patient candidacy, safety, and questions of resource utilization, and it is being increasingly abandoned in the United States. The remote access robotic facelift thyroidectomy overcomes many of the limitations associated with the axillary approach. Robotic-assisted thyroid surgery continues to be refined in several specialized North American centers, and consumer demand for these remote access, hidden-incision approaches remains high among those patients who place a premium on the cosmetic outcomes of thyroid surgery.

References

1. Ohgami M, Ishii S, Arisawa Y, et al. Scarless endoscopic thyroidectomy: breast approach for better cosmesis. Surg Laparosc Percutan Tech. 2000; 10:1–4.
2. Ikeda Y, Takami H, Niimi M, et al. Endoscopic thyroidectomy by the axillary approach. Surg Endosc. 2001;15:1362–4.
3. Park YL, Han WK, Bae WG. 100 cases of endoscopic thyroidectomy: breast approach. Surg Laparosc Percutan Tech. 2003;1:20–5.
4. Ikeda Y, Takami H, Sasaki Y, et al. Clinical benefits in endoscopic thyroidectomy by the axillary approach. J Am Coll Surg. 2003;196:189–95.
5. Shimazu K, Shiba E, Tamaki Y, et al. Endoscopic thyroid surgery through the axillo-bilateral-breast approach. Surg Laparosc Percutan Tech. 2003;13: 196–201.
6. Choe JH, Kim SW, Chung KW, et al. Endoscopic thyroidectomy using a new bilateral axillo-breast approach. World J Surg. 2007;31:601–6.
7. Kang SW, Jeong JJ, Yun JS, et al. Robot-assisted endoscopic surgery for thyroid cancer: experience with the first 100 patients. Surg Endosc. 2009;23: 2399–406.

8. Lobe TE, Wright SK, Irish MS. Novel uses of surgical robotics in head and neck surgery. J Laparoendosc Adv Surg Tech. 2005;15(6):647–52.
9. Kang SW, Lee SC, Lee SH, et al. Robotic thyroid surgery using a gasless, transaxillary approach and the da Vinci S system: the operative outcomes of 338 consecutive patients. Surgery. 2009;146:1048–55.
10. Cadière GB, Himpens J, Germay O, et al. Feasibility of robotic laparoscopic surgery: 146 cases. World J Surg. 2001;25:1467–77.
11. Cabot JC, Lee CR, Brunaud L, et al. Robotic and endoscopic transaxillary thyroidectomies may be cost prohibitive when compared to standard cervical thyroidectomy: a cost analysis. Surgery. 2012;152: 1016–24.
12. Inabnet WB. Robotic thyroidectomy: Must we drive a luxury sedan to arrive at our destination safely? Thyroid. 2012;22:988–90.
13. Perrier ND. Why I, have abandoned robot-assisted transaxillary thyroid surgery. Surgery. 2012;152: 1025–6.
14. Singer MC, Seybt MW, Terris DJ. Robotic facelift thyroidectomy: I. Preclinical simulation and morphometric assessment. Laryngoscope. 2011;121:1631–5.
15. Terris DJ, Singer MC, Seybt MW. Robot facelift thyroidectomy: II. Clinical feasibility and safety. Laryngoscope. 2011;121:1636–41.
16. Li-Tsang CWP, Lau JCM, Chan CCH. Prevalence of hypertrophic scan formation and its characteristics among the Chinese population. Burns. 2005;31: 610–6.
17. McCurdy JA. Considerations in Asian cosmetic surgery. Facial Plast Surg Clin N Am. 2007;15:387–97.
18. Duh QY. Robot-assisted endoscopic thyroidectomy. Has the time come to abandon neck incisions? Ann Surg. 2011;253(6):1067–8.
19. Chung WY. Pros of robotic transaxillary thyroid surgery: its impact on cancer control and surgical quality. Thyroid. 2012;22(10):986–7.
20. Jackson NR, Yao L, Tufano RP, Kandil EH. Safety of robotic thyroidectomy approaches: meta-analysis and systematic review. Head Neck. 2014;36(1):137–43.
21. Kuppersmith RB, Holsinger FC. Robotic thyroid surgery: an initial experience with North American patients. Laryngoscope. 2011;121:521–6.
22. Berber E, Siperstein A. Robotic transaxillary total thyroidectomy using a unilateral approach. Surg Laparosc Endosc Percutan Tech. 2011;21:207–10.
23. Kandil EH, Noureldine SI, Yao L, Slakey DP. Robotic transaxillary thyroidectomy: an examination of the first one hundred cases. J Am Coll Surg. 2012;214: 558–66.
24. Lin HS, Folbe AJ, Carron MA, et al. Single-incision transaxillary robotic thyroidectomy: challenges and limitations in a North American population. Otolaryngol Head Neck Surg. 2012;147(6):1041–6.
25. Gross ND. Is robotic thyroid surgery worth the learning curve? Otolaryngol Head Neck Surg. 2012;147(6):1047–8.
26. Dionigi G. Robotic thyroidectomy: Seoul is not Varese. Otolaryngol Head Neck Surg. 2013;148:178.
27. Kang SW, Lee SH, Ryu HR, et al. Initial experience with robot-assisted modified radical neck dissection for the management of thyroid carcinoma with lateral neck node metastasis. Surgery. 2010;148:1214–21.
28. Ryu HR, Kang SW, Lee SH, et al. Feasibility and safety of a new robotic thyroidectomy through a gasless, transaxillary single-incision approach. J Am Coll Surg. 2010;211(3):e13–9.
29. Tae K, Ji YB, Cho SH, et al. Early surgical outcomes of robotic thyroidectomy by a gasless unilateral axillo-breast or axillary approach for papillary thyroid carcinoma: 2 years' experience. Head Neck. 2012;34: 617–25.
30. Kang SW, Park JH, Jeong JS, et al. Prospects of robotic thyroidectomy using a gasless transaxillary approach for the management of thyroid carcinoma. Surg Laparosc Endosc Percutan Tech. 2011;21: 223–9.
31. Terris DJ, Singer MC. Qualitative and quantitative differences between 2 robotic thyroidectomy techniques. Otolaryngol Head Neck Surg. 2012;147(1): 20–5.
32. Landry C, Grubbs E, Warneke C, et al. Robot-assisted transaxillary thyroid surgery in the United States: is it comparable to open thyroid lobectomy? Ann Surg Oncol. 2012;19:1269–74.
33. Miccoli P, Berti P, Raffaelli M, et al. Minimally invasive video-assisted thyroidectomy. Am J Surg. 2001;181:567–70.
34. Terris D, Singer MC, Seybt MW. Robotic facelift thyroidectomy: patient selection and technical considerations. Surg Laparosc Percutan Tech. 2011;21(4): 237–42.
35. Terris DJ, Singer MC. Robotic facelift thyroidectomy: facilitating remote access surgery. Head Neck. 2012;34:746–7.
36. Stevenson CE, Gardner DF, Grover AC. Patient factors affecting operative times for single-incision transaxillary robotic-assisted (STAR) thyroid lobectomy: does size matter? Ann Surg Oncol. 2012;19:1460–5.
37. WHO Global Database on Body Mass Index. Available at: http://apps.who.int/bmi. Accessed 8 Jan 2014.
38. Kandil E, Noureldine SI, Abbas A, Tufano RP. The impact of surgical volume on patient outcomes following thyroid surgery. Surgery. 2013;154: 1346–53.
39. Perrier ND, Randolph GW, Inabnet III WB, et al. Robotic thyroidectomy: a framework for new technology assessment and safe implementation. Thyroid. 2010;20(12):1327–32.

Robotic Surgery of the Parathyroid Glands

George Garas, Asit Arora, and Neil Tolley

Introduction

In 1925 Felix Mandl successfully performed the first parathyroidectomy in Vienna [1]. Since then, parathyroid surgery has undergone considerable evolution. Traditionally, the treatment for primary hyperparathyroidism (pHPT) involved a collar incision with bilateral cervical exploration to identify all four parathyroid glands with resection of the pathological one(s) [2]. However, as 80–90 % of cases are due to a single adenoma, removal of one gland leads to cure in the majority of cases [2]. This combined with the introduction of new imaging modalities such as high-resolution ultrasound, sestamibi scintigraphy and 4-dimensional computed tomography (4D-CT) allowed for the accurate preoperative localization of the parathyroid adenoma and led to the introduction of the concept of "targeted parathyroidectomy" [2, 3].

The first unilateral approach for the treatment of hyperparathyroidism due to solitary adenoma was reported by Tibblin et al. in 1984 [4]. Following this, a variety of targeted approaches have been described. Examples include radioguided parathyroidectomy, minimally invasive video-assisted parathyroidectomy (MIVAP) and mini-incision focused parathyroidectomy [5–7]. Gagner performed the first endoscopic parathyroidectomy in 1996 [8]. The technique was not adopted widely due to its technical difficulty, long operative time (lasting over 5 h) and complications following gas insufflation [9].

The targeted approach for parathyroidectomy has become the co-gold-standard procedure for pHPT as its results are equivalent to bilateral cervical exploration. As a result, minimal access techniques have replaced bilateral cervical exploration where the adenoma has been localized preoperatively. In non-localized disease, bilateral cervical exploration remains the optimal operation [3]. Despite the numerous techniques described for targeted parathyroidectomy, none has been shown to be overwhelmingly superior [1].

In 2000, Ikeda et al. described an endoscopic approach for performing targeted parathyroidectomy that avoids a neck scar. This used an extra-cervical approach to perform a unilateral neck exploration through an ipsilateral axillary incision [10]. Despite achieving "excellent" cosmetic outcomes due to the absence of a neck scar, the technique was not adopted widely due to the limitations associated with performing endoscopic surgery in a restricted workspace such as the neck [11, 12].

With the introduction of the da Vinci robot (Intuitive Surgical, Inc, Sunnyvale, CA), the advent of robotic-assisted parathyroidectomy

G. Garas, B.Sc., M.B.B.S., M.R.C.S., D.O.H.N.S. (✉)
A. Arora, M.B.B.S., M.R.C.S., D.O.H.N.S.
N. Tolley, M.D., F.R.C.S., D.L.O.
Department of Surgery and Cancer, Imperial College London, St. Mary's Hospital Campus, London W2 1NY, UK
e-mail: g.garas@imperial.ac.uk

G.A. Grillone and S. Jalisi (eds.), *Robotic Surgery of the Head and Neck: A Comprehensive Guide*, DOI 10.1007/978-1-4939-1547-7_13, © Springer Science+Business Media New York 2015

(RAP) was the next logical step. The technique was first described by Tolley et al. in London in 2011 [3].

The Rationale Behind Robotic-Assisted Parathyroidectomy

The introduction of robotic technology has greatly improved and facilitated extracervical endoscopic approaches to the neck. Similar to Robotic-Assisted Thyroidectomy (RAT), the rationale of RAP is to be able to offer carefully selected patients a targeted parathyroidectomy approach that is at least as safe and effective as the conventional (open) approach [13]. In addition to making endoscopic parathyroidectomy less technically challenging, the intention with RAP is to offer patients the possibility of avoiding a neck scar [3, 14, 15]. Although neck scars usually heal well and are associated with high patient satisfaction, this is not always the case. A subset of patients (particularly those with darker skin color) are prone to hypertrophic and/or keloid scarring (Fig. 1). When this happens, scar satisfaction is poor. As the majority of patients suffering from pHPT are women, the issue of satisfaction with scar cosmesis is particularly relevant [16]. RAP may also have an important role to play in patients from certain Asian countries, particularly South Korea and Japan [17]. In those cultures, a horizontal scar in the neck denotes death [16]. As a result, both endoscopic and robotic transaxillary approaches for thyroidectomy were first described there. Moreover, the largest RAT series also originate from South Korea [18, 19]. Early results predict a promising future for RAP and long-term data are currently awaited.

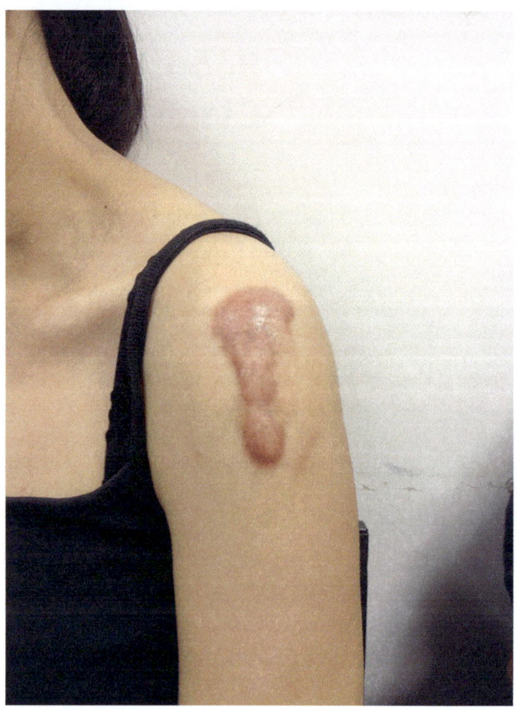

Fig. 1 Keloid scarring on the deltoid area following vaccination. A patient who may have valid reasons for avoiding a visible neck scar

Patient Selection for Robotic-Assisted Parathyroidectomy

As with all surgical operations, careful patient selection is paramount to the successful implementation of RAP. Patients should be carefully evaluated preoperatively and RAP only offered to those considered suitable. Multidisciplinary management with an endocrinologist is essential. The diagnosis of pHPT needs to be confirmed by demonstrating a raised serum calcium and parathyroid hormone (PTH). Vitamin D deficiency and Familial Hypocalciuric Hypercalcemia (FHH) need to be excluded by measuring serum vitamin D levels and 24-h urine calcium:creatinine clearance ratios respectively as these do not require surgical intervention [2].

There are parathyroid specific as well as generic considerations for RAP. With regard to the parathyroid, the indications for RAP are the same as for any targeted parathyroidectomy approach. Hence, RAP should only be offered to patients who have pHPT with a preoperatively localized adenoma. The authors advocate triple modality concordance as a prerequisite using ultrasonography, sestamibi scintigraphy and single-photon emission computed tomography (SPECT-CT) to minimize the risk of failure. However, it is likely that dual modality concordance

Table 1 Contraindications to robotic-assisted parathyroidectomy

Contraindications to robotic-assisted parathyroidectomy
• Large goiter ipsilaterally
• Suspicion of parathyroid carcinoma
• Previous neck surgery
• History of neck irradiation
• A large body habitus (BMI > 30)
• Degenerative shoulder pathology ipsilaterally
• Significant co-morbidity (ASA > 2)

(with ultrasonography and sestamibi scintigraphy) is just as adequate. The accuracy of localizing a single adenoma is reported to be 94–99 % with this modality [2].

There is no limitation to the size of the adenoma, and contrary to thyroid nodules that can reach a very large size, parathyroid adenomas are usually relatively small. RAP should not be offered to patients where there is suspicion of malignant disease, a coexistent large goiter ipsilaterally, history of previous neck surgery or irradiation and to those with a large body habitus. Relative contraindications to RAP include ipsilateral degenerative shoulder pathology or significant co-morbidity placing them in an American Society of Anesthesiologists (ASA) category greater than 2. The contraindications to RAP are summarized in Table 1.

The location of the parathyroid adenoma (including extracervical—ectopic location) is not a contraindication and a robotic-assisted thoracoscopic approach has been described to remove ectopic parathyroid adenoma in the mediastinum [20–23]. This approach is beyond the scope of the chapter.

The ideal RAP patient would be a slim female with a preoperatively localized parathyroid adenoma showing concordance on at least 2 imaging modalities.

Consent for Robotic-Assisted Parathyroidectomy

As with all surgical operations, informed consent is essential and should be undertaken by the attending surgeon. The literature supports that RAP is as safe as conventional parathyroidectomy [2, 3, 16, 17, 24, 25]. The risks associated with RAP are the same as for conventional parathyroidectomy with regard to the recurrent laryngeal nerve, infection, hematoma and hypoparathyroidism. Despite the anaerobic nature of the axilla, the literature does not support an increased infection rate with RAP compared to cervical parathyroidectomy [2, 3, 16, 17, 24, 25]. This "shifting" of the incision does however significantly prolong the operative time as a long subcutaneous flap must be raised to reach the neck and this should be explained to the patient. This may be associated with sensory changes of the overlying skin and higher pain scores and dysesthesia over the area of subcutaneous dissection. These symptoms are usually temporary [2, 16].

The two different approaches should be explained during the consent process. In general, the transaxillary incision is recommended for females because of breast concerns. For males, an infraclavicular incision can be used instead. The approach needs to be decided in conjunction with the patient at the time of obtaining their informed consent.

In the event of a post-operative hematoma, this is less likely to lead to airway obstruction because the potential space for the hematoma to disseminate is so capacious compared to cervical parathyroidectomy.

Another important point that the patient needs to be made aware of is the potential complication of developing a brachial plexus neurapraxia. The postulated mechanism is a traction injury when the ipsilateral arm is raised to reduce the distance between the axilla and anterior neck [26, 27]. This stretch injury is rare and can be prevented by adjusting the position of the ipsilateral arm with the patient awake to assess for comfort [28]. The back of the patient's hand is positioned so that it is touching the central portion of the forehead. This is known as the "extended salute" position.

RAP achieves the objective of "shifting" the incision from the neck to the axilla or infraclavicular area at the expense of an increased operative time. The inpatient stay and time off work are similar to the conventional open technique [3, 16].

Robotic-Assisted Parathyroidectomy: Surgical Technique

Approaches for RAP

There are two distinct approaches for RAP: (1) the transaxillary approach [2, 16, 17, 24, 25] and (2) the infraclavicular approach [3]. The transaxillary incision is preferred for females due to concerns regarding breast scar cosmesis. For male and selected female patients, a 3 cm infraclavicular incision can be used instead as this minimizes the area of subcutaneous dissection when raising the flap. The disadvantage of the infraclavicular approach is that it requires two additional 5 mm trocar skin incisions. These are made high in the anterior axillary line and skin–areolar junction of the nipple whereas the axillary approach requires only one 6 cm incision. Both approaches are described in detail below.

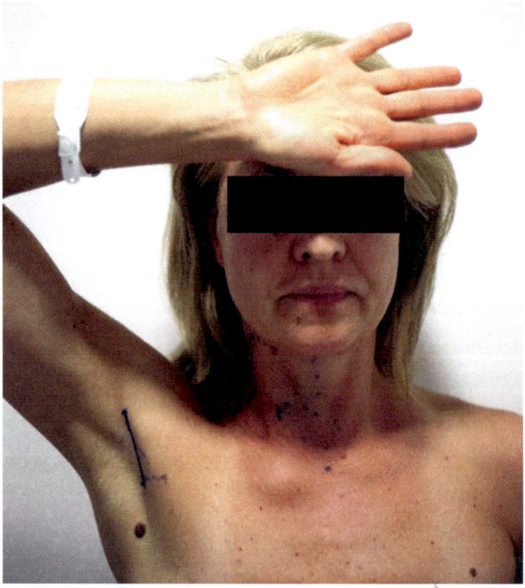

Fig. 2 The "extended salute" position for transaxillary robotic-assisted parathyroidectomy. By adjusting the position of the ipsilateral arm with the patient awake to assess for comfort, the risk of traction injury to the brachial plexus is prevented. Doing so and marking the incision immediately prior to surgery constitute vital components of preoperative planning

Operative Set-up

1. Preoperative Considerations

Team work is essential in the preoperative preparation of the patient and setting up of the operating room (OR). The ipsilateral arm to the parathyroid adenoma must be free of identification bracelets, lines, blood pressure cuffs or ECG leads.

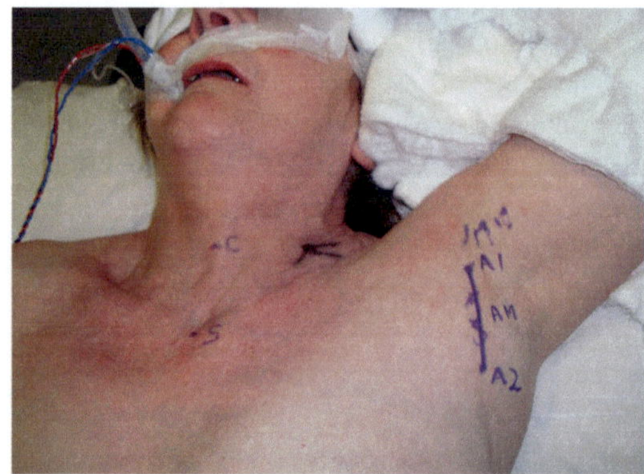

Fig. 3 Surgical position for left transaxillary robotic-assisted parathyroidectomy (laterality pre-marked with arrow). The 5–6 cm axillary incision has been pre-marked and re-checked once the patient is positioned on the operating table as in our experience this is the optimal way to plan where to place the incision to prevent subsequent migration. *C* cricoid cartilage, *S* suprasternal notch, *A1* superior axillary, *AM* mid-axillary, *A2* inferior axillary points of incision

Transaxillary Approach RAP

For the transaxillary approach it is important to position the patient's ipsilateral arm when they are awake in order to ensure comfort and thus minimize the risk of traction on the brachial plexus with subsequent neurapraxia. The arm position involves the back of the patient's hand touching the central portion of the forehead, in an "extended salute" position (Fig. 2). A 5–6 cm axillary incision is also marked at this point as in our experience this is the optimal way to plan where to place the incision to prevent subsequent migration (Fig. 3). The incision may need to be

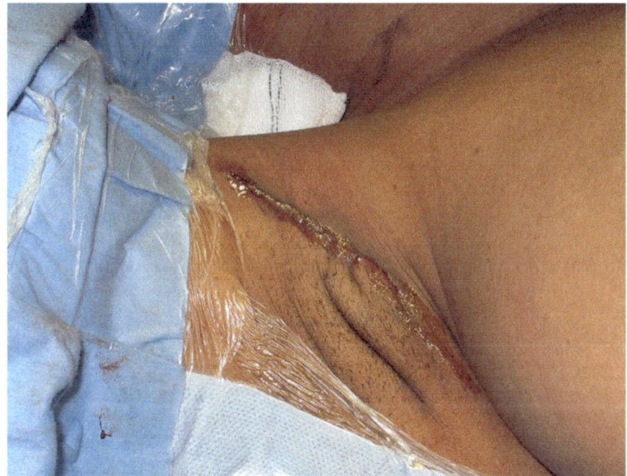

Fig. 4 Axillary incision at the end of right transaxillary robotic-assisted parathyroidectomy. The incision has been extended superiorly in a curvilinear fashion so that it sits in a natural crease. This reduces tension and a tendency towards hypertrophic and pigmented scarring

extended superiorly in a curvilinear fashion so that it sits in a natural crease which reduces tension and a tendency towards hypertrophic and pigmented scarring (Fig. 4).

Infraclavicular Approach RAP

If an infraclavicular approach has been chosen (incision usually 3 cm in length), this is also marked at this stage as are the sites of insertion for the two trocars in the ipsilateral anterior axillary line and periareolar region, respectively. The infraclavicular approach is particularly useful in the muscular male with a hirsute anterior chest wall. With experience and correct planning the incision heals well and becomes almost invisible (Fig. 5).

At this stage, the anesthesiologist intubates the patient and ventilates them via a transoral endotracheal tube with electrodes (NIM EMG Endotracheal Tube, Medtronic, Inc, Jacksonville, FL). The correct positioning of the NIM EMG endotracheal tube with the electrodes at the level of the glottis is confirmed by direct laryngoscopy. Visualization of the electromyographic waveform on the nerve integrity monitor (NIM) following insertion of the stimulator and earth leads serves as additional confirmation. An extended tip of the NIM must be available due to the long distance between the incision (transaxillary or infraclavicular) and neck [17]. At induction, the patient is routinely administered intravenously 1.2 g co-amoxiclav and 4 mg dexamethasone.

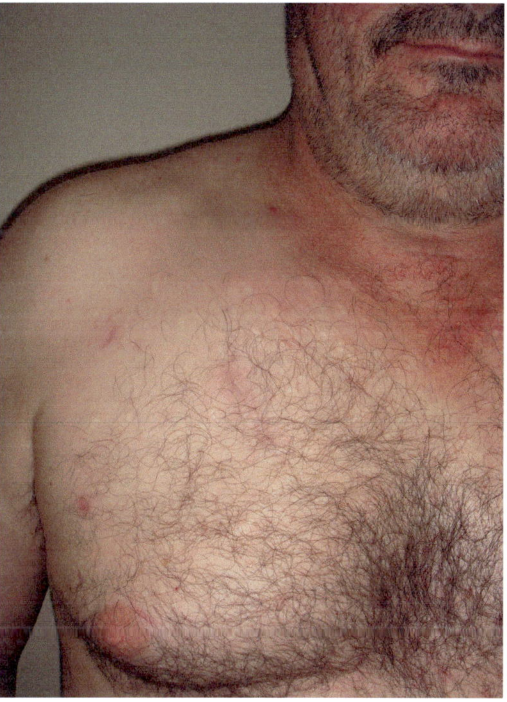

Fig. 5 Patient 4 weeks after right robotic-assisted parathyroidectomy via an infraclavicular approach. The 3 cm infraclavicular incision is barely visible as are the ports of entry for the trocars. With experience and correct planning the incisions heal well and become almost invisible. This approach is particularly useful in the muscular male with a hirsute anterior chest wall

2. Operating Room Set-up

Prior to transfer of the patient to the operating table it is important that all three components of the da Vinci robotic system are appropriately positioned. The cart is placed on the opposite side of the operating table as shown in Fig. 6. The cart is draped and correctly positioned before the patient is moved onto the operating table in preparation for docking. The vision cart is placed to one side of the patient so that the assistant surgeon, scrub nurse and anesthesiologist all have an unobstructed view. The console surgeon can be positioned anywhere in the operating room or even in a remote area (telerobotic surgery). The standard OR configuration used is illustrated in Fig. 7.

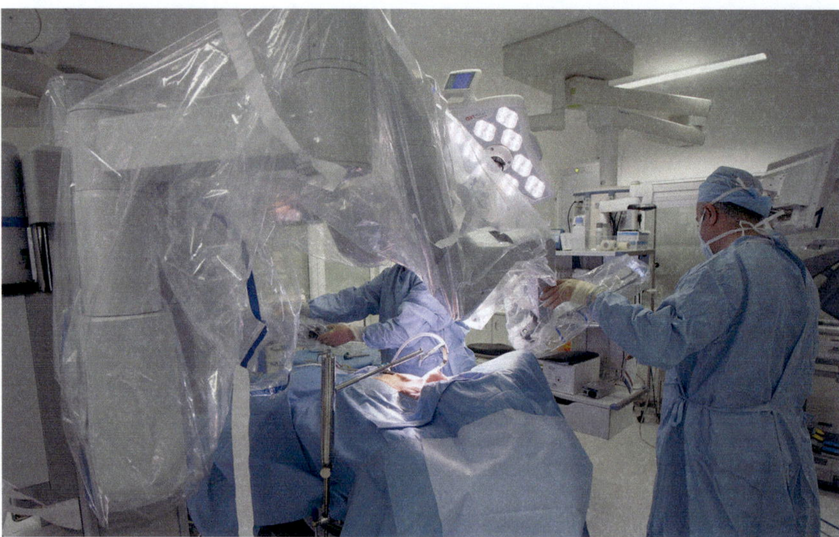

Fig. 6 The patient cart component of the robotic surgical system is covered with sterile drapes and comes in at right angles on the opposite side of the table to the parathyroid adenoma in question

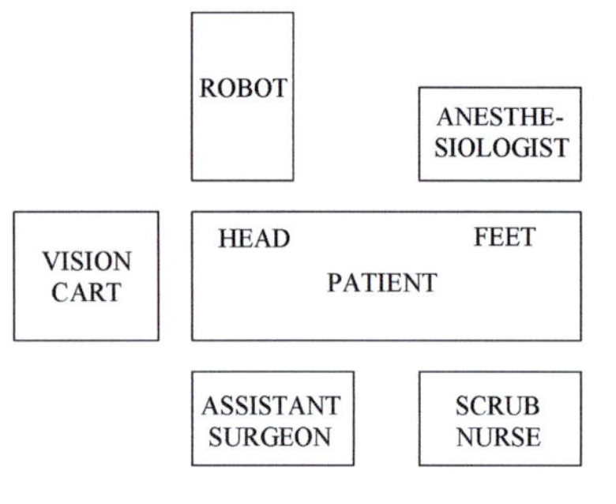

Fig. 7 Operating room configuration for right robotic-assisted parathyroidectomy

Contrary to conventional parathyroid surgery, a shoulder roll is not placed under the shoulders as this has a tendency to hyper-extend the neck and move the superior pole of the thyroid gland away from the robotic instruments. Instead, a pillow is placed under the patient's head and shoulders to provide adequate and comfortable support in a subtle "sniffing the morning air" position. The head of the table is then dropped by about 20° to widen the angle between the arm and the chest.

Transaxillary Approach RAP

For the transaxillary approach, a special arm rest supports the arm which is abducted and flexed with the forearm being pronated so that the back of the hand rests on the central portion of the forehead. A Velcro coin is attached to the hand and forehead to maintain the position (Fig. 8). This position shortens the distance between the incision site and parathyroid adenoma by elevating and externally rotating the clavicle. This is a modification to Chung's method for RAT where the arm is fully extended over the head. We advise against the fully extended arm position as this puts the brachial plexus at risk through traction. We have had no such problems since modifying Chung's method of arm positioning.

Infraclavicular Approach RAP

If the infraclavicular approach is used the ipsilateral arm is maintained in the neutral position.

Once completed, the incision site is infiltrated with 10 ml of 1 % lidocaine and 1:200,000 epinephrine. Skin preparation and draping then take place.

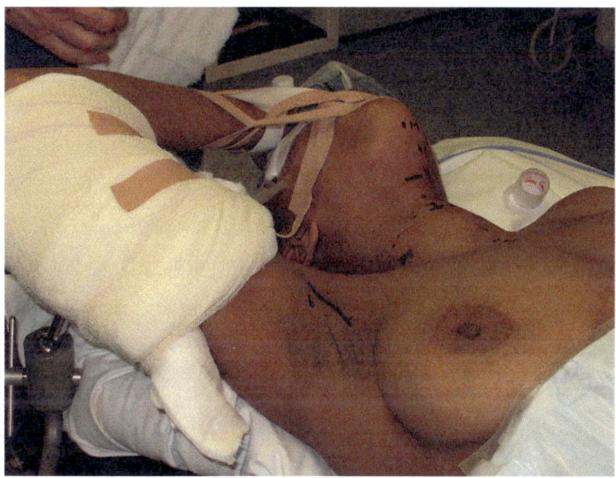

Fig. 8 Transaxillary robotic-assisted parathyroidectomy: a special arm rest supports the arm which is abducted and flexed with the forearm being pronated so that the back of the hand rests on the central portion of the forehead. A Velcro coin is attached to the hand and forehead to maintain the position. This position shortens the distance between the incision site and parathyroid adenoma by elevating and externally rotating the clavicle

The Operation

A. Preparation of the Robotic Field

Transaxillary Approach RAP

Following the axillary incision, a subcutaneous flap is raised anterior to the clavipectoral fascia. The superior and inferior points of the axillary incision are extended to the thyroid cartilage and sternal notch, respectively. The resulting shape of the flap is that of a trapezoid.

In taller patients, if the distance from the axilla to the sternal notch exceeds the limit of the instruments, the robot can be docked in earlier to perform the last (most distal) part of the subcutaneous flap raising. The technique for entering the neck is identical to the one described below but is performed robotically. This modification expands the range of patients to whom transaxillary RAP can be offered [16].

Infraclavicular Approach RAP

If the infraclavicular approach is used, then the flap is raised from the infraclavicular incision to the neck and the two trocars tunneled through small incisions made in the ipsilateral anterior axillary line or periareolar incision for the inferior 5 mm trocar.

Once the subcutaneous flap is raised, dissection is continued above the pectoralis major and over the clavicle. At this point, the sternal and clavicular heads of the sternocleidomastoid muscle are identified and the neck entered through the natural dehiscence between the two. The surgical planes are then developed as in a standard parathyroidectomy. The internal jugular vein, common carotid artery and ipsilateral omohyoid and sternohyoid muscles are exposed. The flap and strap muscles are retracted by a table-mounted self-retaining retractor (Chung, Kuppersmith, Modena or Imperial) to create sufficient working space to access the thyroid lobe laterally. No gas insufflation is required for either transaxillary or infraclavicular RAP. At this point, the da Vinci robot is docked.

B. Docking

The cart is docked at right angles to the operating table.

Transaxillary Approach RAP

All three robotic arms can be placed through the single axillary incision. The 30° down 12 mm stereoscopic endoscope is placed at an angle of 220° and is inserted low laterally extending high and upwards medially towards the thyroid gland. The 4th arm can then be placed under the endoscope which is used to contra-laterally retract the thyroid lobe. Finally, the 1st and 3rd arms are positioned which carry the instruments for dissection and hemostasis. The 4th assistant arm holds the 8 mm Prograsp, while 1st and 3rd arms have a combination of 5 mm Maryland, Debakey and Harmonic shears.

Infraclavicular Approach RAP

If the infraclavicular approach is used, a 30° down 12 mm stereoscopic endoscope is introduced into the operative field via the 3 cm infraclavicular incision. Two 5 mm robotic instruments are used. These are the Maryland and Debakey forceps which are inserted through the superior and periareolar trocars respectively until they come into view in the operative field.

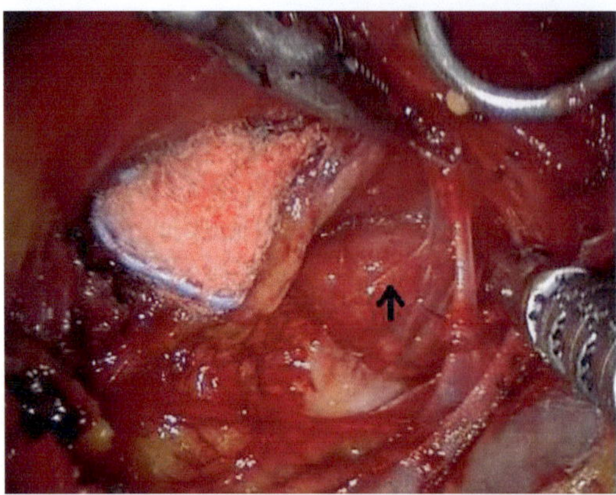

Fig. 9 Intraoperative robotic console surgery to expose the parathyroid adenoma (indicated by *arrow*)

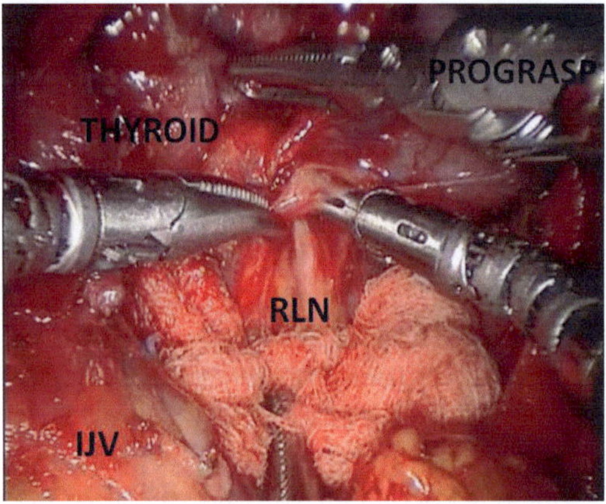

Fig. 10 Intraoperative robotic console surgery to expose the recurrent laryngeal nerve. *RLN* recurrent laryngeal nerve, *IJV* internal jugular vein

C. Robotic Surgery
The robotic dissection begins with exposure of the ipsilateral inferior thyroid pole, trachea, recurrent laryngeal nerve (RLN) and parathyroid adenoma (Figs. 9 and 10). The RLN is stimulated routinely (NIM nerve integrity monitor; Medtronic, Inc). Once the adenoma and its vascular pedicle are delineated, the Debakey dissector is replaced with the 5 mm Harmonic curved shears (Ethicon Endo-Surgery, Inc, Johnson & Johnson, Cincinnati, OH) and the pedicle sealed and divided allowing resection of the adenoma. As with all energy-based hemostatic devices, great care should be taken when using this instrument close to the RLN [29]. We do not routinely use intraoperative quick PTH (iQPTH) monitoring [3].

As with all parathyroid surgery, hemostasis should be meticulous. The anesthesiologist is asked to bring the blood pressure up to normal and a reversed Trendelenburg position and Valsava maneuver applied. Any remaining bleeding points are addressed at this stage to ensure hemostasis. As in conventional parathyroid surgery, no drain is applied. We have found this to be unproblematic.

Following hemostasis, the da Vinci robot is withdrawn and 2-layer closure completed with 4-0 subcuticular Vicryl Rapide sutures (Ethicon Products, Inc, Johnson & Johnson, Cincinnati, OH) followed by application of Dermabond (Ethicon Products, Inc, Johnson & Johnson, Cincinnati, OH) tissue glue on the wound(s). An anterior chest wall compression dressing is applied overnight.

D. Post-operative Care and Follow-Up
Patients are discharged the following morning (<24 h hospital stay). They are advised to wear a sports bra or vest for 2 weeks to provide light compression to the anterior chest wall. Antibiotics (co-amoxiclav 625 mg three times a day) are routinely given for 7 days and analgesia (acetaminophen 1 g four times a day for 7 days) as required. Regular follow-up at 2 weeks, 3, 6, 12 and 18 months allows prospective long-term evaluation.

Review of the Literature: Robotic-Assisted Parathyroidectomy

Similar to the thyroid, the elective nature and consistent anatomy of the parathyroid glands makes targeted parathyroidectomy ideal for a robotic approach [17]. Despite extensive literature on RAT, few studies exist on RAP [3, 16, 17, 24]. These are summarized in Table 2.

The first study from the United Kingdom by Tolley et al. [3] prospectively evaluated 11 patients with pHPT and a preoperatively localized adenoma. Localization was performed with a combination of ultrasound, sestamibi and

Table 2 Studies evaluating robotic-assisted parathyroidectomy

Study: Authors, year, country and type	Level of evidence	Number (n) of patients and approaches evaluated	Approach used, need for CO_2 insufflation	Use of additional equipment to daVinci robot	Key results
Foley et al. [16] 2012 USA Case control study	IIIa	$n=43$ of which: 11 RAT 4 RAP 16 OT (RAT control) 12 OP (RAP control) Mixed cohort of 43 patients: 11 RAT, 4 RAP, 16 OT (RAT control) and 12 OP (RAP control) Hence: 4 RAP (2 focal, 2 unilateral) vs. 12 matched controls (OP) for age, BMI, gender and parathyroid adenoma size	Initially transaxillary combined with small 8 mm incision in chest wall for additional port, chest wall port abandoned and approach converted to single access transaxillary, no CO_2 insufflation used	Intraoperative PTH measurement was used routinely (except for the first RAP case), IONM was not	All RAP patients became eucalcemic post-operatively Total operation time for RAP vs. OP was 186±84.2 min vs. 86±27.9 min ($p=0.001$) A learning curve was demonstrated for RAP In the RAP arm 1 patient developed a wound infection and 1 patient developed a seroma (treated conservatively) Mean incision length was significantly longer for RAP compared to OP
Katz et al. [24] 2012 USA Case report	V	$n=1$ One patient with an atypical parathyroid adenoma that underwent RAP with concomitant RAT (ipsilateral thyroid lobectomy)	Transaxillary (single access), no CO_2 insufflation used	Both IONM and intraoperative PTH measurement were used routinely	The parathyroid adenoma was successfully excised along with the ipsilateral thyroid lobe There were no complications or need for conversion to open surgery Total operative time was 95 min
Landry et al. [17] 2011 USA Individual cohort study	IIb	$n=13$ Prospective study of 13 patients: 11 underwent RAT (one of them also required completion thyroidectomy) and 2 underwent RAP	Transaxillary (single access), no CO_2 insufflation used	Both IONM and intraoperative PTH measurement were used routinely	The parathyroid adenoma was successfully excised in both cases Final pathologic evaluation was consistent with a parathyroid adenoma for both patients There were no complications Total operative times were 115 and 102 min, respectively

(continued)

Table 2 (continued)

Study: Authors, year, country and type	Level of evidence	Number (n) of patients and approaches evaluated	Approach used, need for CO_2 insufflation	Use of additional equipment to daVinci robot	Key results
Tolley et al. [3] (2011) UK Prospective cohort study	IIb	$n=11$ Prospective study of 11 patients who underwent RAP Follow-up: mean 6 months (3–12 months)	Infraclavicular along with three small incisions (one 12 mm and two 5 mm) for trocars in the ipsilateral anterior axillary line If body habitus permitted, the 5 mm inferior trocar was inserted through an ipsilateral periareolar incision No CO_2 insufflation used	IONM was used routinely, intraoperative PTH measurement was not	The parathyroid adenoma was successfully excised in all cases with negligible blood loss (<5 ml) There was one conversion to open surgery (BMI = 33.4) No short-term complications such as RLN palsy, bleeding, hypocalcemia or wound infection There was one failure (persistent pHPT due to double adenoma) Learning curve demonstrated (progressive reduction from 3 h, 10 min to 1 h, 35 min) Excellent cosmetic outcome and patient scar satisfaction (mean VAS score at 1 year was 95 %) Pain scores decreased to 8 % at 2 weeks Significant improvement in QoL

RAT robotic-assisted thyroidectomy, *RAP* robotic-assisted parathyroidectomy, *OT* open thyroidectomy, *OP*, open parathyroidectomy, *pHPT* primary hyperparathyroidism, *US* ultrasonography, *SPECT-CT* single-photon emission computed tomography, *IONM* intraoperative nerve monitoring, *PTH* parathyroid hormone, *PROMs* patient-reported outcome measures, *VAS* visual analog score, *VHI-2* voice handicap index 2, *QoL* quality of life, *EQ-5D* standardized instrument for use as a measure of health outcome (EuroQol Group), *BMI* body mass index

SPECT-CT. Triple modality concordance between these three imaging modalities was an essential prerequisite for study inclusion. Exclusion criteria included patients with a history of significant thyroiditis, bulky thyroid disease, previous neck surgery, or a suspicion of malignancy.

The approach used differed to the one popularized earlier by Chung for RAT [18]. Instead of a transaxillary approach, an infraclavicular incision was made along with two or three small incisions in the ipsilateral anterior axillary line (one 12 mm and two 5 mm). Where body habitus permitted, the 5 mm inferior trocar was inserted through an ipsilateral periareolar incision. Eventually the technique was refined so that only two trocars were inserted in the anterior axillary line and periareolar area with the endoscope transgressing the 3 cm infraclavicular incision. For transaxillary approaches only three robotic arms were required and these all passed through the single incision. There were no complications reported and the parathyroid adenoma was successfully excised in all 11 cases. As with all parathyroid surgery, blood loss was negligible (<5 ml). The RLN was identified and preserved in all cases as evident by pre- and post-operative fiber-optic laryngoscopy. Operative time was longer than for open parathyroidectomy (OP), but a learning curve was demonstrated as a progressive reduction was seen from 3 h, 10 min for the first case to 1 h, 35 min for the last one. One patient suffered persisting hypercalcemia due to undiagnosed MEN I pathology and required ultimately a 4-gland approach to be cured. This however represents a limitation of the preoperative imaging modalities used to localize the adenoma and of targeted parathyroidectomy in general rather than of RAP per se [3, 30]. In one patient, RAP had to be converted to an open approach. This was due to the patient's large body habitus (BMI = 33.4).

The authors conclude that RAP is a safe, feasible alternative to the established targeted parathyroidectomy techniques. By making use of robotic technology, RAP totally avoids a neck scar. This was shown to translate to an excellent cosmetic outcome as evident by the very high patient satisfaction scores with scar cosmesis (mean VAS score at 1 year was 95 %). This study is the largest on RAP although mean follow-up was relatively short (mean follow-up 6 months, range 3–12 months). Prospective evaluation of all relevant Patient-Reported Outcome Measures (PROMs) (pain, scar cosmesis, voice satisfaction and QoL) was conducted at regular time intervals (1 day, 2 weeks, 3, 6 and 12 months post-operatively) and validated assessment tools were used. Limitations include the absence of a control group and the small number of patients ($n = 11$).

Landry et al. [17] prospectively evaluated 13 patients of whom 2 underwent RAP (the remainder underwent RAT). The parathyroid adenoma was localized preoperatively in both patients, and contrary to the technique described by Tolley et al. [3], RAP was performed through a single port via a transaxillary incision. Single port transaxillary RAP was shown to be feasible and safe. Despite the long operative times (115 and 102 min, respectively) there were no complications in the RAP arm and the parathyroid adenoma was successfully excised in both cases. Apart from the advantages of robotic surgical technology such as visual magnification and precise instrumentation, the primary benefit of RAP was superior cosmesis. The authors also reiterate the importance of implementing a team approach. Limitations of the study include the very small number of patients ($n = 2$), the absence of a control group and the lack of PROMs evaluation (the authors failed to report the length of the follow-up period).

Katz et al. [24] published a case report of a patient with an atypical parathyroid adenoma and pHPT who underwent single port transaxillary RAP and RAT (concomitant ipsilateral robotic thyroid lobectomy). The parathyroid adenoma was attached inferiorly to the ipsilateral thyroid lobe and an identifiable plane between the two was not present. Operative time was 95 min. The patient was cured of pHPT and there were no complications or need for conversion to open surgery. Despite the limitation of being a single case report and not formally evaluating PROMs, this study had adequate follow-up (12 months) to ensure biochemical cure and assessment of scar cosmesis, thus confirming the feasibility and safety of RAP.

Foley et al. [16] directly compared 4 RAP patients against 12 matched controls who underwent open parathyroidectomy (OP) in a prospective manner. This is the only study in the literature to directly compare RAP with its open equivalent. All RAP patients were cured of their pHPT, but the operative time for RAP was found to be significantly longer than OP. A learning curve for RAP was once more demonstrated. RAP was thus shown to be feasible and safe in appropriately selected patients with pHPT offering a superior cosmetic outcome over OP. Nevertheless, the authors conclude that improved cosmesis must be weighed against the extent of surgery and increased cost associated with RAP. Limitations comprise of the small number of RAP patients ($n = 4$), the variable follow-up periods (6, 12 and 6 months and 2 weeks, respectively) and the fact that PROMs were not evaluated.

Safety, Effectiveness, Cost and Long-Term Outcomes of Robotic-Assisted Parathyroidectomy

The literature supports that RAP is a safe, feasible alternative to established targeted parathyroidectomy techniques [2, 3, 16, 17, 24, 25]. Its main advantage over existing minimally invasive approaches is the absence of a neck scar. Moreover, the robotic surgical technology that RAP employs overcomes the ergonomic problems associated with conventional endoscopic surgery and avoids the complications of CO_2 insufflation [3]. This combined with the improved visualization offered by the dual channel endoscope increases the surgical efficacy of RAP [24].

In addition to the concealed scar in the axilla or infraclavicular region, benefits include improved visualization and high surgical precision. The post-operative complications associated with RAP are comparable to those of established targeted parathyroidectomy techniques [3, 16, 17, 24]. It is, however, important to mention that RAP is a recent addition to the numerous surgical approaches that exist for targeted parathyroidectomy and, as such, how this technique compares to the most popular minimally invasive approaches is yet to be fully evaluated.

Despite its many advantages, RAP has certain drawbacks. Operative time is significantly longer compared to the conventional approach. Nonetheless, a learning curve does exist with RAP with operative time shown to significantly decrease with consecutive cases [3, 16, 17]. This learning curve phenomenon has been described in several other surgical fields [31, 32]. However, despite the learning curve, RAP still takes considerably longer to perform compared to conventional parathyroidectomy [3, 16, 17].

Another important issue with RAP is the associated cost. This is high due to a combination of factors including the cost of the da Vinci system ($1.4 million), subsequent maintenance costs ($150,000 per annum) and consumable costs ($1,700 per case) and finally the significantly longer operating time incurred [2, 33]. It may be that if patients express a preference for a scarless in the neck RAP approach then they will have to fund such surgery [17].

Attention to the brachial plexus is mandated with RAP. Although brachial plexus neurapraxia has not yet been reported following RAP, this "new" complication is an important factor to consider when implementing RAP. Traction injury to the brachial plexus is a rare but well-described complication of RAT [28]. Potential injury to other structures not normally associated with conventional parathyroid surgery is also possible including the trachea, carotid artery, internal jugular and axillary vein. Fortunately these complications are very rare and have only been reported with RAT [17, 28]. Nevertheless, the axillary approach followed in RAP is identical to that in RAT and therefore these complications are possible with either procedure. It is likely that the significantly higher number of RAT cases performed universally compared to RAP accounts for the reason why these complications have not yet been encountered with RAP.

For now, and until long-term data regarding its effectiveness and outcomes are published, RAP should be reserved for high-volume parathyroid surgeons [17]. Although the technique may be particularly appealing to a well-recognized subset of patients, namely those with a propensity towards hypertrophic or keloid scarring [34] and/or those patients where the cosmetic impact of a neck scar carries significant social stigma [16], there are several issues associated with RAP that need addressing before this procedure is employed on a wider scale. These include its high cost, longer operative time and additional complications not associated with conventional parathyroid surgery [17]. As with every surgical technique, patient selection remains the key and more long-term prospective comparative studies are needed to clarify the role of RAP in the management of patients with pHPT.

The Future of RAP

It is likely that the introduction of new systems in the market (e.g. Amadeus™ Robotic Surgical System, Titan Medical Inc., Toronto, ON) will create competition as the existing climate is a monopoly limited by high cost and the need for expensive training [35]. Nevertheless, RAP is not for every patient, surgeon or hospital. Careful patient selection is vital to optimize surgical results and minimize conversion rates. RAP should be undertaken by appropriately trained surgeons with sufficient experience in endocrine surgery and employed at institutions where the nursing staff are familiar with robotic surgery and where the necessary equipment and technical support is readily available. Early results predict a promising future for RAP. Nonetheless, the long-term results of prospective comparative studies (currently in progress) are awaited to elucidate the exact role that RAP will attain in the field of endocrine surgery.

Conclusion

RAP offers a viable but expensive alternative to other forms of minimally invasive parathyroidectomy in patients where even the smallest and most cosmetic scar is not an option. At present it can only be justified on a self-pay basis in patients who have cultural or biological considerations to avoid a neck scar and, as such, RAP is likely to occupy a role in a niche capacity.

Keypoints

- Robotic-assisted parathyroidectomy (RAP) constitutes the latest addition to the plethora of surgical approaches that exist for targeted parathyroidectomy.
- RAP permits an extracervical approach for targeted parathyroidectomy that avoids a neck scar with equivalent results to conventional parathyroidectomy.
- RAP offers a viable but expensive alternative to other forms of minimally invasive parathyroidectomy in patients when a neck scar is not an option.
- How RAP compares to the most popular minimally invasive approaches is yet to be fully established.
- Early results predict a promising future for RAP and long-term data are currently awaited.

References

1. Palazzo FF, Delbridge LW. Minimal-access/minimally invasive parathyroidectomy for primary hyperparathyroidism. Surg Clin North Am. 2004;84(3):717–34.
2. Noureldine SK, Kandil E. Robotic transaxillary parathyroidectomy: surgical technique and pearls. Oper Techn Otolaryng. 2013;24:126–30.
3. Tolley N, Arora A, Palazzo F, Garas G, Dhawan R, Cox J, Darzi A. Robotic-assisted parathyroidectomy: a feasibility study. Otolaryngol Head Neck Surg. 2011;144(6):859–66.
4. Tibblin S, Bondeson AG, Bondeson L, Ljungberg O. Surgical strategy in hyperparathyroidism due to solitary adenoma. Ann Surg. 1984;200(6):776–84.
5. Agarwal G, Barraclough BH, Reeve TS, Delbridge LW. Minimally invasive parathyroidectomy using the 'focused' lateral approach. II. Surgical technique. ANZ J Surg. 2002;72(2):147–51.
6. Costello D, Norman J. Minimally invasive radioguided parathyroidectomy. Surg Oncol Clin N Am. 1999;8(3):555–64.
7. Miccoli P, Bendinelli C, Berti P, Vignali E, Pinchera A, Marcocci C. Video-assisted versus conventional parathyroidectomy in primary hyperparathyroidism: a prospective randomized study. Surgery. 1999;126(6):1117–21. discussion 1121-1112.
8. Gagner M. Endoscopic subtotal parathyroidectomy in patients with primary hyperparathyroidism. Br J Surg. 1996;83(6):875.
9. Gottlieb A, Sprung J, Zheng XM, Gagner M. Massive subcutaneous emphysema and severe hypercarbia in a patient during endoscopic transcervical parathyroidectomy using carbon dioxide insufflation. Anesth Analg. 1997;84(5):1154–6.
10. Ikeda Y, Takami H. Endoscopic parathyroidectomy. Biomed Pharmacother. 2000;54 Suppl 1:52s–6s.
11. Ikeda Y, Takami H, Niimi M, Kan S, Sasaki Y, Takayama J. Endoscopic thyroidectomy and parathyroidectomy by the axillary approach. A preliminary report. Surg Endosc. 2002;16(1):92–5.
12. Ikeda Y, Takami H, Sasaki Y, Kan S, Niimi M. Endoscopic neck surgery by the axillary approach. J Am Coll Surg. 2000;191(3):336–40.
13. Lee J, Nah KY, Kim RM, Ahn YH, Soh EY, Chung WY. Differences in postoperative outcomes, function, and cosmesis: open versus robotic thyroidectomy. Surg Endosc. 2010;24(12):3186–94.
14. Chang EH, Lobe TE, Wright SK. Our initial experience of the transaxillary totally endoscopic approach for hemithyroidectomy. Otolaryngol Head Neck Surg. 2009;141(3):335–9.
15. Ikeda Y, Takami H, Sasaki Y, Takayama J, Kurihara H. Are there significant benefits of minimally invasive endoscopic thyroidectomy? World J Surg. 2004;28(11):1075–8.
16. Foley CS, Agcaoglu O, Siperstein AE, Berber E. Robotic transaxillary endocrine surgery: a comparison with conventional open technique. Surg Endosc. 2012;26(8):2259–66.

17. Landry CS, Grubbs EG, Morris GS, Turner NS, Holsinger FC, Lee JE, Perrier ND. Robot assisted transaxillary surgery (RATS) for the removal of thyroid and parathyroid glands. Surgery. 2011;149(4): 549–55.
18. Kang SW, Jeong JJ, Yun JS, Sung TY, Lee SC, Lee YS, Nam KH, Chang HS, Chung WY, Park CS. Robot-assisted endoscopic surgery for thyroid cancer: experience with the first 100 patients. Surg Endosc. 2009;23(11):2399–406.
19. Lee J, Yun JH, Nam KH, Choi UJ, Chung WY, Soh EY. Perioperative clinical outcomes after robotic thyroidectomy for thyroid carcinoma: a multicenter study. Surg Endosc. 2011;25(3):906–12.
20. Bodner J, Profanter C, Prommegger R, Greiner A, Margreiter R, Schmid T. Mediastinal parathyroidectomy with the da Vinci robot: presentation of a new technique. J Thorac Cardiovasc Surg. 2004;127(6): 1831–2.
21. Chan AP, Wan IY, Wong RH, Hsin MK, Underwood MJ. Robot-assisted excision of ectopic mediastinal parathyroid adenoma. Asian Cardiovasc Thorac Ann. 2010;18(1):65–7.
22. Ismail M, Maza S, Swierzy M, Tsilimparis N, Rogalla P, Sandrock D, Ruckert RI, Muller JM, Ruckert JC. Resection of ectopic mediastinal parathyroid glands with the da Vinci robotic system. Br J Surg. 2010;97(3):337–43.
23. Van Dessel E, Hendriks JM, Lauwers P, Ysebaert D, Ruyssers Jr N, Van Schil PE. Mediastinal parathyroidectomy with the da Vinci robot. Innovations (Phila). 2011;6(4):262–4.
24. Katz L, Abdel Khalek M, Crawford B, Kandil E. Robotic-assisted transaxillary parathyroidectomy of an atypical adenoma. Minim Invasive Ther Allied Technol. 2012;21(3):201–5.
25. Li XM, Massasati SA, Kandil E. Single incision robotic transaxillary approach to perform parathyroidectomy. Gland Surg. 2012;1(3):169–70.
26. Kang SW, Lee SC, Lee SH, Lee KY, Jeong JJ, Lee YS, Nam KH, Chang HS, Chung WY, Park CS. Robotic thyroid surgery using a gasless, transaxillary approach and the da Vinci S system: the operative outcomes of 338 consecutive patients. Surgery. 2009;146(6): 1048–55.
27. Luginbuhl A, Schwartz DM, Sestokas AK, Cognetti D, Pribitkin E. Detection of evolving injury to the brachial plexus during transaxillary robotic thyroidectomy. Laryngoscope. 2012;122(1):110–5.
28. Chung WY. Pros of robotic transaxillary thyroid surgery: its impact on cancer control and surgical quality. Thyroid. 2012;22(10):986–7.
29. Garas G, Okabayashi K, Ashrafian H, Shetty K, Palazzo F, Tolley N, Darzi A, Athanasiou T, Zacharakis E. Which hemostatic device in thyroid surgery? A network meta-analysis of surgical technologies. Thyroid. 2013;23(9):1138–50.
30. Miccoli P, Berti P, Materazzi G, Massi M, Picone A, Minuto MN. Results of video-assisted parathyroidectomy: single institution's six-year experience. World J Surg. 2004;28(12):1216–8.
31. Heemskerk J, van Gemert WG, de Vries J, Greve J, Bouvy ND. Learning curves of robot-assisted laparoscopic surgery compared with conventional laparoscopic surgery: an experimental study evaluating skill acquisition of robot-assisted laparoscopic tasks compared with conventional laparoscopic tasks in inexperienced users. Surg Laparosc Endosc Percutan Tech. 2007;17(3):171–4.
32. Kaul S, Shah NL, Menon M. Learning curve using robotic surgery. Curr Urol Rep. 2006;7(2):125–9.
33. Garas G, Ibrahim A, Ashrafian H, Ahmed K, Patel V, Okabayashi K, Skapinakis P, Darzi A, Athanasiou T. Evidence-based surgery: barriers, solutions, and the role of evidence synthesis. World J Surg. 2012;36(8): 1723–31.
34. Allah KC, Yeo S, Kossoko H, Assi Dje Bi Dje V, Richard Kadio M. Keloid scars on black skin: myth or reality. Ann Chir Plast Esthet. 2013;58(2): 115–22.
35. Trehan A, Dunn TJ. The robotic surgery monopoly is a poor deal. BMJ. 2013;347:f7470.

Experimental Approaches and Future Applications of Robotic Surgery in the Head and Neck

Christopher Brook and Gregory A. Grillone

Benign Neck Masses and Salivary Gland Procedures

Several authors have published on experimental robotics approaches for benign entities of the neck. One group reported on the use of the robot for removal of a series of benign masses [1]. They reported a successful approach via a retroauricular incision for second branchial cleft cysts as well as a single submental lymph node in level I of the neck. They also reported retroauricular submandibular gland removal in six patients with benign pathology. Through use of the robotic modified facelift approach, the authors reported high cosmetic satisfaction with the procedures and no significant intraoperative or postoperative complications. Specifically they reported no nerve palsies including the marginal mandibular branch of the facial nerve [1].

Other authors have reported on the use of the robot via a retroauricular approach for removal of a benign isolated thyroglossal duct cyst [2]. They were able to dissect out the thyroglossal duct cyst from under the strap muscles, and remove the central portion of the hyoid bone through a retroauricular incision. They reported no evidence of a tract superior to the hyoid bone and were able to remove the specimen en bloc through the incision site. The only non-robotic assistance during the case was the introduction of a bone cutter through the incision site for resection of the hyoid bone [2].

Neck Dissection

Initial experience with robotic neck dissection has occurred primarily in the area of lateral neck dissection in patients with metastatic well-differentiated thyroid cancer. These patients are often young, female, and interested in the cosmetic appearance of their surgical incision [3]. Because initial experience with robotic neck dissection was focused on areas of metastasis common to thyroid cancer (levels 2–5), it did not focus on levels, 1, 2b, or 5a [3]. Subsequent papers have demonstrated the technical feasibility of performing this procedure through combined transaxillary/retroauricular approach (Fig. 1) [4], pre- and post-auricular incision [5], and modified facelift incision [6].

In addition to technical feasibility, outcomes of robotic neck dissection have been compared to those of conventional techniques in patients with papillary thyroid cancer [7]. In general, there are longer operative times, shorter hospital stays, equivalent complication rates, and equivalent lymph node yields when using robot approaches. Notably though, the robotic arm of the study had significantly younger patients with lower staged disease [7].

C. Brook, M.D. • G.A. Grillone, M.D. (✉)
Department of Otolaryngology—Head and Neck Surgery, Boston University School of Medicine, Boston Medical Center, Boston, MA, USA
e-mail: Gregory.Grillone@bmc.org

G.A. Grillone and S. Jalisi (eds.), *Robotic Surgery of the Head and Neck: A Comprehensive Guide*,
DOI 10.1007/978-1-4939-1547-7_14, © Springer Science+Business Media New York 2015

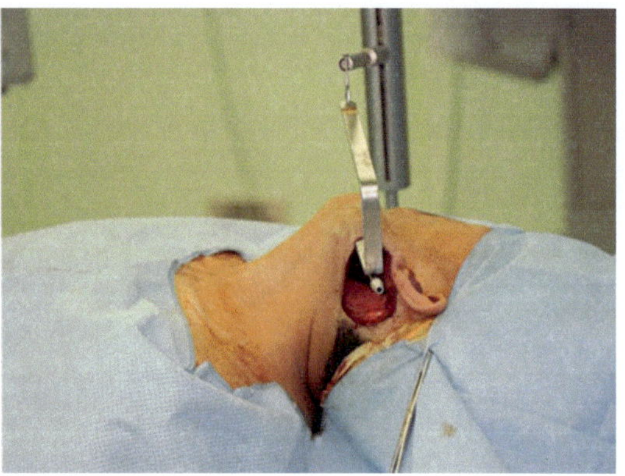

Fig. 1 Robotic neck dissection performed through a retroauricular incision

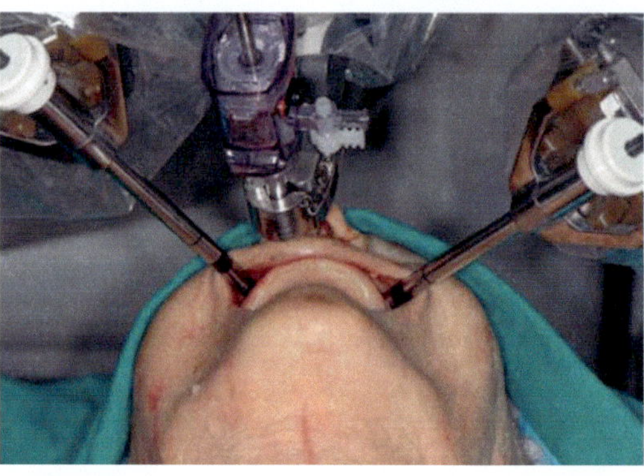

Fig. 2 Robotic Trocars placed through Caldwell-Luc maxillary antrostomies and camera placement through the right side of the nose

Robotic neck dissection for primary tumors other than thyroid has also been studied. Several authors have reported on the use of robotic neck dissection via the modified facelift approach for parotid tumors [6, 8], submandibular cancer [9], oral cavity cancers [10–12], and laryngopharyngeal cancer [12, 13]. The authors of these studies endorsed the technical feasibility of this procedure for low stage neck disease, and almost all patients in these studies had preoperative cN0 disease. Outcomes data was provided for robotic neck dissection and conventional neck dissection, demonstrating similar findings to the studies done comparing these approaches for neck dissection done for thyroid cancer [7, 12]. The authors found that operative times were longer in the robotic group but that hospital stay, lymph node yield, and complications were equivalent [10]. Taken together, the literature suggests that robotic transaxillary or modified facelift approaches for neck dissection are technically feasible, oncologically sound, and cosmetically superior procedures for thyroid disease and low N stage head and neck cancers.

Sellar and Parasellar Applications

One of the most logical applications of robotic surgery within the head and neck is in the sellar and parasellar region. Although it is remote from the nasal vestibule, there are multiple endoscopic approaches already described to build upon. Several authors have detailed robotic techniques used to approach the sella with varying degrees of success. The da Vinci robot from Intuitive Surgical, which has traditionally been used in the head and neck for transoral approaches, now commonly referred to as transoral robotic surgery (TORS), has been applied to surgical approaches in this region. Additionally, several authors have described novel robotic systems for use in sellar or parasellar surgery.

One group described using the da Vinci robot to access the skull base through nasal placement of the camera, and bilateral sublabial incisions with anterior and medial maxillary antrostomies (Fig. 2) [14]. The surgical corridors were then joined posterior to the nasal septum, providing good access to the sellar, parasellar, clival, and anterior skull base regions. The authors commented that the three-dimensional view and precision of the robot allowed for meticulous dural closure as well [14]. The obvious limitation with this technique is the invasive nature of the approach involving bilateral anterior maxillary antrostomies through a vestibular incision.

Another group described using the da Vinci robot to access the sella and parasellar regions through a combined oral and transcervical approach on cadavers [15]. The authors pointed out that the limitation of traditional TORS in skull base surgery is access of the mechanical instruments, even though reasonable visualization can be achieved using an angled camera. Therefore the authors placed the camera transorally and the arms of the da Vinci were placed transcervically through a blind introduction of trocars posterior to the submandibular glands. Using this technique the authors reported adequate surgical access to the sella, sphenoid, clivus, nasopharynx, and suprasellar anterior fossa [15]. Again, the limitation stems from the invasive nature of placement of the robotic arms..

Other researchers have reported the development of novel robots for assistance with sellar surgery. Nathan et al. reported the use of a robotic endoscope holder named the Automated Endoscope System for Optimal Positioning (AESOP). This robotic scope holder assists the surgeon and can be activated by voice commands to move or return to set positions. In a cadaveric study, the authors report improvement in visualization and tremor reduction, with the additional benefit of freeing the surgeon's second hand for another instrument [16]. Another team modified a robotic endoscope holder used for ventriculostomies, the Evolution 1 from Universal Robotic Systems, for use in sellar surgery [17]. Similarly to the AESOP design, this robot is designed to free up more hands for traditional endoscopic surgery. The robotic-held endoscope is controlled from a remote joystick, and the authors reported successful two handed surgery with the scope in place [17].

Aside from the da Vinci system and the robotic endoscope holders, another group has developed a novel surgical robot, the A73, based on the RV-1a automated arms robot from Mitsubishi Electric. The robot has an arm with visualization capabilities and multiple functions, including drilling, suctioning, and flushing, and has been designed to perform automated resection of the anterior sphenoid wall. The robot integrates preoperative imaging into its surgical plan and removes the anterior sphenoid face without deep penetration in the sphenoid or into lateral structures. In a series of cadaveric heads, the robot successfully removed the anterior sphenoid wall without damage to surrounding structures in five specimens [18, 19]. Before widespread adoption of an automated surgical robot, though, large trials will need to demonstrate its reliability and safety.

Anterior Cranial Fossa Applications

The approaches previously described for the sella and parasellar regions have also been used to operate in the anterior cranial fossa on cadaveric specimens. Hanna et al described the sublabial incisions with anterior and medial maxillectomies for robotic arm placement and intranasal camera placement, and described this for use in the anterior cranial fossa as well [14]. They noted with this approach that they had excellent exposure of the cribriform plate, fovea ethmoidalis, medial orbit, and planum sphenoidale in all four cadaveric specimens experimented on. In addition they noted that the greatest advantage they perceived with this technique was magnified, tremor free closure, and suturing of dural defects [14]. Another group described a combined unilateral transmaxillary and endonasal approach to the skull base [20]. The authors reported that the endonasal portion of the surgery could be constricted and sometimes benefitted from release of the medial crural nasal cartilages from the caudal septum for increased room to maneuver. The investigators noted adequate dissection of the anterior skull base back to the region of the pituitary, allowing pituitary dissection, although they suffered from more frequent robotic instrument collisions anteriorly. The transmaxillary window was created with an osteoplastic flap that could be replaced at the end of the case [20]. The authors of these studies worked with the da Vinci robot and both noted that there was a lack of tools designed for boney work, necessitating an assistant to perform this part of the resection [14, 20].

Infratemporal Fossa and Paraphayrngeal Space Applications

Dissection of the intratemporal fossa and parapharyngeal space has also been described with robotic surgery or robotic-assisted techniques. One group described entirely transoral approaches to the parapharyngeal space and the infratemporal fossa using the da Vinci robot [8]. They were able to perform this technique on two cadaveric

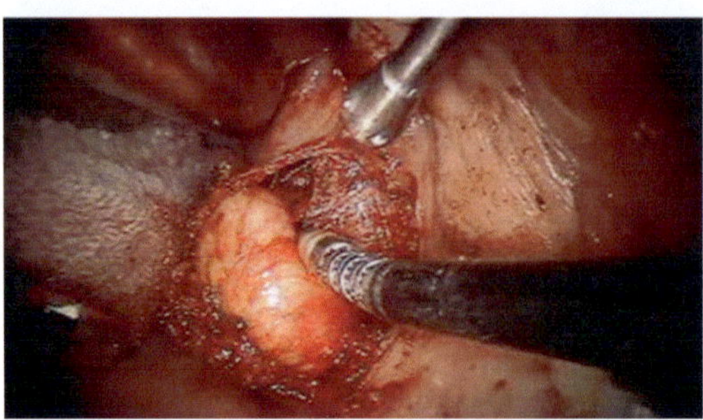

Fig. 3 Transoral resection of parapharyngeal space tumor

and one live canine specimen, with adequate access to the internal and external carotid, jugular vein, cranial nerves IX, X, XI, and XII. The authors then followed up their preclinical discussion with a report of robotic dissection and removal of a benign cystic parapharyngeal mass in a living patient. The dissection was described without complication and the wound was closed intraorally [20].

One paper described successful resection of three tumors of the parapharyngeal space via a completely transoral (TORS) approach (Fig. 3) [21]. They were successful in removal of a pleomorphic adenoma, parapharyngeal lipoma and an adenoid cystic carcinoma from paraphayngeal locations via this technique. The authors noted that the main limitations in this approach were inadequate oral access, involvement of the carotid artery, or cervical spine instability [21].

Another group described a combined transoral and suprahyoid transcervical approach to the infratemporal fossa using the da Vinci robot [23]. While this approach also utilized a transoral camera and robotic arm placement, it was combined with a suprahyoid pharyngotomy into the vallecula for placement of the second robotic arm. The authors noted excellent visualization of the infratemporal fossa and the limits of dissection were listed as the lower cranial nerves and jugular foramen posteriorly, the pterygoid space anteriorly, the temporomandibular joint and mandibule ramus laterally, and foramen ovale medially [23].

A different approach described using a transmaxillary placement of the da Vinci robot for cadaveric dissection [20]. The authors required an assistant to perform boney removal of the anterior osteoplastic flap, as well as the removal of the boney medial and posterior walls of the maxillary sinus. They then reported on dissection of the infratemporal fossa using the robot, noting excellent visualization for anatomic dissection [20].

It seems that dissection of the infratemporal fossa and parapharyngeal space can be achieved from a completely transoral route, although more invasive camera and arm placement have been described. Future research will need to focus on limitations of these approaches and outcomes when using this approach.

Clivus, Nasopharynx and Craniocervical Junction Applications

Robotic surgical approaches to the nasopharynx, clivus, and craniocervical junction have been described using the da Vinci surgical robot. For nasopharyngectomy a preclinical study on cadavers compared a strictly transoral (TORS) approach to a combined transnasal and transoral approach [24]. In the traditional TORS procedure all of the robotic arms were placed transorally, while in the combined procedure investigators placed the camera transnasally and the robotic working arms transorally. The authors noted improved visualization of the surgical field with the combined approach, although they also noted that the procedure could be accomplished from either route. Additionally the authors noted that the cadaveric study was performed in an edentulous patient, and they felt the presence of teeth would limit transoral robotic arm placement. The authors then described a transcervical placement of the robotic working arms posterior to the submandibular gland with transnasal camera placement based on the cervical TORS (C-TORS) technique (Fig. 4) [22, 24].

Similarly, other researchers reported on a comparison of several techniques of robotic nasopharyngectomy [25]. The camera arm was placed either transnasally, transpalatally, or transorally with the working robotic arms placed either through the palate, oral cavity, or transcervically. The authors found that the best visualization

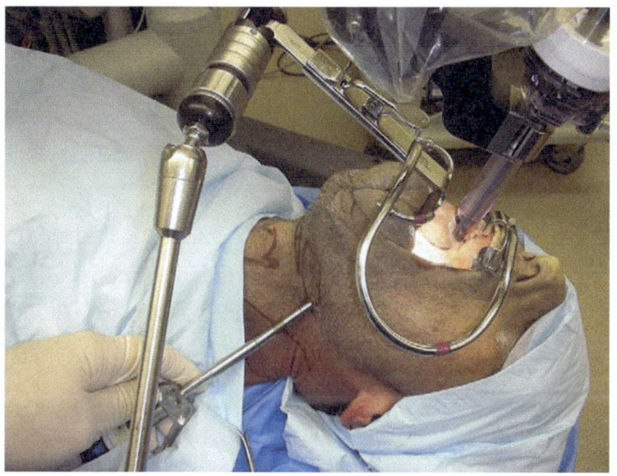

Fig. 4 Cervical TORS techniques with transcerical and transoral placement of instruments

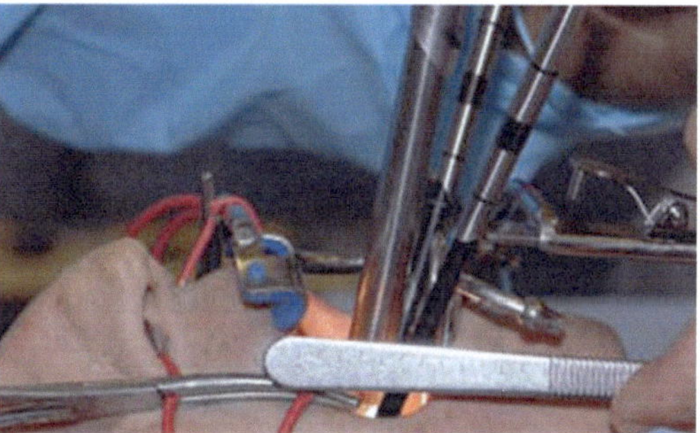

Fig. 5 Completely transoral placement of robotic arms for approaches to the craniocervical junction and atlanto-axial spine

was achieved with transnasal or transpalatal placement of the camera arm, and that the instruments had better maneuverability with the transcervical compared to the transoral route, and still better maneuverability with the transpalatal route [25]. They therefore concluded that the transpalatal route for both camera arm and working arms provided an optimal corridor for working and visualization [25].

Other studies reported combined endonasal and TORS procedures for resection of lesions of the nasopharynx, clivus, or craniocervical junction [26, 27], and one study demonstrated the use of this technique for recurrent nasopharyngeal carcinoma after radiation failure in a live patient [27]. The da Vinci system was used in this case for soft tissue dissection of the nasopharynx, while a traditional endonasal approach was required for boney work in the region of the sphenoid sinus. The authors were successful with the resection of the basisphenoid and achieved negative margins [27].

In approaching strictly the clivus and craniocervical junction, one group described transoral access based on their experience with TORS for head and neck cancer [28]. Initially they performed several cadaveric transoral approaches with a 30° endoscope, noting that the strictly oral route provided access to the middle and lower clivus, as well as excellent visualization for suturing dura; however, this technique was limited in more superior and anterior directions [28]. In a similar paper the same group tested the feasibility of decompression of the craniocervical junction using the da Vinci robot [29]. They found that using red rubber catheters to retract the palate and with completely transoral placement of the robotic arms they had adequate access to the lower clivus, the first cervical vertebrae, and the odontoid process (Fig. 5). They described successful odontoidectomy in a cadaveric study and thought this approach would be suitable for intra and extradural tumors of this region as well. Of note, this technique involved boney work using a handheld drill that was operated by an assistant due to a lack of instrumentation for bone available on the da Vinci platform, and therefore was deemed robotic-assisted surgery [29].

Overall it seems that resection of the nasopharynx, clivus, and craniocervical junction can be achieved via transoral placement of the robotic arms with or without nasal placement of the camera arm. More superior dissection in the nasopharynx is best achieved from transnasal or transpalatal camera arm placement with either transpalatal or transcervical working arm placement.

Conclusions

Experimental surgical approaches using robotic technology for surgery of the head and neck and skull base surgery are evolving rapidly as innovative approaches and new robotic technology are developed. Benign and malignant neck disease is being treated with transaxillary, retroauricular, and modified facelift approaches. Using these techniques, removal of salivary glands, congential cysts, and lymph nodes is possible, especially for limited disease. Further research will need to delineate the limitations of this type of surgery, and where its advantages and disadvantages lie when compared with traditional open surgical techniques.

Several robotic surgical approaches or robotic-assisted approaches have been described for skull base surgery. At this point there are no standardized approaches and there is limited data on living patients other than case reports or small series. Additionally, the largest robotic platform, the da Vinci robot, lacks instrumentation suitable for major boney work. Future research will need to identify the standard approaches for different regions, potential complications, as well as data on living patients before these techniques become widespread.

References

1. Park YM, Byeon HK, Chung HP, Rho KJ, Kim SH. Robotic resection of benign neck masses via a retroauricular approach. J Laparoendosc Adv Surg Tech A. 2013;23(7):578–83.
2. Kim CH, Byeon HK, Shin YS, Koh YW, Choi EC. Robot-assisted sistrunk's operation via a retroauricular approach for thyroglossal duct cyst. Head Neck. 2014;36:456–8.
3. Kang SW, Lee SH, Ryu HR, Lee KY, Jeong JJ, Nam KH, et al. Initial experience with robot-assisted modified radical neck dissection for the management of thyroid carcinoma with lateral neck node metastasis. Surgery. 2010;148(6):1214–21.
4. Kim WS, Lee HS, Kang SM, Hong HJ, Koh YW, Lee HY, et al. Feasibility of robot-assisted neck dissections via a transaxillary and retroauricular ("TARA") approach in head and neck cancer: preliminary results. Ann Surg Oncol. 2012;19(3):1009–17.
5. Blanco RG, Ha PK, Califano JA, Fakry C, Richmon J, et al. Robotic-assisted neck dissection through a pre- and post-auricular hairline incision: preclinical study. J Laparoendosc Adv Surg Tech A. 2012;22(8):791–6.
6. Kim CH, Chang JW, Choi EC, Shin YS, Koh YW. Robotically assisted selective neck dissection in parotid gland cancer: preliminary report. Laryngoscope. 2013;123(3):646–50.
7. Kang SW, Lee SH, Park JH, Jeong JS, Park S, Lee CR, et al. A comparative study of the surgical outcomes of robotic and conventional open modified radicalneck dissection for papillary thyroid carcinoma with lateral neck node metastasis. Surg Endosc. 2012;26(11):3251–7.
8. Shin YS, Choi EC, Kim CH, Koh YW. Robot-assisted selective neck dissection combined with facelift parotidectomy in parotid cancer. Head Neck. 2014;36:592–5.
9. Kim CH, Koh YW, Kim D, Chang JW, Choi EC, Shin YS. Robotic-assisted neck dissection in submandibular gland cancer: preliminary report. J Oral Maxillofac Surg. 2013;71(8):1450–7.
10. Lee HS, Kim WS, Hong HJ, Ban MJ, Lee D, Koh YW, et al. Robot-assisted Supraomohyoid neck dissection via a modified face-lift or retroauricular approach in early-stage cN0 squamous cell carcinoma of the oral cavity: a comparative study with conventional technique. Ann Surg Oncol. 2012; 19(12):3871–8.
11. Tae K, Ji YB, Song CM, Min HJ, Kim KR, Park CW. Robotic selective neck dissection using a gasless postauricular facelift approach for early head and neck cancer: technical feasibility and safety. J Laparoendosc Adv Surg Tech A. 2013;23(3):240–5.
12. Tae K, Ji YB, Song CM, Jeong JH, Cho SH, Lee SH. Robotic selective neck dissection by a postauricular facelift approach: comparison with conventional neck dissection. Otolaryngol Head Neck Surg. 2014;150(3):394–400.
13. Park YM, Holsinger FC, Kim WS, Park SC, Lee EJ, Choi EC, et al. Robot-assisted selective neck dissection of levels II to V via a modified facelift or retroauricular approach. Otolaryngol Head Neck Surg. 2013; 148(5):778–85.
14. Hanna EY, Holsinger C, DeMonte F, Kupferman M. Robotic endoscopicsurgery of the skull base: a novel surgical approach. Arch Otolaryngol Head Neck Surg. 2007;133:1209–14.
15. O'Malley Jr BW, Weinstein GS. Robotic anterior and midline skull base surgery: preclinical investigations. Int J Radiat Oncol Biol Phys. 2007;69(2 Suppl): S125–8.
16. Nathan CO, Chakradeo V, Malhotra K, D'Agostino H, Patwardhan R. The voice-controlled robotic assist scope holder AESOP for the endoscopic approach to the sella. Skull Base. 2006;16(3):123–31.
17. Nimsky C, Rachinger J, Iro H, Fahlbusch R. Adaptation of a hexapod-based robotic system for extended endoscope-assisted transsphenoidal skull base surgery. Minim Invasive Neurosurg. 2004;47(1): 41–6.
18. Steinhart H, Bumm K, Wurm J, Vogele M, Iro H. Surgical application of a new robotic system for paranasal sinus surgery. Ann Otol Rhinol Laryngol. 2004;113(4):303–9.
19. Bumm K, Wurm J, Rachinger J, Dannenmann T, Bohr C, Fahlbusch R, et al. An automated robotic approach with redundant navigation for minimal invasive extended transsphenoidal skull base surgery. Minim Invasive Neurosurg. 2005;48(3):159–64.

20. Blanco RG, Boahene K. Robotic-assisted skull base surgery: preclinical study. J Laparoendosc Adv Surg Tech A. 2013;23(9):776–82.
21. Arshad H, Durmus K, Ozer E. Transoral robotic resection of selected parapharyngeal space tumors. Eur Arch Otorhinolaryngol. 2013;270(5):1737–40.
22. O'Malley Jr BW, Weinstein GS. Robotic skull base surgery: preclinical investigations to human clinical application. Arch Otolaryngol Head Neck Surg. 2007;133(12):1215–9.
23. McCool RR, Warren FM, Wiggins 3rd RH, Hunt JP. Robotic surgery of the infratemporal fossa utilizing novel suprahyoid port. Laryngoscope. 2010;120(9):1738–43. doi:10.1002/lary.21020.
24. Dallan I, Castelnuovo P, Montevecchi F, Battaglia P, Cerchiai N, Seccia V, et al. Combined transoral transnasal robotic-assisted nasopharyngectomy: a cadaveric feasibility study. Eur Arch Otorhinolaryngol. 2012; 269:235–9.
25. Ozer E, Durmus K, Carrau RL, de Lara D, Ditzel Filho LF, Prevedello DM, et al. Applications of transoral, transcervical, transnasal, and transpalatal corridors for robotic surgery of the skull base. Laryngoscope. 2013;123(9):2176–9.
26. Carrau RL, Prevedello DM, de Lara D, Durmus K, Ozer E. Combined transoral robotic surgery and endoscopic endonasal approach for the resection of extensive malignancies of the skull base. Head Neck. 2013;35:E351–8.
27. Yin Tsang RK, Ho WK, Wei WI. Combined transnasal endoscopic andtransoral robotic resection of recurrent nasopharyngeal carcinoma. Head Neck. 2012;34:1190–3.
28. Lee JYK, O'Malley Jr BW, Newman JG, Weinstein GS, Lega B, Diaz J, et al. Transoralrobotic surgery of the skull base: a cadaver and feasi-bility study. ORL J Otorhinolaryngol Relat Spec. 2010;72:181–7.
29. Lee JY, O'Malley BW, Newman JG, Weinstein GS, Lega B, Diaz J, Grady MS. Transoral robotic surgery of craniocervical junction and atlantoaxial spine: a cadaveric study. J Neurosurg Spine. 2010;1 2(1):13–8.

Index

G.A. Grillone and S. Jalisi (eds.), *Robotic Surgery of the Head and Neck: A Comprehensive Guide*, DOI 10.1007/978-1-4939-1547-7, © Springer Science+Business Media New York 2015

O

P

R

S

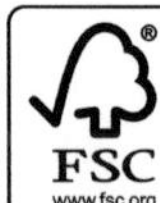

MIX
Papier aus verantwortungsvollen Quellen
Paper from responsible sources
FSC® C105338

If you have any concerns about our products,
you can contact us on
ProductSafety@springernature.com

In case Publisher is established outside the EU,
the EU authorized representative is:
Springer Nature Customer Service Center GmbH
Europaplatz 3, 69115 Heidelberg, Germany

Printed by Libri Plureos GmbH
in Hamburg, Germany